Interpreting Complex Arrhythmias: Part III

Editors

GIUSEPPE BAGLIANI
ROBERTO DE PONTI
FABIO M. LEONELLI

CARDIAC ELECTROPHYSIOLOGY CLINICS

www.cardiacEP.theclinics.com

Consulting Editors
RANJAN K. THAKUR
ANDREA NATALE

June 2019 • Volume 11 • Number 2

ELSEVIER

1600 John F. Kennedy Boulevard • Suite 1800 • Philadelphia, Pennsylvania, 19103-2899

http://www.theclinics.com

CARDIAC ELECTROPHYSIOLOGY CLINICS Volume 11, Number 2
June 2019 ISSN 1877-9182, ISBN-13: 978-0-323-68113-1

Editor: Stacy Eastman
Developmental Editor: Donald Mumford

Cardiac Electrophysiology Clinics (ISSN 1877-9182) is published quarterly by Elsevier Inc., 360 Park Avenue South, New York, NY 10010-1710. Months of issue are March, June, September, and December. Subscription prices are $224.00 per year for US individuals, $366.00 per year for US institutions, $249.00 per year for Canadian individuals, $413.00 per year for Canadian institutions, $303.00 per year for international individuals, $442.00 per year for international institutions and $100.00 per year for US, Canadian and international students/residents. To receive student/resident rate, orders must be accompanied by name of affiliated institution, date of term, and the signature of program/residency coordinator on institution letterhead. Orders will be billed at individual rate until proof of status is received. Foreign air speed delivery is included in all Clinics subscription prices. All prices are subject to change without notice. **POSTMASTER:** Send address changes to Cardiac Electrophysiology Clinics, Elsevier Health Sciences Division, Subscription Customer Service, 3251 Riverport Lane, Maryland Heights, MO 63043. **Customer Service: 1-800-654-2452 (US and Canada). From outside of the US and Canada, call 314-477-8871. Fax: 314-447-8029. E-mail: JournalsCustomerService-usa@elsevier.com (for print support); JournalsOnlineSupport-usa@elsevier.com (for online support).**

Reprints. For copies of 100 or more of articles in this publication, please contact the Commercial Reprints Department, Elsevier Inc., 360 Park Avenue South, New York, NY 10010-1710. Tel.: 212-633-3874; Fax: 212-633-3820; E-mail: reprints@elsevier.com.

Cardiac Electrophysiology Clinics is covered in *MEDLINE/PubMed (Index Medicus).*

Contributors

CONSULTING EDITORS

RANJAN K. THAKUR, MD, MPH, MBA, FHRS
Professor of Medicine and Director, Arrhythmia Service, Thoracic and Cardiovascular Institute, Sparrow Health System, Michigan State University, Lansing, Michigan, USA

ANDREA NATALE, MD, FACC, FHRS
Executive Medical Director, Texas Cardiac Arrhythmia Institute, St. David's Medical Center, Austin, Texas; Consulting Professor, Division of Cardiology, Stanford University, Palo Alto, California; Adjunct Professor of Medicine, Heart and Vascular Center, Case Western Reserve University, Cleveland, Ohio; Director, Interventional Electrophysiology, Scripps Clinic, San Diego, California; Senior Clinical Director, EP Services, California Pacific Medical Center, San Francisco, California

EDITORS

GIUSEPPE BAGLIANI, MD
Arrhythmology Unit, Cardiology Department, Foligno General Hospital, Foligno, Perugia, Italy; Cardiovascular Disease Department, University of Perugia, Perugia, Italy

ROBERTO DE PONTI, MD, FHRS
Associate Professor, Department of Cardiology, School of Medicine, Department of Heart and Vessels, Ospedale di Circolo and Macchi Foundation, University of Insubria, Varese, Italy

FABIO M. LEONELLI, MD
Staff Electrophysiologist and Director, Center Clinical Research, Cardiology Department, James A. Haley Veterans' Hospital, Associate Professor of Medicine, University South Florida, Tampa, Florida, USA

AUTHORS

ANWAR BABAN, MD, PhD
Pediatric Cardiology and Cardiac Arrhythmias Complex Unit, Department of Pediatric Cardiology and Cardiac Surgery, Bambino Gesù Children's Hospital and Research Institute, Rome, Italy

GIUSEPPE BAGLIANI, MD
Arrhythmology Unit, Cardiology Department, Foligno General Hospital, Cardiovascular Disease Department, University of Perugia, Perugia, Italy

PAOLA BERNE, MD
Cardiology Department, Nuoro General Hospital, Nuoro, Italy

SERGE BOVEDA, MD, PhD
Cardiac Arrhythmia Management Department, Clinique Pasteur, Toulouse, France

JOSEP BRUGADA, MD
Hospital Clinic, University of Barcelona, Barcelona, Spain

FABRIZIO CARAVATI, MD
Department of Heart and Vessels, Ospedale di Circolo and Macchi Foundation, University of Insubria, Varese, Italy

GIOVANNI CARRERAS, MD
Arrhythmology Unit, Cardiology Department, Terni Hospital, Terni, Italy

FRANCO CECCHI, MD
Heart and Vessels Department, University of Florence, Florence, Italy; IRCCS Auxologico, Milano, Cardiovascular San Luca Hospital, Studio Cardiologico Locati, Milano, Italy

ALFREDO CHAUCA-TAPIA, MD
Texas Cardiac Arrhythmia Institute, St. David's Medical Center, Austin, Texas, USA

QIONG CHEN, MD
Texas Cardiac Arrhythmia Institute, St. David's Medical Center, Austin, Texas, USA; Henan Provincial People's Hospital, Zhengzhou, Henan Province, China

DANIEL CORTEZ, MD
Pediatric and Adult Congenital Cardiology, Department of Pediatric Cardiology and Cardiac Surgery, University of Minnesota/Masonic Children's Hospital, Minneapolis, Minnesota, USA

MATTEO CRIPPA, MD
Department of Heart and Vessels, Ospedale di Circolo and Macchi Foundation, University of Insubria, Varese, Italy

ROBERTO DE PONTI, MD, FHRS
Associate Professor, Department of Cardiology, School of Medicine, Department of Heart and Vessels, Ospedale di Circolo and Macchi Foundation, University of Insubria, Varese, Italy

DOMENICO G. DELLA ROCCA, MD
Texas Cardiac Arrhythmia Institute, St. David's Medical Center, Austin, Texas, USA

LUIGI DI BIASE, MD, PhD
Texas Cardiac Arrhythmia Institute, St. David's Medical Center, Department of Internal Medicine, Dell Medical School, Department of Biomedical Engineering, Cockrell School of Engineering, University of Texas, Austin,

Texas, USA; Arrhythmia Services, Department of Medicine, Montefiore Medical Center, Albert Einstein College of Medicine, Bronx, New York, USA; Department of Clinical and Experimental Medicine, University of Foggia, Foggia, Italy

STEFANO DONZELLI, MD
Arrhythmology Unit, Cardiology Department, Terni Hospital, Terni, Italy

FABRIZIO DRAGO, MD
Pediatric Cardiology and Cardiac Arrhythmias Complex Unit, Department of Pediatric Cardiology and Cardiac Surgery, Bambino Gesù Children's Hospital and Research Institute, Rome, Italy

ALESSIO GASPERETTI, MD
Texas Cardiac Arrhythmia Institute, St. David's Medical Center, Austin, Texas, USA

OMER GEDIKLI, MD
Texas Cardiac Arrhythmia Institute, St. David's Medical Center, Austin, Texas, USA

MASSIMO GRISELLI, MD
Pediatric and Adult Congenital Cardiology, Department of Pediatric Cardiology and Cardiac Surgery, University of Minnesota/Masonic Children's Hospital, Minneapolis, Minnesota, USA

ZEYNAB JEBBERI, MD
Cardiac Arrhythmia Management Department, Clinique Pasteur, Toulouse, France

HELOU JOHNY, MD
Cardiology Department, Arrhythmology Unit, Foligno General Hospital, Foligno, Italy

LUDOVICO LAZZARI, MD
Arrhythmology Unit, Cardiology Department, Terni Hospital, Terni, Italy

FABIO M. LEONELLI, MD
Staff Electrophysiologist and Director, Center Clinical Research, Cardiology Department, James A. Haley Veterans' Hospital, Associate Professor of Medicine, University South Florida, Tampa, Florida

EMANUELA T. LOCATI, MD, PhD
Department of Arryhmology, IRCCS
San Donato Hospital, Studio Cardiologico
Locati, Electrophysiology Unit, Cardiovascular
Department, Niguarda Hospital, Milano,
Italy

MAURIZIO LUNATI, MD
Cardiothoracovascular Department,
Electrophysiology Unit, Niguarda Hospital,
Milano, Italy

JACOPO MARAZZATO, MD
Department of Heart and Vessels, Ospedale di
Circolo and Macchi Foundation, University of
Insubria, Varese, Italy

RAFFAELLA MARAZZI, MD
Department of Heart and Vessels, Ospedale
di Circolo and Macchi Foundation, University
of Insubria, Varese, Italy

CHIARA MARINI, MD
Arrhythmology Unit, Cardiology Department,
Terni Hospital, Terni, Italy

SANGHAMITRA MOHANTY, MD
Texas Cardiac Arrhythmia Institute,
St. David's Medical Center, Austin,
Texas, USA

ILARIA MY, MD
Department of Heart and Vessels, Ospedale di
Circolo and Macchi Foundation, University of
Insubria, Varese, Italy

ANDREA NATALE, MD, FACC, FHRS
Executive Medical Director, Texas Cardiac
Arrhythmia Institute, St. David's Medical
Center, Austin, Texas; Consulting Professor,
Division of Cardiology, Stanford University,
Palo Alto, California; Adjunct Professor
of Medicine, Heart and Vascular Center,
Case Western Reserve University, Cleveland,
Ohio; Director, Interventional
Electrophysiology, Scripps Clinic, San Diego,
California; Senior Clinical Director, EP
Services, California Pacific Medical Center,
San Francisco, California

MARTINA NESTI, MD
Cardiovascular and Neurological
Department, Ospedale San Donato, Arezzo,
Italy

MARGHERITA PADELETTI, MD, PhD
Cardiology Unit, Mugello Hospital, Florence,
Italy

ZEFFERINO PALAMÀ, MD
Cardiology Unit, Ospedale SS. Annunziata,
Taranto, Italy

CARLO PAPPONE, MD
Department of Arryhmology, IRCCS San
Donato Hospital, Milano, Italy

MARCO M. PIRRAMI, MD
Arrhythmology Unit, Cardiology Department,
Terni Hospital, Terni, Italy

ANDREA POZZOLINI, MD
Department of Cardiology, Azienda
Ospedaliera Marche Nord, Pesaro, Italy

TERESA RIO, MD
Department of Cardiology, Azienda
Ospedaliera Marche Nord, Pesaro, Italy

LUIGI SCIARRA, MD
Cardiology Unit, Policlinico Casilino, Rome,
Italy

ALESSANDRA TORDINI, MD
Arrhythmology Unit, Cardiology Department,
Terni Hospital, Terni, Italy

CHINTAN TRIVEDI, MD
Texas Cardiac Arrhythmia Institute, St. David's
Medical Center, Austin, Texas, USA

MANOLA VILOTTA, EPTech
Department of Heart and Vessels, Ospedale di
Circolo and Macchi Foundation, University of
Insubria, Varese, Italy

GRAZIANA VIOLA, MD
Cardiology Department, Nuoro General
Hospital, Nuoro, Italy

EMANUELA T. LOCATI, MD, PhD
Department of Arrhythmology (IRCCS)
San Donato Hospital, Studio Cardiologico
Locati, Electrophysiology Unit, Dermatofarmar
Dermatological Sisinae Hospital, Milano,
Italy

MAURIZIO LUNATI, MD
Cardiac Intravascular Department,
Electrophysiology Unit, Niguarda Hospital,
Milan, Italy

JACOPO MARAZZATO, MD
Department of Heart and Vessels, Ospedale di
Circolo and Macchi Foundation, University of
Insubria, Varese, Italy

RAFFAELLA MARAZZI, MD
Department of Heart and Vessels, Ospedale
di Circolo and Macchi Foundation, University
of Insubria, Varese, Italy

CHIARA MARINI, MD
Arrhythmology Unit, Cardiology Department,
Terni Hospital, Terni, Italy

SANGHAMITRA MOHANTY, MD
Texas Cardiac Arrhythmia Institute,
St. David's Medical Center, Austin,
Texas, USA

ILARIA MY, MD
Department of Heart and Vessels, Ospedale di
Circolo and Macchi Foundation, University of
Insubria, Varese, Italy

ANDREA NATALE, MD, FACC, FHRS
Executive Medical Director, Texas Cardiac
Arrhythmia Institute, St. David's Medical
Center, Austin, Texas; Consulting Professor,
Division of Cardiology, Stanford University,
Palo Alto, California; Adjunct Professor
of Medicine, Heart and Vascular Center,
Case Western Reserve University, Cleveland,
Ohio; Director, Interventional
Electrophysiology, Scripps Clinic, San Diego,
California; Senior Clinical Director, EP
Services, California Pacific Medical Center,
San Francisco, California

MARTINA NESTI, MD
Cardiovascular and Neurological
Department, Ospedale San Donato, Arezzo,
Italy

MARGHERITA PADELETTI, MD, PhD
Cardiology Unit, Mugello Hospital, Florence,
Italy

ZEFFERINO PALAMÀ, MD
Cardiology Unit, Ospedale SS. Annunziata,
Taranto, Italy

CARLO PAPPONE, MD
Department of Arrhythmology, IRCCS San
Donato Hospital, Milano, Italy

MARCO M. PIRRAMI, MD
Arrhythmology Unit, Cardiology Department,
Terni Hospital, Terni, Italy

ANDREA POZZOLINI, MD
Department of Cardiology, Azienda
Ospedaliera Marche Nord, Pesaro, Italy

TERESA RIO, MD
Department of Cardiology, Azienda
Ospedaliera Marche Nord, Pesaro, Italy

LUIGI SCIARRA, MD
Cardiology Unit, Policlinico Casilino, Roma,
Italy

ALESSANDRA TORDINI, MD
Arrhythmology Unit, Cardiology Department,
Terni Hospital, Terni, Italy

CHINTAN TRIVEDI, MD
Texas Cardiac Arrhythmia Institute, St. David's
Medical Center, Austin, Texas, USA

MANOLA VILOTTA, RPT/ech
Department of Heart and Vessels, Ospedale di
Circolo and Macchi Foundation, University of
Insubria, Varese, Italy

GRAZIANA VIOLA, MD
Cardiology Department, Nuoro General
Hospital, Nuoro, Italy

Contents

Precision Electrocardiology: A Rational Approach for Simple and Complex Arrhythmias   175

Giuseppe Bagliani, Roberto De Ponti, and Fabio M. Leonelli

Electrocardiography (ECG) in all its forms, from 12-lead ECG to long-term monitoring, is considered, an old and increasingly irrelevant test in this high technology era. This article reviews the clinical utility of this tool and argues that the obsolescence is due to an increasing inability to read electrocardiographic tracings. The usual interpretative pitfalls are discussed and a logical approach is proposed with illustrative examples. Finally, the concept of precision ECG is presented and its meaning reviewed.

Surface Electrocardiogram Recording: Baseline 12-lead and Ambulatory Electrocardiogram Monitoring   189

Margherita Padeletti, Giuseppe Bagliani, Roberto De Ponti, Fabio M. Leonelli, and Emanuela T. Locati

The 12-lead standard electrocardiogram (ECG) is a 10 second recording of human myocytes electrical activity. Filters and oversampling are necessary in order to acquire a smooth signal without distortion. ECG recordings may display ongoing arrhythmias, and some leads may be helpful in formulating the diagnosis. Advanced modalities of baseline ECG recording can be used to extract additional information with significant prognostic value. Ambulatory ECG (AECG) recording is a long-term and low-cost external recording obtained with 1 to 12 leads lasting from 24 to 30 days. For patient comfort, longer AECG recordings use fewer leads.

Advanced Cardiac Signal Recording   203

Roberto De Ponti, Ilaria My, Manola Vilotta, Fabrizio Caravati, Jacopo Marazzato, Giuseppe Bagliani, and Fabio M. Leonelli

Implantable loop recorders allow prolonged and continuous single-lead electrocardiogram recording, with the pivotal addition of remote monitoring. They have significantly shortened time to electrocardiographic diagnosis and appropriate therapy of many bradyarrhythmias/tachyarrhythmias and proved helpful in arrhythmia burden definition, offering invaluable information in the diagnostic workup for syncope and atrial fibrillation. Advanced cardiac signal recording is also possible by transesophageal catheters. They have been used to orient diagnosis during wide and narrow QRS complex tachycardias and also to perform minimally invasive pacing. Intracardiac electrophysiologic study remains, however, essential for diagnosis of several arrhythmias in the perspective of curative catheter ablation.

Owing to the rapid development of new electrophysiologic techniques, our understanding of arrhythmias and their underlying mechanisms has reached unprecedented levels. In some cases, baseline ECG alterations can be identified before arrhythmia development; early recognition of these alterations is of utmost importance to start appropriate preventive therapies and stratify the risk according to patients' outcomes. Hereby, we report a systematic revision of main baseline ECG abnormalities and their implications on clinical outcomes.

When faced with an electrocardiographic recoding of a complex arrhythmia, we often use inflexible algorithms or try to recall patterns already seen, which is often insufficient to explain the mechanisms of difficult bradycardias and tachycardias. We propose an approach to these situations where, starting from basic observations, the behavior of the different components of the arrhythmia is reconstructed using logical deductions. The extensive use of laddergrams faithfully illustrates how analysis of timing of each visible event, P and QRS, clarifies their relationship and dictates the behavior of electrocardiographic silent cardiac structures (sinus node and atrioventricular node).

Sinus node dysfunction or atrioventricular blocks are the causes of bradycardias. Diagnosis and management begin with evaluation of patient's hemodynamic status and diagnosis of bradycardia's cause. This is followed by an in depth evaluation of pathophysiology of the arrhythmia, its severity, and likelihood of progression. Implementing emergent measures depends on the presence of subsidiary pace makers maintaining cardiac output. Many of these decisions are greatly helped by 12 lead electrocardiogram, because its tracings are often diagnostic of the cause of the bradycardia and help to assess its persistence and progression and to evaluate the presence and reliability of subsidiary pacemakers.

Several arrhythmogenic substrates may generate narrow QRS complex tachycardia, frequently encountered in clinical practice. Some narrow QRS complex tachycardias, however, are sustained by an uncommon arrhythmogenic mechanism. Although rare, these forms should be taken into account in the differential diagnosis to avoid misdiagnosis and improper patient management. Dual atrioventricular node physiology can be responsible for different uncommon forms of narrow QRS complex tachycardia, also nonreentrant in mechanism. A ventricular origin also is possible, if the tachycardia site is located in the upper ventricular septum with fast ventricular propagation to the specific conduction system and narrowing of the QRS complex.

Alessandra Tordini, Fabio M. Leonelli, Roberto De Ponti, Giuseppe Bagliani, Stefano Donzelli, Ludovico Lazzari, Chiara Marini, Marco M. Pirrami, and Giovanni Carreras

Electrocardiographic algorithms are particularly useful to differentiate, in the presence of a wide complex tachycardia, between supraventricular aberrancy and ventricular tachycardias (VT). There are numerous limitations to the sensitivity and specificity of these algorithms including the presence of accessory pathways, use of antiarrhythmic drugs, congenital heart diseases, electrolytes impairments, and artificial pacing. Once the diagnosis of VT has been reached, other algorithms can help in localizing the origin of the ventricular arrhythmia. These approaches are also limited by the anatomic structure of where the arrhythmia originates. This article illustrates the difficulties in applying common algorithms in many clinical circumstances.

Giuseppe Bagliani, Josep Brugada, Roberto De Ponti, Graziana Viola, Paola Berne, and Fabio M. Leonelli

Electrocardiogram (ECG) analysis trying to understand the mechanisms of QRS widening is often problematic. During WCTs, identification of P waves and atrioventricular relationship is often difficult and increasingly so if the number of recording leads available for examination is limited. For this reason, it is necessary to use every information available in an ECG tracing. The goal of this article is to focus on the reasons for QRS variations occurring during tachycardia. Correct interpretation of these data can offer the key to understand the arrhythmia mechanism.

Zeynab Jebberi, Jacopo Marazzato, Roberto De Ponti, Giuseppe Bagliani, Fabio M. Leonelli, and Serge Boveda

Polymorphic wide QRS complex tachycardia is defined as a tachyarrhythmia showing variable and frequently alternating morphologies of the QRS complex with irregular R-R intervals. It may present with a specific and reproducible pattern including torsade de pointes and bidirectional ventricular tachycardia or with a nonspecific and very irregular pattern, different from ventricular fibrillation. Polymorphic ventricular tachycardia is a challenging diagnosis and is associated with a high risk for sudden cardiac death. Although rare, preexcited atrial fibrillation over multiple accessory pathways can also generate a polymorphic wide QRS complex tachycardia mimicking polymorphic ventricular tachycardia.

Emanuela T. Locati, Giuseppe Bagliani, Franco Cecchi, Helou Johny, Maurizio Lunati, and Carlo Pappone

Several acquired and congenital disease conditions and many cardiac and noncardiac drugs affect ventricular repolarization and increase susceptibility to ventricular arrhythmias. Abnormal ventricular repolarization can be reflected on the surface ECG by prolonged or shortened QT interval, early repolarization, and abnormal T-wave configuration. Reduced outward K+ currents and abnormal or increased sodium or calcium currents increase the vulnerability to ventricular arrhythmias. Multiple mechanisms give rise to ventricular arrhythmias in conditions of congenital or acquired abnormal ventricular repolarization. Ventricular arrhythmias associated with abnormalities of ventricular repolarization typically are rapid, usually polymorphic, ventricular tachycardia or torsades de pointes, often degenerating into ventricular fibrillation.

Pacemakers, cardioverter/defibrillators, and implantable loop recorders with their continuously improved diagnostic capabilities offer detailed information that can help interpreting a cardiac arrhythmia in implanted patients. Nevertheless, in some cases, analysis of the electrical signals stored in the device memory may not be easy. An accurate knowledge of the company-specific software and the meaning of the different markers used are necessary to correctly interpret the arrhythmia or diagnose an inappropriate device intervention due to under- or oversensing. This new technology does not replace the "old" surface electrocardiogram but supplements it to improve arrhythmia diagnosis.

Abnormalities in cardiac rhythm are caused by disorders of impulse generation, conduction, or a combination of the 2, and may be life-threatening because of a reduction in cardiac output or myocardial oxygenation. Cardiac arrhythmias are commonly classified as tachycardias (supraventricular or ventricular) or bradycardias. Bradycardias are uncommon in the critically ill patient and often are caused by an underlying reversible disorder (eg, hyperkalemia, drug toxicity). Supraventricular and ventricular tachycardias are more often encountered in the critically ill patient and often have underlying treatable disorders that precipitate their development (eg, hypokalemia, hypomagnesemia, antiarrhythmic proarrhythmia, myocardial ischemia).

Classic ECG interpretation is based on identification of waveforms and deductive analysis of the electrical events the waveforms represent. The more in depth the understanding of electrophysiologic cellular interactions, the more precise the interpretation of ECG tracing. Surface ECG has limitations; yet, it is accurate in representing myocytes' pathologic behaviors. Recent advances have improved understanding of arrhythmias by reconstructing their mechanisms of induction and maintenance and exploring cellular channel dysfunction. Translating this knowledge to ECG analysis will create the link that allows ECG interpretation to reach the level of precision electrocardiology. This article presents cases illustrating new techniques for electrophysiologists.

CARDIAC ELECTROPHYSIOLOGY CLINICS

SERIES OF RELATED INTEREST

Cardiology Clinics
Available at: https://www.cardiology.theclinics.com/

THE CLINICS ARE AVAILABLE ONLINE!
Access your subscription at:
www.theclinics.com

Foreword
Electrocardiographic Trilogy

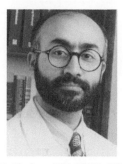 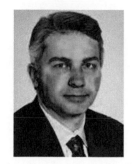

Ranjan K. Thakur, MD, MPH, MBA, FHRS   Andrea Natale, MD, FACC, FHRS
Consulting Editors

We are pleased to introduce this issue of *Cardiac Electrophysiology Clinics* devoted to interpretation of complex arrhythmias. This is the third issue of a trilogy on interpretation of the 12-lead electrocardiogram (ECG). Dr Luigi Padeletti started this project, but he passed away unexpectedly while working on the second issue. We appreciate and congratulate his colleagues, Drs Giuseppe Bagliani, Roberto De Ponti, and Fabio Leonelli, for bringing Luigi's dream to fruition by completing the trilogy.

The first issue in this series (September 2017, volume 9, issue 3) focused on basic electrocardiography in normal and diseased hearts. It took a unique approach to discussing electrocardiography of arrhythmias. It first detailed what can be learned about physiology, pathology, and neural control from each wave and interval of the ECG and then built on that to discuss arrhythmias originating in each cardiac structure. The second issue (June 2018, volume 10, issue 2) focused on electrocardiography of various arrhythmias: bradycardias, tachycardias, and some specific arrhythmias. This issue focuses on interpretation of complex arrhythmias due to problematic ECGs or intricate arrhythmia mechanisms.

Again, we congratulate the editors for fulfilling the vision of one of their colleagues. It speaks to their love and admiration for Dr Luigi Padeletti. We hope the readers will dust off the previous issues in this trilogy and enjoy reading all three volumes together.

Ranjan K. Thakur, MD, MPH, MBA, FHRS
Sparrow Thoracic and Cardiovascular Institute
Michigan State University
1200 East Michigan Avenue, Suite 580
Lansing, MI 48912, USA

Andrea Natale, MD, FACC, FHRS
Texas Cardiac Arrhythmia Institute
Center for Atrial Fibrillation at
St. David's Medical Center
1015 East 32nd Street, Suite 516
Austin, TX 78705, USA

E-mail addresses:
thakur@msu.edu (R.K. Thakur)
andrea.natale@stdavids.com (A. Natale)

Preface
Complex Arrhythmias: A Systematic Approach Toward a "Precision Electrocardiology" Horizon

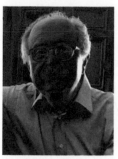
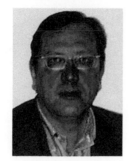
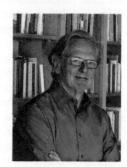

Giuseppe Bagliani, MD   Roberto De Ponti, MD, FHRS   Fabio M. Leonelli, MD

Editors

"Interpreting Complex Arrhythmias" is the third in a series of issues dealing with electrocardiographic analysis published in *Cardiac Electrophysiology Clinics*.

Our thanks to Drs Ranjan K. Thakur and Andrea Natale for their continuous support of our long-lasting passion for the surface electrocardiogram (ECG) behind the compilation of these three issues.

We also need to thank Professor Luigi Padeletti, friend, inspirer, and leader in this endeavour, who, from the beginning of this effort, reminded us that the interpretation of an electrocardiographic tracing is not just a mere diagnostic tool to guide clinical choices but also an instrument to advance our knowledge of the normal and pathologic cardiac electrical properties.

Part I of this series, "Normal Electrophysiology, Substrates, and the Electrocardiographic Diagnosis of Cardiac Arrhythmias," explored the links between basic anatomic and electrophysiologic concepts and the electrocardiographic manifestations of arrhythmias. The second issue, "Bradycardias, Complex Tachycardias, and Clinical Arrhythmias: The Role of Electrocardiography,"

dealt with brady-tachyarrhythmias and their clinical context, while this third issue, "Interpreting Complex Arrhythmias," approaches arrhythmias of higher complexity either because of problematic ECG interpretation or because of intricate electrophysiologic mechanisms. Following the approach of the previous issues, ECG tracings are logically analyzed to obtain fundamental clinical information guiding patient management. Within this issue, the article by Bagliani and colleagues stresses the need for a correct interpretation analysis; articles by Padeletti and colleagues and De Ponti and colleagues compare the simple and complex acquisition of the electrocardiographic recording; and articles by Chen and colleagues and Leonelli and colleagues describe the overall method of arrhythmia's analysis. Having provided the interpretative tools, the reader is introduced to a deeper analysis of complex arrhythmias: bradycardias in the article by Leonelli and colleagues, narrow complex tachycardias in the article by De Ponti and colleagues, and wide complex tachycardias in the article by Tordini and colleagues.

Card Electrophysiol Clin 11 (2019) xv–xvi
https://doi.org/10.1016/j.ccep.2019.04.001
1877-9182/19/© 2019 Published by Elsevier Inc.

In the article by Bagliani and colleagues, subtle variations of ECG morphology are discussed; these cannot be overlooked, representing the key to the interpretation of the arrhythmia's mechanism. Articles by Jebberi and colleagues, Locati and colleagues, Sciarra and colleagues, and Pozzolini and colleagues deal with four complex arrhythmologic problems: polymorphic wide QRS complex tachycardias; inherited and acquired abnormalities of ventricular repolarization; arrhythmias in patients with implantable devices; and complex arrhythmias due to reversible causes.

The article by Leonelli and colleagues describes representative cases of hidden complexity in routine adult and pediatric arrhythmia interpretation and introduces the concept of "precision electrocardiology." This defines a deeper knowledge of the arrhythmic electrophysiologic mechanisms obtained by correlating electrocardiographic tracing with data obtained with 3D catheter mapping, genetic analysis, or diverse cardiac imaging. The end result should be a complete understanding of each component of an ECG recording.

We hope that this issue of *Cardiac Electrophysiology Clinics*, a compendium of years of study and clinical observations, becomes a useful instrument in the hands of students, clinical cardiologists, electrophysiologists, and scientists.

For ourselves, we wish to continue in the path marked by our teachers.

Giuseppe Bagliani, MD
Arrhythmology Unit
Cardiology Department
Foligno General Hospital
Via Massimo Arcamone, Foligno
Perugia 06034, Italy

Cardiovascular Disease Department
University of Perugia
Perugia, Italy

Roberto De Ponti, MD, FHRS
Department of Cardiology
School of Medicine
University of Insubria
Viale Borri, 57, Varese
Varese 21100, Italy

Fabio M. Leonelli, MD
Center Clinical Research
James A. Haley Veterans Administration Hospital
University South Florida
13000 Bruce B Down Boulevard
Tampa, FL 33612, USA

E-mail addresses:
giuseppe.bagliani@tim.it (G. Bagliani)
roberto.deponti@uninsubria.it (R. De Ponti)
fabio.leonelli@va.org (F.M. Leonelli)

Precision Electrocardiology
A Rational Approach for Simple and Complex Arrhythmias

Giuseppe Bagliani, MD[a,b,*], Roberto De Ponti, MD, FHRS[c],
Fabio M. Leonelli, MD[d]

KEYWORDS

• ECG • Precision electrocardiology • Arrhythmias • Interpretative method

KEY POINTS

- The electrocardiography (ECG) interpretation is particularly difficult in arrhythmias potentially presenting with a myriad of variations.
- The need for a logical approach is fundamental to interpreting an electrocardiographic tracing, to understanding tachycardia's mechanism, and for preventing common interpretative pitfalls.
- This approach is described step by step, reinforcing the importance of the laddergram.
- A new role for the ECG is suggested in the optics of precision medicine.

INTRODUCTION

The diagnosis of arrhythmia is among the most fascinating areas of medicine and cardiology. The ability to generate an electrical gradient across a cellular membrane is a unique feature of living organisms.

In the myocytes, the cyclic contractions are correlated with the transmembrane inversion of polarity, which generates electrical currents and are faithfully registered by the electrocardiogram. The electrocardiography (ECG) interpretation, therefore, represents a challenge to understanding the cellular mechanisms closely related to cardiac function and mechanisms maintaining life. From its beginning, surface ECG has been constrained by the limitations of recording the miniscule amount of current generated by the cardiac structures: some of the current produced by atria and ventricles can be recorded but the potentials created by the specialized cellular structures deputed to the generation and conduction of the electrical impulse cannot be registered.

The interpretative challenge of ECG becomes extremely difficult when an abnormal cardiac activation (arrhythmia) takes the place of sinus rhythm with normal propagation.

Despite its schematic classification, arrhythmias can present on the ECG recording with thousands of variations. The loss of a regular activation sequence creates overlapping signals that are completely different from the well-defined waveforms observed during sinus rhythm.

Loss of electrical signals, abnormal waveform morphologies, or fusion of simultaneous electrical events creates the difficulties surrounding arrhythmia's diagnosis. This is a situation akin the quest to understand, in a complex musical symphony,

The authors have no relevant conflicts to disclose.
[a] Cardiology Department, Arrhythmology Unit, Foligno General Hospital, Foligno, Italy; [b] Cardiovascular Diseases Department, University of Perugia, Perugia, Italy; [c] Cardiology Department, University of Insubria, Varese 21100, Italy; [d] Cardiology Department, James A. Haley Veterans' Hospital, University of South Florida, 13000 Bruce B. Downs Boulevard, Tampa, FL 33612, USA
* Corresponding author. Via Centrale Umbra 17, Spello, Perugia 06038, Italy.
E-mail address: giuseppe.bagliani@tim.it

Card Electrophysiol Clin 11 (2019) 175–187
https://doi.org/10.1016/j.ccep.2019.01.003
1877-9182/19/© 2019 Elsevier Inc. All rights reserved.

not only the instrument's role but even their individual musical score.

For this reason, the study of cardiac arrhythmias in medicine has never been considered a simple task. In many ways it is comparable to the study of mathematics in the universal curriculum of studies. As mathematics requires a logical mechanism to be understood, so arrhythmia's comprehension needs a systemic, deductive approach that offers the keys to solve an apparently impossible quest.

Teaching is essential to reach this level of knowledge. A teacher transfers his or her knowledge to students while remaining ready to accept new knowledge coming from this encounter.

To simultaneously be the teacher and the student is not always easy. This is what the authors of this article would like to be able to do: share their knowledge while learning from others' clinical experience.

SIMPLE AND COMPLEX: FOOLED BY APPEARANCES

A complex arrhythmia does not lend itself to an immediate mechanistic interpretation[1,2] and it usually generates multiple diagnostic possibilities (case 1 A, B, C). Equally, arrhythmias that are considered to be simple may, if not analyzed in depth, be interpreted too simplistically or even incorrectly (case 2 A, B, C). Therefore, subdividing arrhythmias into simple or complex may lead to a misconstrued diagnosis in the former and a premature interpretative surrender due to the perceived complexities in the latter.

The level of complexity of an arrhythmic ECG tracing does not always match the complexity of its electrophysiological mechanism. Often, tachycardias with convoluted ECGs have simple electrophysiological explanations, whereas some straightforward tracings are the result of complicated mechanisms.[3] In the first case, experience guides attentive analysis of the waveforms based on selection of specific leads in which P and QRS are best represented and identification of all the waveforms when they are easily visible or overlapping 1 into the other. To find a P buried into a T wave (case 2 A) or to imagine it hiding within the QRS (case 1) is an historic achievement!

Other times, everything appears obvious: P is clear, QRS evident, and ST-T distinguishable. In this apparent simplicity, subtle but important electrophysiological phenomena may be overlooked: PR variability, fusion of different activation wavefronts, or expression of variable His-Purkinje system delay.

Therefore, to correctly diagnose an arrhythmia, experience in evaluating the ECG tracing and an in-depth knowledge of their electrophysiological mechanisms are both necessary.

A correct analysis of a simple test such as the ECG allows not just straightforward diagnosis but also gives valuable insights to guide more complex procedures.[4]

A Rational Approach Against Diagnostic Irrational Forces

ECG analysis of arrhythmia requires a rigorous rational approach to avoid the risk of falling into irrational perspectives that can be summarized as follows:

- Instinctive approach: the diagnosis is not based on careful observation of the tracing but driven by the recognition of similar ECG seen in the past. A classic example is the misinterpretation of an AT with highly irregular QRS mimicking AF.
- Clinical preconditioning: choosing first most likely diagnosis and falling in love with it. This is the case of a diagnosis based on the subconscious desire to confirm a specific type of arrhythmia that fits particularly well in a certain clinical situation. These snap diagnoses are mostly based on an irrational approach and are often incorrect. In fact, once formulated, the diagnosis initiates a search to find often minor confirmatory elements that are acquired despite their lack of logical cohesion and are forced together to confirm an erroneous initial diagnosis. Snap diagnosis are almost always risky unless the presenting arrhythmia is so obvious that does not leave any other possible interpretation.
- Diagnostic one-upmanship: when in a group of colleagues, the desire to show superior interpretative skills by identifying subtle but fundamental details gone unnoticed in an ECG tracing. The desire to shine often leads to the surprising discovery of irrelevant electrocardiographic abnormalities rendered important by faulty deductions lacking a proper logical sequence.

CERTAIN OR LIKELY DIAGNOSIS?

Surface ECG is a bird's eye vision of cardiac electrical events. The relationship between the electrocardiographic waveform and the electrical event represented could be affected by a large number of factors, some known and some unknown. Furthermore, ECG does not record activation potentials of common His and its bundles, and provides no detailed information on arrhythmia propagation. These limitations can be partially overcome by a solid knowledge of electrophysiological properties of normal and abnormal cardiac tissue, as well as the mechanisms of arrhythmias.

Because tachycardias do not occur in a vacuum, the first step in ECG diagnosis of an arrhythmia is to be well-informed of the patient's clinical status, including cardiac pathologic conditions, comorbidities, and drug therapy, as well as any available electrocardiographic tracings.

Identification of each electrocardiographic waveform is the next step in an attempt to recreate the progression of cardiac activation in the different heart chambers.

From collected observations, the analysis proceeds to deduction of diagnostic keys that can generate a corollary of differential diagnosis. In this final process, awareness of the pitfalls of interpretation previously expressed is obviously fundamental.

It is not surprising that, given the limitations previously illustrated, it is not always possible to reach certain diagnosis of an arrhythmia with ECG. Despite the use of subtle logic supplemented by experience and knowledge, there are situations in which a differential diagnosis is narrowed down to 2 possibilities. More extensive observations of the arrhythmia behavior on telemetry strips or Holter monitoring can often help to identify the most likely diagnosis but prolonged data collections may not always be possible.

It is, therefore, more accurate to consider any ECG arrhythmia diagnosis in terms of likelihood instead of certainty. For some tracings, the likelihood can be extremely high and, for others, there will be more than 1 possibility competing for the highest degree of likelihood.

A Solid Working Approach: Building a Laddergram

In the current clinical ECG interpretation of arrhythmias, several criteria are used that are not diagnostic, although frequently observed in specific arrhythmias; for example, irregular R-R during atrial fibrillation (AF) and wide complex tachycardia (WCT) in ventricular tachycardia (VT):

1. Total R-R irregularity, particularly if there is atrial activity, is not obvious at first glance and leads to an immediate diagnosis of AF,[5] contributing to cursory analysis of atrial depolarization. A valid differential diagnosis should include several atrial arrhythmias due to abnormal automaticity (cases 3 and 4).
2. Wide QRS and diagnosis of VT: although it is correct to associate a wide QRS with a rhythm originating in the ventricles propagating with

slow saltatory conduction within the ventricles (case 5), very wide QRSs are also observed in other conditions, such as supraventricular rhythms with bundle branch block, maximal pre-excitation, and artificial ventricular stimulation.[6,7] These 2 examples are similar to many others that present difficulties in identification of ECG waveforms or their correlation. To approach an arrhythmia, therefore, it is necessary to have a working method aimed at graphically representing the arrhythmia's mechanism and based on

a. Identification of the electrocardiographic waveforms representing atrial and ventricular depolarization
b. Formulation of probable diagnostic hypotheses, most frequently 3 or more, among which the correct hypothesis is included. These hypotheses require an in-depth knowledge of the electrophysiological properties of the cardiac tissues and their electrocardiographic representation.
c. A search for the diagnostic key: this depends greatly on the observer's specific knowledge and allows the identification of the diagnostic elements leading, in the specific clinical scenario, to the irrefutable diagnosis of arrhythmia.

This entire process is greatly aided by the construction of a laddergram that graphically shows all this information and allows relating them to each other in a logical manner. Classic examples of diagnostic keys are the identification of fibrillatory waveforms during AF or identification of asynchronous sinus rhythm during WCT tantamount to diagnosis of VT. It is at this stage of the analysis that it may be necessary to compare the ECG with arrhythmia in previous ECGs, or even consider the use of drugs or special maneuvers.

The interpretative effort should not be cut short just because the answer could be obtained by performing an invasive electrophysiology study (EPS). This is in itself an intellectual defeat and a full understanding of the arrhythmia could spare the patient the risks of an invasive procedure and provide much useful information should an EPS be required.

Phenotype-Genotype Precision Electrocardiology in the Era of Precision Medicine: the Strength of Electrocardiography Diagnosis

The initial analysis of an electrocardiographic tracing based on interpretation of surface leads can, if approached with a solid knowledge background, provide valuable information on the pattern of cardiac activation. Correlating atrial and ventricular activation can be particularly useful in the diagnosis of VT (case 5).

Case 1 compounds several electrophysiological observations on the 3 fundamental cardiac structures: atria, conduction system, and ventricles. It shows

- Three different types of atrial activation (sinus node, ectopic, and retrograde)
- Two different modalities of Atrio Ventricular (AV) conduction corresponding to 2 distinct Atrio Ventricular Node (AVN) pathways: the fast pathway situated in the superoanterior portion of the AVN with consistent expression of Sino atrial Node (SA) channels and, therefore, fast propagation of the impulse but prolonged refractory period, and the slow pathway located inferiorly with slower conduction but shorter refractory period. This arrangement is probably present in most individuals but when the normal electrophysiological equilibrium is altered, conditions for emergence of a reentrant circuit are set.
- Two-level of block in the conduction system: at the His bundle level (transient 2:1 conduction or His alternans)[8] and its branch (due to prematurity in a sequence known as the Ashman phenomenon).[6]

These numerous observations should stimulate reflection on the possibility of a precision diagnosis in electrocardiology which, based on surface recordings (phenotypes), enable clarification of the function and malfunction of specific ionic channels associated with specific anatomic structures (genotypes).

Surface ECG can precisely diagnose both macroscopic abnormalities, in reality phenotic, and ionic cellular derangements, appropriately defined as phenotypic.

This reasoning is exemplified in case 7 in which a patient presents with a normal rhythm but a clear abnormality in cardiac repolarization due to altered K channels function.[9] This is the substrate responsible for triggering Ventricular Premature Contractions (VPCs) that, by occurring in profoundly electrically inhomogeneous ventricles, trigger torsade de pointe (TdP), the partonomic VF associated with these anomalies.

This is an arrhythmogenic model produced by the combination of a substrate genetically or anatomically altered that can, in specific conditions, such as hypokalemia, dysautonomia, drug exposure, and so forth, trigger a ventricular arrhythmia with characteristic ECG tracing.

CLINICAL CASES
Case 1

The need for detailed analysis
Clinical presentation: A 12-year-old boy is investigated for frequent episodes of palpitations of variable intensity. Holter monitoring demonstrates a symptomatic episode of sudden doubling of heart rate from 100 to 200 beats per minute (bpm) (Fig. 1A).

Observation (Fig. 1B): Initial sinus rhythm, an supra ventricular tachycardia (SVT) of 100 bpm with long PR, and 3 wide complex QRS, is followed by a narrow complex tachycardia rate 200 bpm with subtle change in QRS morphology. After the third premature atrial beat (P′), an abrupt prolongation of the PR interval, a jump strongly suggests a sudden change in anterograde AVN conduction from the fast to slow pathway.

Wide QRS analysis shows a progressive narrowing of the QRS and R-R interval of the 3 beats is identical to following R-R of faster tachycardia.

Heart rate acceleration occurs following 3 beats of wide QRS with change in narrow QRS morphology; during faster tachycardia no P wave is visible.

Differential diagnosis: There is initial sinus tachycardia with reentrant SVT induced by VPCs. There is a doubling of the ventricular rate of tachycardia with initial aberrancy, followed by accommodation and normalization of QRS. Slight changes in QRS morphology occur as the rate doubles and a small notch is visible at QRS end during faster rates. This notch is not visible during sinus rhythm.

Diagnostic keys: The laddergram clearly shows the diagnostic keys (Fig. 1C). Key observations are the exact doubling of heart rate, which leads to the question of the mechanism of arrhythmia. There should be, during the initial tachycardia, 100 bpm, a second hidden within the QRS. Searching and finding the hidden P is the second diagnostic key.

Case 2

Simple but not that simple
Clinical presentation: A 65-year-old woman presents with periods of profound weakness and bradycardia; in view of presentation and findings a pace maker was considered (Fig. 2A).

Observations: This tracing appears to be a very straightforward ECG. Sinus bradycardia, heart rate 38 bpm, with normal conduction. In view of the symptoms, this appears to be inappropriate, suggesting a diagnosis of sick sinus syndrome. A second ECG (Fig. 2B) is, at first glance, very similar to the initial ECG except that the rate is 65 bpm. A second relevant difference between the 2 tracings is the different T-wave morphology (Fig. 2C).

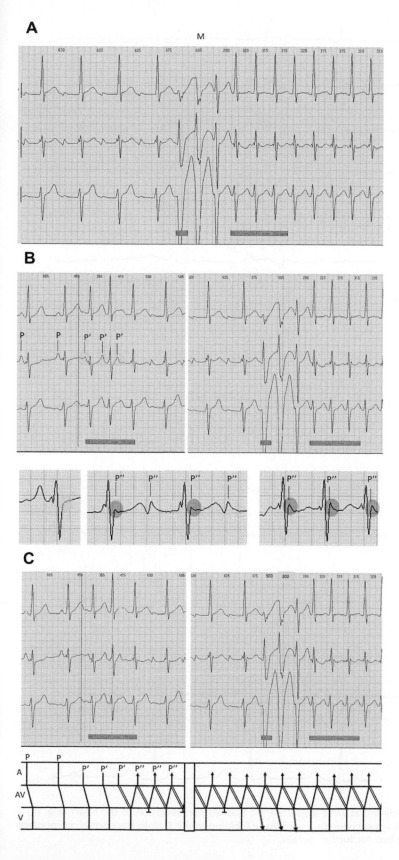

Fig. 1. Clinical case 1. (*A*) Holter monitoring demonstrates a symptomatic marker (M) episode of sudden doubling of heart rate from 100 (*left*) to 200 (*right*) bpm. See text for further details. (*B*) The search for reading keys. Upper left sinus rhythm and start of tachycardia; at the top right the doubling of the heart rate. Below: the search for waves P. See text for further details. (*C*) The laddergram: After a particularly premature atrial beat (P′), an abrupt prolongation of the PR interval happens (jump) suggests a change in anterograde AVN conduction from fast (*single line*) to slow (*double line*) pathway. Doubling of ventricular rate of tachycardia with initial 3 aberrant QRS. In conclusion: AVN reentry tachycardia with transient 2:1 AV block and aberrant right bundle branch block. See text for further details.

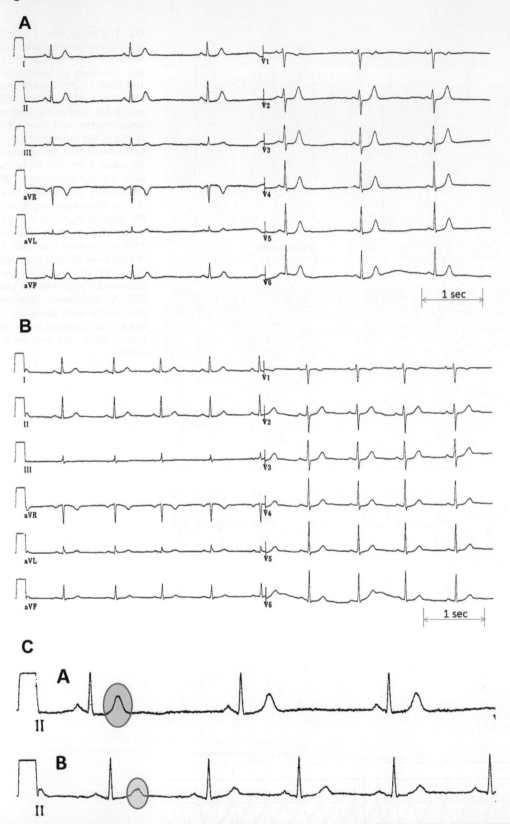

Fig. 2. Clinical case 2. (*A*) Sinus bradycardias were suspected. (*B*) Sudden normalization of the heart rate. (*C*) A picked T wave in the tracing A (*red*) appears due to a premature P hiding in the T. Note the normal morphology of the T wave in the tracing B. See text for further details.

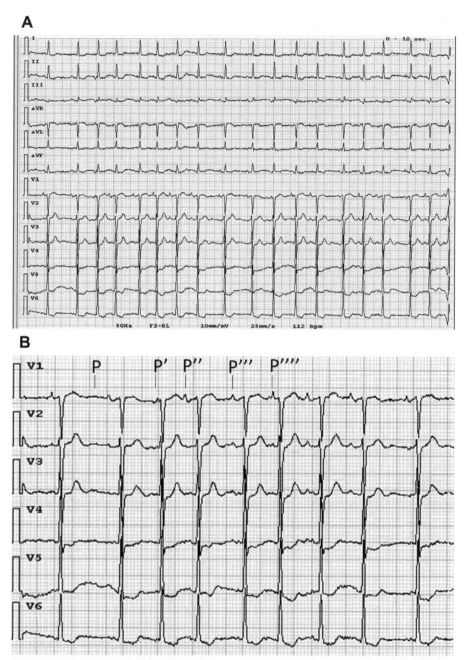

Fig. 3. Clinical case 3. (A) Highly irregular R-R intervals are highly suggestive of AF. (B) This type of R-R behavior is due to 4 different P-wave morphologies, which are due to multifocal automatic atrial tachycardia.

Diagnostic keys: The alteration of the T, which in tracing A appears to be bifid and clearly peaked, is due to a premature P hiding in the T.

The second diagnostic observation is the P (premature) to P (sinus) timing in tracing A, which is almost identical to P-P in sinus rhythm; this is in keeping with sinus node resetting due to premature penetration and discharge by the APC.

Case 3

When memory may fail

Clinical presentation: A 75-year-old man presents with palpitations.

Observations: There is a narrow QRS with highly irregular with R-R with not so obvious P waves, in part due to a baseline artifact. Using a pattern recognition approach, this type of irregularity is

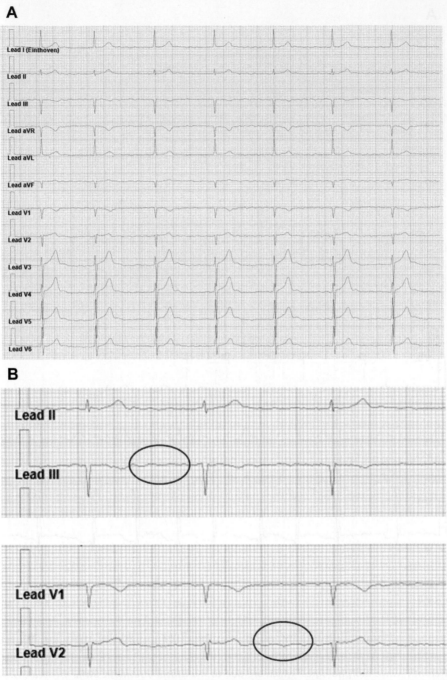

Fig. 4. Clinical case 4. (*A*) Regular narrow complex R-R was observed. (*B*) AF is present (*red circles*) and the almost identical R-R is diagnostic of complete AVN block.

highly suggestive of AF (**Fig. 3**A). A busy observer can easily reach this conclusion and move to next ECG. A closer analysis (**Fig. 3**B) shows P waves of different morphologies with rare sinus P waves.

Diagnostic key: Understand that this type of R-R behavior in a case of narrow QRS represents AVN response to an irregular atrial rhythm.

Not all irregular atrial rhythms are necessarily AF and distinguishing between the different possibilities is necessary to implement a correct therapy.

Ancillary point: There are at least 4 different P-wave morphologies due to multifocal automatic discharges probably coming from both

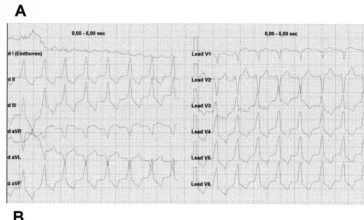

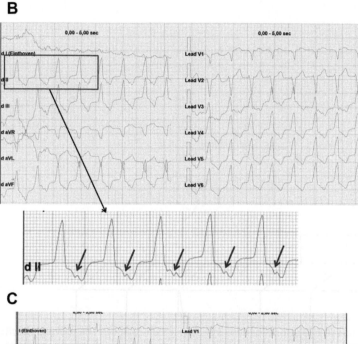

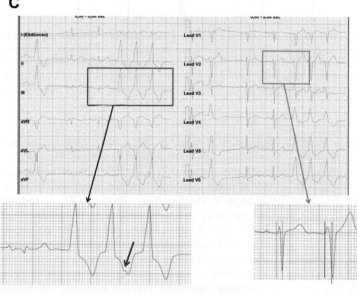

Fig. 5. Clinical case 5. (*A*) WCT with LBBB morphology. (*B*) The same WCT with 1:1 V-A ratio (*red arrows*). (*C*) Nonsustained episodes of the same tachycardia with 2:1 A-V ratio (*red arrows*). On the right (*green arrow*), the morphology of normal and wide QRS. LBBB, left bundle branch block. See text for further details.

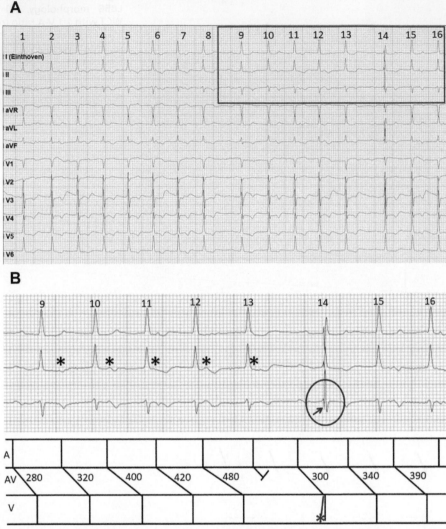

Fig. 6. Clinical case 6. (*A*) Irregular R-R intervals in 3 distinct periods interspersed by 2 pauses. The fourteenth QRS is of a different morphology. (*B*) Diagnostic key: P waves (*asterisk*) buried in the T wave. P-P interval is 500 ms. Every P is followed by a QRS with the exception of the ninth and fifteenth. The fourteenth QRS is of a different morphology being narrower due to fusion with a wavefront generated by a pacemaker (*red circle* and *arrow*). The PR varies explaining R-R irregularity. Diagnostic key: sinus rhythm with atypical Wenckebach. See text for further details.

atria (see different polarities of P wave in V1). Therapy for this condition is different from management of AF.

Case 4

Always consider the electrophysiological properties of each cardiac tissue

Clinical presentation: A 78-year-old man presents with long-standing persistent AF with sudden disappearance of palpitations.

Observations: There is an absence of reproducible P waves and a fibrillatory low-voltage baseline in keeping with clinical history. Regular narrow complex R-R was observed (**Fig. 4**A).

Diagnostic key: Regularization of AVN response to a highly irregular rhythm suggests either a change in rhythm (from irregular AF to regular SR or AFL) or development of complete heart block. AF is still present as can be observed from the fibrillatory atrial activity (**Fig. 4**B) and the almost identical R-R is diagnostic of complete AVN block.

Ancillary observations: Full evaluation of clinical severity of CHB is necessary. Implantation of ppm may be necessary.

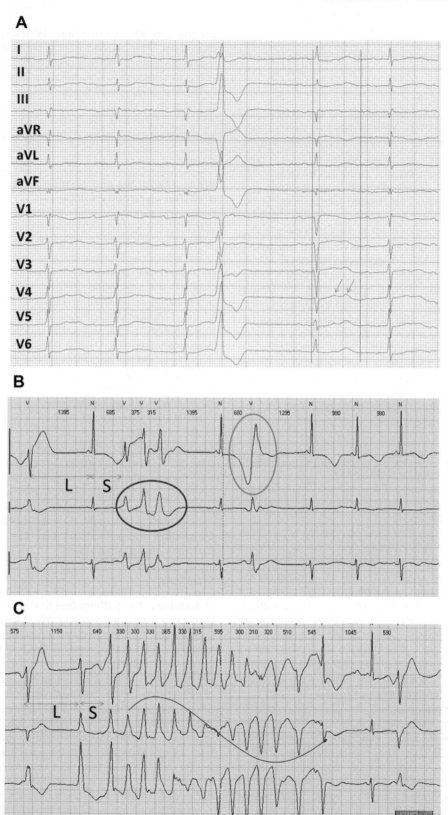

Fig. 7. Clinical case 7. (*A*) Sinus bradycardia rate 50 bpm, with a single VPC. Prolonged QT 660 ms with a bifid morphology (*arrows*) suggestive of LQTS 2. (*B*) Long-short sequences induce single VPCs (*green circle*) and polymorphic nonsustained VT (*red circle*). (*C*) Long-short sequences induce run of TdPs (*red line*), occurring at the end of T wave in keeping with early after depolarizations. TdPs, Torsade de Pointes; See text for further details.

Case 5

Building diagnosis from different observations

Clinical presentation: A 45-year-old woman presents with episodic palpitations and normal cardiovascular system.

Observations: Presenting ECG demonstrates a WCT with QRS duration of 130 ms, normal axis, and precordial progression (**Figs. 5**A and **Fig. 6**). The differential diagnosis appears to be helped by the observation of P waves associated with QRS in a 1:1 relation (**Fig. 5**B) suggesting an SVT with aberrancy. The P-wave morphology is not clear and possibly includes an initial negative deflection. None of these findings are diagnostic.

Diagnostic key: The observation of the beginning of the WCT not preceded by atrial activity and, more importantly, with intermittent P wave following the QRS. Demonstrating Ventriculo-Atrial dissociation excluded the diagnosis of SVT with aberrancy (**Fig. 5**C). Note the slurring of the initial portion, which is suggestive of slow propagation in keeping with VT.

Ancillary observations: The morphology of the QRS suggests a VT origin, probably in the septal right ventricular outflow tract. These arrhythmias tend to respond well to beta blockers and are not difficult radio frequency ablation targets.

Case 6

The importance of laddergram

Clinical presentation: A 64-year-old asymptomatic woman presents with hypertension at regular cardiology follow-up visit.

Observations: The most obvious finding is an irregularity of R-R intervals occurring in 3 distinct periods interspersed by a longer pause. The pause is interrupted by a clear wide P wave, duration 160 ms, with sinus morphology. The search for following Ps leads to observe T-wave variations with a few evident Ps buried in the T wave. P-P interval is, therefore, defined at 500 ms and found to be regular. Every P is followed by a QRS with an incomplete LBBB (duration 120 ms, absent septal vector in V1-V2 and V5-V6) with the exception of the ninth and fifteenth. The fourteenth QRS is of a different morphology, being narrower due to fusion with a wavefront generated by a pacemaker. The PR varies, explaining R-R irregularity.

Diagnostic keys: The P to R relationship, when plotted in a laddergram, is diagnostic of sinus rhythm with atypical Wenckebach. A Mobitz type I is first suspected when the repetition of periods of AV conduction is interrupted by a single nonconducted P in an arrangement called group beating. Measuring the P-R shows a different behavior from typical Wenckebach in which progressive PR prolongation is followed by a drop beat. The second conducted PR prolongs maximally with a minor increase in the following P-R and constant P-R to the drop beat.

The first conducted PR after the pause is always the shorter of the last conducted. Group beating and a progressive lengthening of conduction, albeit nontypical, are the diagnostic keys.

Case 7

When phenotype and genotype meet: toward precision electrophysiology

Clinical presentation: A 36-year-old man presents with frequent episodes of presyncope, normal cardiovascular evaluation, and unclear family history.

Observations: There is a sinus bradycardia rate of 50 bpm, with a single VPC. The obvious abnormality is the prolonged QT (660 ms) with a bifid morphology suggestive of LQTS 2. Lengthening of the R-R interval produces a more marked QT prolongation (780 ms) and deformation with profoundly inverted T wave (**Fig. 7**A). Long-short sequences induce single VPCs (**Fig. 7**B), polymorphic nonsustained VT (**Fig. 7**B), or runs of TdPs (**Fig. 7**C), occurring at the end of a T wave, in keeping with early after depolarizations.

Ancillary observations: The phenotypical abnormality observed in SR and accentuated during bradycardia (either stable or episodic, such as in periodic R-R prolongation) corresponds to a specific genetic alteration coding for an abnormal K channel. This correspondence between phenotype (ECG alteration) and specific pathologic findings (genetic, anatomic, or electrophysiological) constitutes, the authors believe, the concept of precision electrophysiology.

SUMMARY

In summary, the authors feel that analysis of 12-lead ECG remains an ideal clinical tool, in which knowledge and reasoning come together to solve very relevant questions: What is the mechanism of the tachycardia? What are its clinical implications? The miniscule cost, the absolute noninvasiveness of this test, and the ease and speed of acquisition of the large amount of data contained in the tracings are, however, inversely correlated with the dedication and analytic skills necessary to extract and reach diagnostic conclusions from this information. In an era in which difficult clinical tasks are often bypassed, and clinicians increasingly rely on new and more powerful technology, the 12-lead ECG is becoming an almost obsolete test, along with other noninvasive tools such as cardiac auscultation, patient observation, full clinical examination, and so on. The ability to interpret complex sets of data is at risk, which might represent a global view of a clinical scenario, favoring instead a very precise, albeit very narrow, assessment of a single organ. Going from general to particular, constructing a differential diagnosis based on a complex analysis is a far more successful clinical approach than trying to put together very precise but small pieces of information. In the first case, the authors use deduction and induction comparison, as well as all the other logic instruments at our disposal. In the second, we try to interpret clinical information obtained from increasingly sensitive diagnostic tools but we may be unable to assess their clinical relevance or place them correctly in the general clinical framework.

This article is an attempt to underline the persisting value of the 12-lead ECG as a clinical tool. The authors have presented the wealth of data hidden in any tracing and offered a method to unlock and connect them to reach a final diagnosis.

Furthermore, this old and humble device is a fundamental instrument in the classification of a large number diseases, providing us with a precise insight into the pathophysiology of electrophysiological disease. From a 12-lead ECG, it is possible to reconstruct the alterations present at the microscopic level, implicating cellular structures such as channels or gap junctions. The genetic variations related to the LQTS represent a clear demonstration of the close link between the electrocardiographic phenotype and the genetic derangement. This information is particularly helpful in classifying individuals into subpopulations at risk for specific diseases, assessing their prognosis, and individualizing their treatment. It is, therefore, not too whimsical to talk of precision electrocardiology based on the interpretation of ECG data.

The tracings presented are an initial test of the reader's skills and an introduction to a journey that the authors hope will last a long time.

REFERENCES

1. Antzelevitch C, Burashnikov A. Overview of basic mechanisms of cardiac arrhythmia. Card Electrophysiol Clin 2011;3:23–45.
2. Jalife J, Delmar M, Anumonwo J, et al. Basic mechanisms of cardiac arrhythmias. Basic cardiac electrophysiology for the clinician. 2nd edition. New Jersey: Wiley-Blackwell; 2009.
3. Padeletti L, Bagliani G. General Introduction, classification and Electrocardiographic diagnosis of cardiac arrhythmias. Card Electrophysiol Clin 2017;9:345–63.
4. Savino K, Bagliani G, Crusco F, et al. Electrocardiogram and imaging: an integrated approach to arrhythmogenic cardiomyopathies. Card Electrophysiol Clin 2018;10:413–29.
5. Leonelli F, Bagliani G, Boriani G, et al. Arrhythmias originating in the atria. Card Electrophysiol Clin 2017;9:383–409.
6. De Ponti R, Bagliani G, Padeletti L, et al. General approach to a wide QRS complex. Card Electrophysiol Clin 2017;9:461–85.
7. De Ponti R, Marazzato J, Bagliani G, et al. Peculiar electrocardiographic aspects of wide QRS complex tachycardia: when differential diagnosis is difficult. Card Electrophysiol Clin 2018;10:317–32.
8. Bagliani G, Della Rocca DG, Di Biase L, et al. PR interval and junctional zone. Card Electrophysiol Clin 2017;9:411–33.
9. Locati ET, Bagliani G, Padeletti L. Normal and abnormal ventricular repolarization. QT interval: ionic background, measurements and modifiers. Card Electrophysiol Clin 2017;9:487–513.

Surface Electrocardiogram Recording
Baseline 12-lead and Ambulatory Electrocardiogram Monitoring

Margherita Padeletti, MD, PhD[a],*, Giuseppe Bagliani, MD[b,c],
Roberto De Ponti, MD, FHRS[d], Fabio M. Leonelli, MD[e],
Emanuela T. Locati, MD, PhD[f]

KEYWORDS

- Standard ECG • Vectorcardiography • Body surface mapping • Ambulatory ECG recording

KEY POINTS

- Standard electrocardiogram (ECG) is a 12-lead electric signal recording of with a velocity 25 mm/s and 10 mm/mV of amplitude.
- D2, aVR, and V1 are particularly useful to differentiate between ventricular or supraventricular arrhythmia's origin.
- Vectorcardiography, body surface mapping, and signal-averaged ECG are advanced modalities of surface ECG recordings.
- Ambulatory ECG recording is a long-term recording lasting from 24 to 30 days.

STANDARD BASELINE ELECTROCARDIOGRAM RECORDING
Modalities and Characteristics of 12-Lead Recording

The 12-lead standard electrocardiogram (ECG) is a 10-second recording of human low-intensity electrical current originating from cells in the upper part of the right atrium and propagating through the ventricles.

The Standard Electrocardiogram

The technology of the ECG recorder has changed over the decades. Initial observations were made in 1791, when Galvani first recorded electricity from a frog. The instrument that recorded that signal was called the galvanometer. The standard principle of the galvanometer recording is that when current flows toward the positive electrode of the bipolar lead it generates a signal with positive deflection from isoelectric line, whereas when it flows away it inscribes a negative deflection under the isoelectric line. This principle has remained unchanged over the centuries. The galvanometer was initially used to record human electricity in early 1900s when Einthoven developed a 270 kg recorder able to register through Einthoven derivations (standard D1, D2, and D3 bipolar derivations). This was achieved with the patient immersing the both arms and a foot in 3

[a] Cardiology Unit, Mugello Hospital, Viale della Resistenza, 60, Borgo San Lorenzo, Florence 50032, Italy;
[b] Arrhythmology Unit, Cardiology Department, Foligno General Hospital, Via Massimo Arcamone, Foligno, Perugia 06034, Italy; [c] Cardiovascular Disease Department, University of Perugia, Piazza Menghini 1, Perugia 06129, Italy; [d] Department of Cardiology, School of Medicine, University of Insubria, Viale Borri, 57, Varese 21100, Italy; [e] Cardiology Department, James A. Haley Veterans' Hospital, University South Florida, Tampa, FL, USA; [f] Electrophysiology Unit, Cardiovascular Department, Niguarda Hospital, Milan, Italy
* Corresponding author. Arrhythmology Unit, Cardiology Department, Foligno General Hospital, Via Massimo Arcamone, Foligno, Perugia 06034, Italy.
E-mail address: marghepadeletti@gmail.com

Card Electrophysiol Clin 11 (2019) 189–201
https://doi.org/10.1016/j.ccep.2019.01.004
1877-9182/19/© 2019 Elsevier Inc. All rights reserved.

buckets filled with normal saline. The unipolar derivations V1 to V6 were subsequently introduced by Wilson in 1938. Finally, in 1942 the unipolar leads aVR, aVF, and aVL were introduced by Goldberger.

Since then, the standard ECG is an electric signal recording of 12 leads with a velocity 25 mm/s and 10 mm/mV of amplitude.

The ECG trace should always be completed using speed and amplitude reference to read all 12 leads. Rhythm description, axis deviation, duration of the conduction, and final interpretation of the recording should be included in every report (**Table 1**).

How to Maximize the Information from Baseline 12-Lead Electrocardiogram Recording

The ECG is currently based on a processed digital signal, whereas formerly the signal was analogic. The digital signal has advantages because the single beat is analyzed at the same time in 12 leads, whereas the analogic signal was continuous.

Oversampling

To process a smooth signal of the 12-lead ECG recording, oversampling is a technique that improves the resolution of the signal and decreases the noise by a significant multiple of the upper-frequency cutoff to provide the recommended bandwidth in the digitized signal.

On the other hand, the presence of oversampling hides pacemaker (PM) artifacts, especially when the electrical stimulus is delivered bipolarly. Artificially enhancing the PM outputs in the tracing is not helpful because it only deforms the recorded ECG.

If necessary, unipolar output can be programmed in PMs to visualize the spike of the stimulus in the ECG.[1]

Filters

Low-frequency filters The human heart signal recorded by an electrocardiograph is about 10 Hz. To avoid noise and baseline drift during respiration, low-frequency filters less than 0.05 Hz are normally applied in analogical ECG recorders; this is the lowest filter than can be used without the distortion of the ECG created by ST segment depression, especially when ECG is displayed on monitors. In digital devices, however, low-frequency filters can be up to 0.67 Hz without any ST distortion.[1]

High-frequency filters The correct detection of rapid upstroke velocity, peak amplitude, and waves of small duration are measured more accurately if the digital signal is filtered as high as possible. The standard high filter setting is 150 Hz for adults and up to 250 Hz for children. Setting the filter cutoff below that standard falsifies all amplitude ECG signal measurements.

In addition, a monitor display greater than or equal to 500 dpi should be used during the ECG continuous recording to avoid QRS disruption.[1]

Table 1
Standard electrocardiogram measurements in adults

	Normal Value	Hints
P	<120 ms; 0.25 mV; angle = 60°.	Check all leads, generally in DII and V1; positive in D2
P-Q	120–200 ms	From the beginning of the P to the beginning of the QRS
QRS	80–110 ms (adults) Prolonged ≥120 ms	Generally positive in D1 and aVF, negative in V1 an positive in V6 (transition leads V3-V4).
QT/QTc	410–440 ms men 410–460 ms women	From the beginning of the QRS at the end of the T wave generally measure in lead II T wave ends at the tangent of the steepest point of the downslope to the isoelectric line QT at 60 bpm <360 is considered short
T	Limb leads: <0.5 mV (<5 mm) Precordial leads: <1.5 mV (15 mm)	T wave is inverted in aVR; upright or inverted in leads aVL, III, and V1; and upright in leads I and II and in chest leads V3 through V6.
Heart Rate	60–100 bpm	Interval among of each RR spike (300/big square)
Frontal axis	0°-90°	Left axis deviation 0° and −90° Right axis deviation 90°-180° Indefinite 180°and −90°

More Informative Leads for the Differential Diagnosis of Arrhythmias

ECG recordings may display ongoing arrhythmias, and some leads may help in formulating the diagnosis.

D2

The bipolar lead D2 is optimal in detecting atrial activation because its axis is parallel to the atria wave front. The positive P deflection inscribed in D2 in an ECG recording represents the classic top-down left and right atria activation. The switching from positive to negative (P) wave in D2 during an arrhythmia can be due to an ectopic focus or represent reentry. During a paroxysmal tachycardia, positive P waves in D2 are due to ectopic tachycardia ruling out retrograde atrial activation due to atrioventricular nodal tachycardia (AVNRT) or atrioventricular reentrant tachycardia (AVRT) (**Fig. 1**).

During typical atrial flutter, the P waves are replaced in all leads by the classic sawtooth wave shape, which are negative in the D2, whereas during atrial fibrillation P waves are replaced by fibrillation waves (**Figs. 2 and 3**).

In addition, a Lewis lead may improve the detection of P waves on the ECG and help in the differential diagnosis of the atrial flutter or atrial fibrillation.

A Lewis lead is a bipolar chest lead with the right-arm electrode applied to the right side of the sternum at the second intercostal space and the left-arm electrode applied to the right fourth intercostal space adjacent to the sternum, with a caliper of 1 mV equals 20 mm. This particular nonstandard lead can be displayed in D1.

V1

V1, as previously described, is a lead that records the initial weak current of septal depolarization.

This initial current can be hidden inside the QRS, especially when there is a δ (delta) wave suggesting preexcitation of the ventricle. The preexcitation current, which represents the current passing through the accessory pathway, can bypass the septal current, preventing its inscription in V1. If the δ is positive in V1 it identifies a left accessory pathway, whereas if it is negative it identifies a right accessory pathway[2] (**Fig. 4**).

During AVNRT, V1 shows the particular pseudo-R′ pattern along with the pseudo-S in the inferior leads[2] (**Fig. 5**).

A wide complex tachycardia (WCT) can be difficult to diagnose because sometimes the origin of the arrhythmia can be uncertain (**Fig. 6**).

V1 analysis is helpful during a WCT of uncertain origin. In particular, the initial r in V1 is inscribed by septal depolarization and its preservation is keeping with normal septal activation and consequently confirms the supraventricular origin of the WCT. On the other hand, its absence suggests abnormal

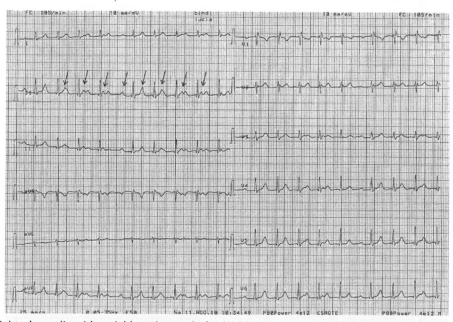

Fig. 1. Atrial tachycardia with variable atrioventricular (AV) block. P waves with P-P interval of 425 ms are clearly visible in lead II. Red arrow identifies a nonconducted P during a long R-R interval. The black arrows correspond to P waves.

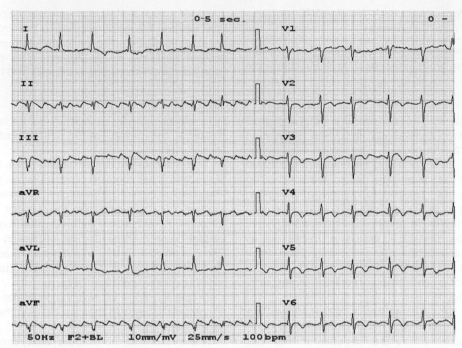

Fig. 2. Typical atrial flutter with sawtooth wave in D2 and a 2:1 or 3:1 AV conduction. Flutter waves are mainly negative in the inferior leads with a slow, downsloping component followed by a steeper upsloping branch of the waveform.

septal activation as observed in arrhythmias originating in the ventricle.

From a practical standpoint, WCTs are defined as having a right bundle branch block (RBBB) morphology in the presence of mostly positive V1 or left bundle branch block (LBBB) if V1 is mainly negative.

In WCT with RBBB morphology, notching on the upstroke (rabbit ears) suggests aberrancy if the sequence is rR' (left ear smaller than right)

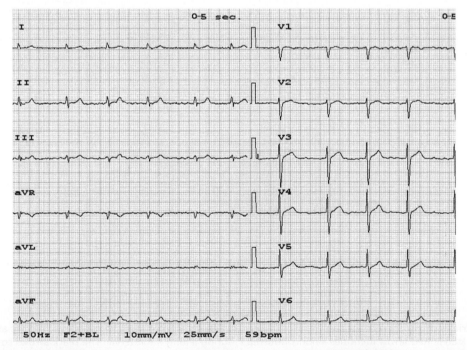

Fig. 3. Clear-cut fibrillatory waves in every lead. Ventricular response is irregular with highly variable R-R intervals.

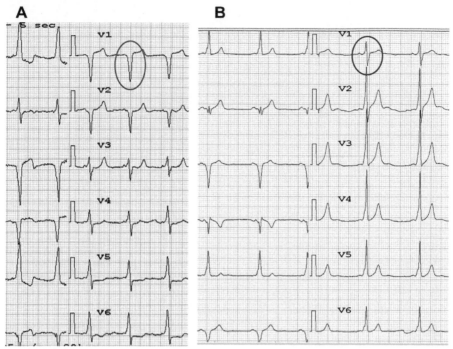

Fig. 4. Wolf-Parkinson-White syndrome. (*A*) The blue circle identifies a negative delta wave in V1, LBBB morphology, typical of right-sided accessory pathway location. (*B*) Red circle shows a positive delta wave in V1, RBBB morphology, present in left-sided accessory pathways.

because septal activation vector remains unaltered (**Fig. 7**). The opposite sequence (Rr'), monophasic R, or qR combinations are all due to a loss of normal septal activation and,

therefore, more diagnostic of ventricular tachycardia (VT) (**Fig. 8**).

Features suggestive of abnormal septal activation during LBBB morphology are an r wider than

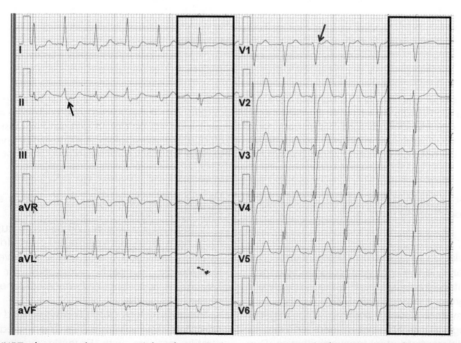

Fig. 5. AVNRT: almost synchronous atrial and ventricular activation; terminal component of a retrograde P wave is visible in lead II (*black arrow*). In V1, the retrograde P inscribes a small pseudo-r' (*red arrow*). Compare this tracing with ECG in sinus rhythm (*black boxes*).

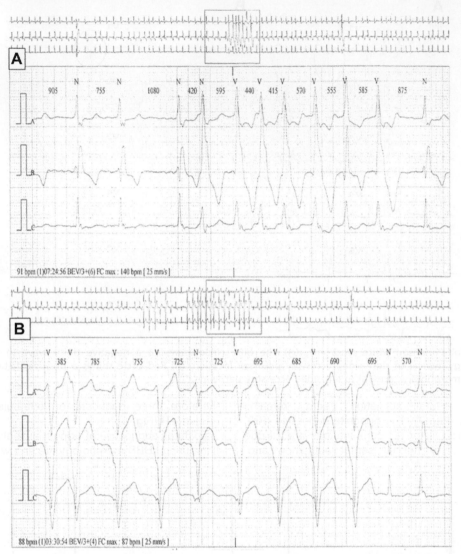

Fig. 6. A 24-hour ambulatory ECG (AECG) recording of an 85-year-old man with ischemic cardiomyopathy, permanent atrial fibrillation, and a right bundle branch block (RBBB). (*A*) shows 7 ventricular beats with an abrupt increase in rate and a morphology change from rSR′ to Rsr′, which is diagnostic of an episode of nonsustained VT. (*B*) 9-beat run of nonsustained VT with left bundle branch block (LBBB) morphology at a rate of 110 bpm. Typical of VTs are the notched descending branch and a fusion beat (the fifth QRS complex starting from the left).

30 ms and a notched downstroke of the S wave lasting more than 60 ms (**Fig. 9**).[3]

aVR

The unipolar lead aVR explores the right upper part of the heart and the right ventricular outflow tract.

In the standard ECG, the P wave is negative in aVR, whereas it is positive in D2.

The switch from positive to negative morphology of the P wave in lead aVR can be used to differentiate atrial tachyarrhythmias. During a narrow QRS tachycardia, a positive P wave in aVR and in aVL, and a negative P wave in the inferior lead, suggests an AVRT with a septal or paraseptal origin.

A negative P wave in aVR can also suggests a focal right atrial tachycardia (AT). In addition, ST segment elevation in aVR during supraventricular tachycardia suggests atrioventricular reentry through an accessory pathway as the mechanism of the tachycardia.

The morphology of the R wave in lead aVR, the so-called Brugada sign, has been used to risk-stratify patients with Brugada syndrome. The aVR sign was defined as an R wave greater than or equal to 0.3 mV or R/q greater than or equal to

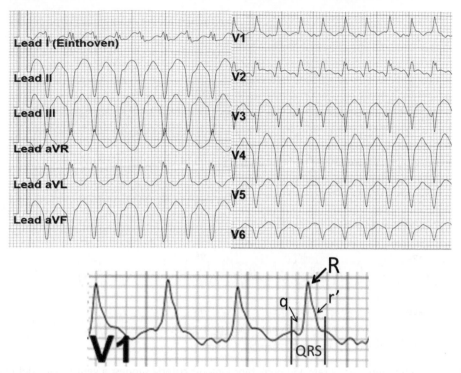

Fig. 7. WCT with RBBB morphology rate 250 bpm. VT is diagnosed based on completely positive aVR (Vereckei criteria), qRr' in V1, atrioventricular dissociation, and retrograde 2:1 conduction (*arrows*), noticeable in V1.

to 0.75 in lead aVR. The prominent R wave in lead aVR may reflect more right ventricular conduction delay and electrical heterogeneity, which it may responsible for a higher risk of arrhythmia.[4] It has

become a crucial lead to discriminate the origin of the WCT and the Vereckei algorithm is based solely on this lead. The initial ventricular activation wavefront during supraventricular tachycardia

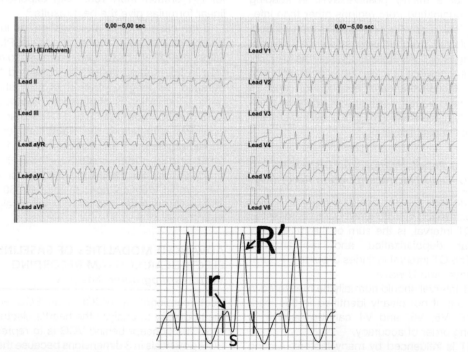

Fig. 8. WCT with RBBB morphology rate 200 bpm. In V1 an rsR' is in keeping with an aberrantly conducted supraventricular arrhythmia.

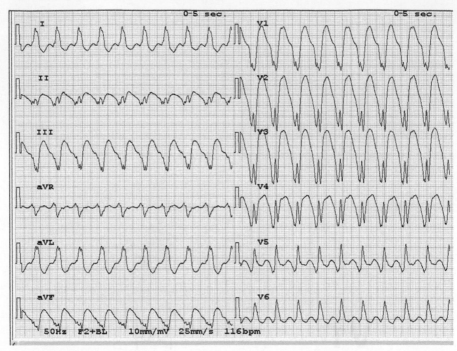

Fig. 9. WCT with LBBB morphology rate 150 bpm. Morphologic criteria suggest a ventricular origin (see text).

(SVT) and sinus rhythm should go away from lead aVR, yielding a negative QRS complex. Thus, an initial dominant R wave suggests a ventricular origin of the cardiac electrical impulse, whereas if it is supraventricular it should be negative. In the absence of a mainly positive aVR, in keeping with VTs originating from regions other than inferior or apical, a small r or q greater than 40 sec, or a low slurred, notched downstroke, can alternatively suggest VT. All these ECG patterns are due, in VT, to impairment of initial septal activation with a slower initial ventricular propagation and an initial upward vector component. While in presence of SVT, the initial part in the aVR is steeper due to fast septal activation.[4]

Ventricular Repolarization and Dispersion from a 12-Lead Electrocardiogram Recording

Repolarization

The repolarization in a standard ECG, represented by the QT interval, is the sum of the duration of ventricular depolarization and repolarization waves. The QT interval includes J-point, ST duration, T wave, and U wave.

The QT interval should normally be measured in lead DII but, if not clearly identified in this lead, aVR, aVF, V5, V6, and V4 can be used in a decreasing order of accuracy.

The QT is influenced by many factors. Among these are age; gender; and, more substantially, heart rate (HR). This is the reason QT duration

has to be corrected for these variables. Within normal HR range, every formula (Bazett, Fridericia, linear, exponential) give more or less equivalent results. In the case of HR less than 40 beats per minute (bpm), the linear formula is preferable, whereas for HR greater than 100, both exponential and linear formulas give the best results.[5]

In the case of QRS prolongation, as in bundle branch blocks, hemiblocks, or artificial PM stimulation, the QT will prolonged. Formulas to measure QTc in this setting should be corrected for QRS duration. JT length rather than QTc should be used. JT duration is obtained by subtracting the QRS duration from the QTc. If QTc is used in artificial PM stimulation, the Rautaharju correction should applied: QT (RR, QRS) = QT − 155 × (60 / HR − 1) − 0.93 × (QRS − 139) + k, with k = −22 ms for men and −34 ms for women, with almost identical normal limits at 460 ms and 450 ms for women and men, respectively, as for the QTc.[5,6]

ADVANCED MODALITIES OF BASELINE ELECTROCARDIOGRAM RECORDING
Vectorcardiographic Analysis

Vectorcardiography (VCG) is an ECG advanced methodology to analyze the heart's electrical vectors. The concept behind VCG is to represent the ECG potentials in 3 dimensions because the human body is three-dimensional. The VCG standard configuration was developed by Frank. The Frank leads are represented by right-left axis (X), head-to-feet axis (Y), and front-back (anteroposterior) axis (Z), and all are derived from a 12-lead ECG.

VCG represents the heart vector through the cardiac cycles as loops. The QRS loop represents depolarization, whereas the T loop represents repolarization. The spatial angle between depolarization and repolarization is the QRS-T angle. The normal value of the QRS-T angle depends on gender: in female patients it is 20° to 116° and in male patients it is 30° to 130°. A widened QRS-T angle correlates with sudden cardiac death (SCD) and predicts ventricular arrhythmias.[7]

Body Surface Mapping

Body surface mapping (BSM) is another extension of the concept of 12-lead ECG, which, by increasing the number of the unipolar leads, allows noninvasive mapping of cardiac electrical activity. In early 1990s, a BSM of 140 electrodes, 105 electrodes over the anterior part of the thorax and 35 on the back, was developed to map potentials in patients with idiopathic long QT syndrome (LQTS). In this early study, body surface potentials in patients with LQTS often showed an anterior thoracic area of negative potentials larger than normal during repolarization and a multipeak potential distribution more complex than normal, suggesting regional electrical disparities in the ventricular recovery process, which may in part account for the high susceptibility to malignant arrhythmias in these patients.[8]

A further development of the method is the electrocardiographic mapping (ECM), which is a 3-dimensional, noninvasive, beat-by-beat mapping system that facilitates the diagnosis of AT. The ECM consists of a 252-electrode vest that records body surface electrograms when placed on the torso; all this information is combined with computed tomography scan–based biatrial anatomy (CardioInsight Inc, Cleveland, OH, USA), which accurately diagnoses the mechanism of AT and the location of focal arrhythmias.[8,9]

Signal-Averaged Electrocardiogram

Signal-averaged electrocardiography (SAECG) is a special electrocardiographic technique in which multiple electric signals from the heart are

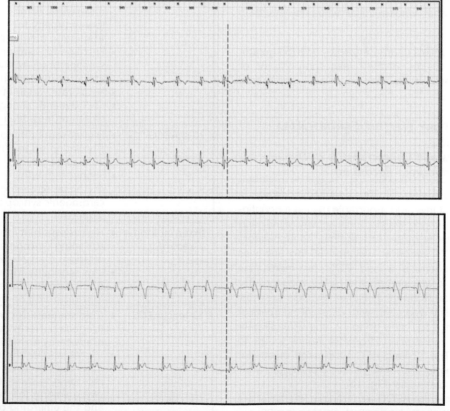

Fig. 10. A 60-year-old man with history of recurrent syncope and ventricular fibrillation at anesthesia induction for hepatic transplant. AECG tracing showing incomplete RBBB conduction in the square above, and in the square below the onset of a clear Brugada pattern I.

averaged to remove interference and magnified to reveal small variations at the end of the QRS average complex, known as late potentials. Late potentials are generated by scar or damaged tissues that prolong the normal conduction through the myocardium.

The diagnosis of late potentials documented in dilated cardiomyopathies, postischemic cardiomyopathies, arrhythmogenic right ventricular dysplasia, and Brugada syndrome showed significant correlation with increased SCD.

Normally, late potentials cannot be observed by naked eye analysis of standard ECG.

The registration of SAECG is based on 3 leads, X, Y, and Z, and requires up to 10 minutes to average 400 heart beats, from baseline QRS, which are synchronized, amplified, and then summarized in a plot.

Parameters of SAECG are

- Total QRS duration (QRSd), which includes late potentials is the total ventricular activation time
- Root mean square voltage of the terminal at 40 ms (RMS40) represents the relative amplitude of the late potential component
- Low-amplitude signal (LAS) is the duration of the signal whose initial value is less than 40 µV.

Late potentials characterized by a QRSd greater than 114 ms or RMS40 less than 20 µV or LAS greater than 38 ms are considered pathologic.[10]

AMBULATORY ELECTROCARDIOGRAM RECORDING
Modalities and Characteristics of Dynamic Electrocardiogram Recording

At the beginning of the twentieth century, a biophysicist invented a portable device for continuously monitoring the electrical activity of the heart for 24 hours or more. At that time, an ambulatory ECG (AECG) recorder weighed 85 Kg and was able to record a 3-lead ECG for more than 24 hours. It was named the Holter monitor after his inventor Norman J. Holter. AECGs are now lighter; easily wearable; with different numbers of leads, from 1 to 3 and up to 12; and with different length of registration, from 24 hours to up to 30 days. The 12-lead AECG are used mostly for Brugada pattern identification and brady-tachy arrhythmias diagnosis (**Fig. 10**).

The longer the AECG recording is, the fewer are the leads that can be applied, as seen in a 30-day AECG recording, which has only 1 or 2 leads. In addition, some devices for long-term recording

can also function as external loop recording by recording the ECG trace on demand during symptoms.

AECGs have different fields of applications and indications **Table 2**.

The most common electrode positions to record are the 3 bipolar leads (I, II, and III) and, eventually, 1 unipolar lead with 3 to 5 electrodes is standard with the right arm and left arm at the third intercostal right and left space, with the midclavicular line as the left leg and the right leg at the end of the twelfth costal bone of the chest, and a fifth on the right fourth intercostal space.[11]

Ambulatory Electrocardiogram Analysis and Interpretations

AECGs have different programs to facilitate their reading and help arrhythmias identification. Processing algorithms detect and document

Table 2 Ambulatory electrocardiogram recording indications	
24–72 h AECG	• First line for palpitations differential diagnosis, but low sensibility for atrial fibrillation diagnosis • First line for cardiogenic syncope brady-tachy arrhythmias screening • Heart rate variability • ST–T dynamic changes for screening possible ischemia
30 d AECG	• Higher sensibility for atrial fibrillation up to 50% vs 20% of 24 h AECG • Higher sensibility for arrhythmias screening when cardiogenic syncope is suspected
External loop recorder	• Higher sensibility for screening syncope and palpitations than 24–72 h AECG • Low sensibility for atrial fibrillation for the intermittent recording on demand
12-lead AECG	• Gold standard for searching Brugada patterns and brady-tachy arrhythmias • V1, V2, and V3 should be observed closely all over the recording to check the swing among the patterns and the emerging of pattern I during nighttime and or exercise

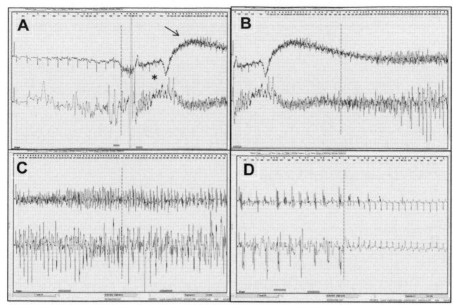

Fig. 11. A 24-hour AECG recording of a 45-year-old man investigated for episodes of syncope. The tracing was recorded during one of the syncopal episodes when the patient experienced a grand mal seizure attack. During the tonic phase (*arrow*), myopotential artifacts are recorded with regular R-R intervals still present (*asterisk*) (*A*). This period is followed by a clonic phase with higher voltage myopotential recording and an undulating baseline (*B,C*). At the end of the seizure, normal ECG is again visible (*D*).

abnormal rhythms or conduction abnormalities. Correct identification of bradycardias and/or tachyarrhythmias is essential in formulating the final report with a quantitative analysis of the total arrhythmic burden of the patient. In addition, depending on the programs' facilities, algorithms can also analyze other multiple parameters, such as ST–T segment shift, HR variability, QT

dynamics and T-wave variability, T-wave alternans, and HR turbulence.

To avoid AECG misinterpretation, there are some tips and tricks reported to help in formulating the final report (**Figs. 11** and **12**):

1. Read the AECG recording as a whole, including artifacts that may hide an arrhythmia.

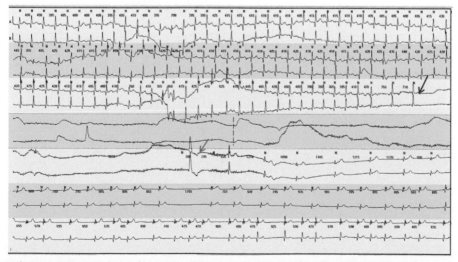

Fig. 12. A 24-hour AECG recording of a 2-year-old boy with history of recurrent syncope and suspected seizure. Tracing shows a period of sinus arrest (*red arrow*) lasting 26 seconds terminated with a ventricular beat (*blue arrow*) and resumption of sinus bradycardia with cycle length 1216 ms.

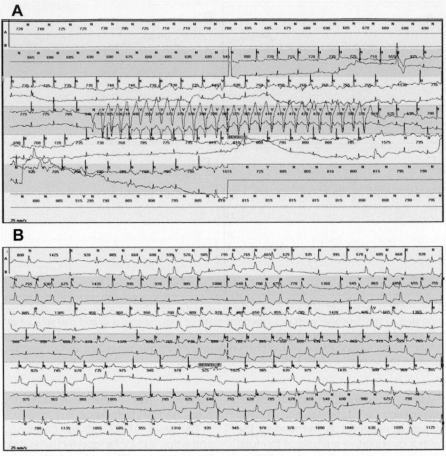

Fig. 13. A 24-hour AECG recording of a 54-year-old with a suspected myocardial sarcoidosis. (*A*) A run of non sustained ventricular tachycardia of likely RV origin. (*B*) Multiple simple and complex ventricular ectopic beats of probable LV origin. Further clinical investigations demonstrated a multiple myeloma infiltrating both ventricles.

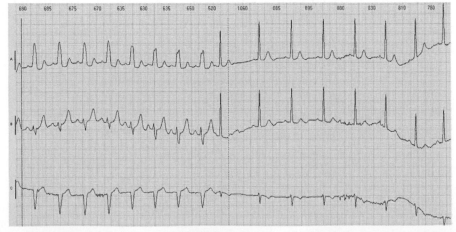

Fig. 14. At the beginning of the tracing, 8 beats of AT conducted with LBBB aberrancy. The ninth beat is an atrial premature contraction, restores normal conduction, and terminates the tachycardia. Sinus rhythm with normal conduction resumes following arrhythmia termination.

Multichannel ECG may help in recognizing real artifacts from genuine arrhythmias.

2. Check HR graph to observe circadian HR, onset or offset of an arrhythmia, and average RR interval.
   - In the presence of highly variable rate, graph suspect the presence of atrial fibrillation.
   - If there is a steep sudden increase of the average HR graph (>100 bpm) followed by a plateau terminated by an equally sudden decrease of HR back to average, consider onset or offset of a supraventricular or ventricular sustained tachycardia (**Figs. 13** and **14**)
3. Check beat-by-beat ECG morphology to diagnose intermittent preexcitation. In case of a 12-lead AECG, focus on the V1, V2, and V3 to check for diagnostic changes in Brugada patients

The AECG final report should include rhythm description during day and night, atrioventricular and interventricular conduction, sinus pauses, number of supraventricular and ventricular beats, isolated and/or complex arrhythmias, and ST–T segment description.

REFERENCES

1. Kligfield P, Gettes LS, Bailey JJ, et al, American Heart Association Electrocardiography and Arrhythmias Committee, Council on Clinical Cardiology, American College of Cardiology Foundation, Heart Rhythm Society. Recommendations for the standardization and interpretation of the electrocardiogram: part I: the electrocardiogram and its technology a scientific statement from the American Heart Association Electrocardiography and Arrhythmias Committee, Council on Clinical Cardiology; the American College of Cardiology Foundation; and the Heart Rhythm Society endorsed by the International Society for Computerized Electrocardiology. J Am Coll Cardiol 2007;49:1109–27.

2. Di Biase L, Gianni C, Bagliani G, et al. Arrhythmias involving the atrioventricular junction. Card Electrophysiol Clin 2017;9:435–52.

3. De Ponti R, Bagliani G, Padeletti L, et al. General approach to a wide QRS complex. Card Electrophysiol Clin 2017;9(3):461–85.

4. George A, Arumugham PS, Figueredo VM. aVR - the forgotten lead. Exp Clin Cardiol 2010;15:e36–44.

5. Locati ET, Bagliani G, Padeletti L. Normal ventricular repolarization and QT interval: ionic background, modifiers, and measurements. Card Electrophysiol Clin 2017;9:487–513.

6. Rautaharju PM, Zhang ZM, Prineas R, et al. Assessment of prolonged QT and JT intervals in ventricular conduction defects. Am J Cardiol 2004;93:1017–21.

7. Scherptong RW, Henkens IR, Man SC, et al. Normal limits of the spatial QRS-T angle and ventricular gradient in 12-lead electrocardiograms of young adults: dependence on sex and heart rate. J Electrocardiol 2008;41:648–55.

8. De Ambroggi L, Bertoni T, Locati E, et al. Mapping of body surface potentials in patients with the idiopathic long QT syndrome. Circulation 1986;74:1334–45.

9. Shah AJ, Hocini M, Xhaet O, et al. Validation of novel 3-dimensional electrocardiographic mapping of atrial tachycardias by invasive mapping and ablation: a multicenter study. J Am Coll Cardiol 2013;62:889–97.

10. Dinov B, Bode K, Koenig S, et al. Signal-averaged electrocardiography as a noninvasive tool for evaluating the outcomes after radiofrequency catheter ablation of ventricular tachycardia in patients with ischemic heart disease: reassessment of an old tool. Circ Arrhythm Electrophysiol 2016;9 [pii: e003673].

11. Steinberg JS, Varma N, Cygankiewicz I, et al. 2017 ISHNE-HRS expert consensus statement on ambulatory ECG and external cardiac monitoring/telemetry. Heart Rhythm 2017;14:e55–96.

Advanced Cardiac Signal Recording

Roberto De Ponti, MD, FHRS[a],*, Ilaria My, MD[a], Manola Vilotta, EPTech[a], Fabrizio Caravati, MD[a], Jacopo Marazzato, MD[a], Giuseppe Bagliani, MD[b,c], Fabio M. Leonelli, MD[d]

KEYWORDS

- Implantable loop recorder • Syncope • Atrial fibrillation • Transesophageal electrophysiologic study
- Wide QRS complex Tachycardia • Intracardiac electrophysiologic study

KEY POINTS

- Implantable loop recorders allow prolonged and continuous single-lead electrocardiogram recording, with the invaluable option of remote monitoring.
- Since the advent of implantable loop recorders, time to electrocardiographic diagnosis and appropriate therapy is significantly shortened in the diagnostic workup for syncope and atrial fibrillation.
- High sensitivity algorithms and good quality of the recorded P- and R-waves are instrumental in detection and burden quantification by implantable loop recorders of many bradyarrhythmias and tachyarrhythmias.
- Transesophageal catheters enable to efficiently record atrial and, in some cases, ventricular signals. Minimally invasive pacing is also doable.
- Esophageal recordings can help guide intracardiac mapping and atrial fibrillation ablation procedures. Intracardiac electrophysiologic study remains essential for diagnosis and catheter ablation of several cardiac arrhythmias.

INTRODUCTION

The standard 12-lead electrocardiogram (ECG) is currently complemented by innovative technologies that render possible recording of the cardiac electrical signals in different conditions. Although the surface ECG has a key role to initially orient the patients management, in specific subsets of patients it may not be enough and advanced cardiac signal recording is necessary. This can be done by newer technologies, such as the implantable loop recorder (ILR), or using an older methodology, such as transesophageal recording. Undoubtedly, the most complete evaluation of a given arrhythmia is performed by an invasive electrophysiology study (EPS), during which sophisticated arrhythmia mapping can also be performed by 3-dimensional systems. This article reviews the current use of these methodologies, excluding signals recorded and stored in pacemakers and implantable cardioverter/defibrillator, which are described elsewhere in this issue.

Conflicts of Interest: Dr R. De Ponti received lectures fees from Biosense Webster and Biotronik, and educational grants from Biosense Webster, Biotronik, Medtronic, Abbott, and Boston Scientific; none for the other authors.

[a] Department of Heart and Vessels, Ospedale di Circolo and Macchi Foundation–University of Insubria, Viale Borri, 57, 21100 Varese, Italy; [b] Arrhythmology Unit, Cardiology Department, Foligno General Hospital, Via Massimo Arcamone, Foligno, 06034 Perugia, Italy; [c] Cardiovascular Disease Department, University of Perugia, Piazza Menghini 1, 06129 Perugia, Italy; [d] Cardiology Department, James A. Haley Veterans' Hospital, University of South Florida, 13000 Bruce B Down Boulevard, Tampa, FL 33612, USA
* Corresponding author. Department of Heart and Vessels, Ospedale di Circolo and Macchi Foundation, University of Insubria-Varese, Viale Borri, 57, 21100 Varese, Italy.
E-mail address: roberto.deponti@uninsubria.it

Card Electrophysiol Clin 11 (2019) 203–217
https://doi.org/10.1016/j.ccep.2019.01.005

IMPLANTABLE LOOP RECORDER
General Considerations

The first ILRs were inserted subcutaneously in patients with syncope of unknown origin in the mid-1990s,[1] roughly 35 years after the introduction of Holter monitoring. This technology was hailed as the one that would start a new age in electrocardiography.[2] Over the years, the implantation of a loop recorder has represented an alternative, advanced, and useful method to continuously record a surface electrocardiographic lead. Having a pair of sensing electrodes on its shell, this device is implanted subcutaneously, usually in the left subclavicular or left parasternal area through a small skin incision. The optimal site and device orientation for each patient is identified by preimplantation mapping of the site where all the surface electrocardiographic waves can be clearly and distinctly recorded, which is crucial for correct tracing interpretation during arrhythmias. Recently, implantation in the axillary position, at the fourth/fifth intercostal space in the anterior axillary line, has been tested for different device technologies, with a horizontal[3] or 45° inclination to the midaxillary line.[4] This position, which ideally has a good alignment with the cardiac electrical vector, allows for a good quality of electrocardiographic recordings, comparable with the one obtained in the standard position and can be better accepted by some subjects, such as young patients and women.[4]

The structural characteristics and technical capabilities of the commercially available loop recorders are listed in **Table 1**. Among those capabilities, remote monitoring is of great importance. When this feature is combined with well-defined institutional protocols, including data analysis every working day,[5] the elapsed time from the arrhythmia event to the appropriate therapy is minimized to 2.4 days. This is particularly crucial in cases of asymptomatic arrhythmia episodes, in which automatic recording by the ILR and remote monitoring trigger the appropriate intervention well in advance (3.8 months, on average) to the next scheduled in-office device interrogation.[5]

Type and Quality of the Electrical Signal

A wide variety of bradyarrhythmias and tachyarrhythmias has been reported in patients undergoing implantation of a loop recorder, including atrial fibrillation (AF), atrial tachycardia/flutter, nonsustained or sustained supraventricular or ventricular arrhythmias, premature beats, different degrees of atrioventricular block, and sinus pauses.[5–8] Although automatic capture of asymptomatic episodes depends on device programming and detection algorithms, a good quality of the recorded ECG is essential for the correct interpretation of every recorded episode. Moreover, correlation between patient symptoms and electrocardiographic recordings is instrumental in the correct classification of each event. In fact, when the patients reports symptoms possibly related to a cardiac dysrhythmia, but the corresponding ECG shows no arrhythmia, the episode can be classified as noncardiovascular in origin.

Automatic arrhythmia detection critically relays on R-wave sensing and an amplitude greater than 0.3 mV is recommended by the company that first developed this technology. Besides the site of implant and body position, R-wave amplitude depends on the interelectrode spacing, which therefore depends on the structural characteristics of the device. The R-wave amplitude is affected also by body mass index, which can prevent appropriate sensing if it is greater than 35 kg/m^2.[9] As mentioned, good quality of all the electrographic waves is essential for tracing interpretation. Specifically, a clearly distinguishable P-wave during both sinus rhythm and a supraventricular arrhythmia helps to make an accurate diagnosis and has the potential to decrease the burden of inappropriate data at remote monitoring. In addition to the variables that can affect the sensing of the R-wave, P-wave amplitude may vary also according to respiratory movements[4,10] and to movements of the left arm.[3] However, a clear P-wave can be recorded in 60% to 70% of the patients in the supine and upright positions,[3,4,10] and this percentage can increase to more than 90% if the definition of a visible P-wave is less strict.[10] In clinical practice, the patient's underlying disease can play a major role in the P-wave amplitude and, therefore, limits the ability of the device to record a well visible P-wave. **Fig. 1** shows the tracing of an older patient with hypertensive cardiomyopathy and atrial electrical disease, in whom the P-wave is more visible in an atrial premature complex than during sinus rhythm. **Fig. 2** remarks the importance of well visible P-waves for a correct diagnosis: 4 blocked P-waves allow for a diagnosis of paroxysmal complete atrioventricular block in this patient with recurrent syncope. A complete absence of P-waves with chaotic atrial electrical activity and irregular R-R intervals is evident in a case of AF (**Fig. 3**A, B). When, in the same patient, the AF organizes in atrial flutter (**Fig. 4**A, B), regular F-waves appear and the ventricular rate becomes regular at 150 beats per minute. Although the clinical history of this patient and the tracings shown in

Table 1
Structural characteristics and technical capabilities of commercially available loop recorders

	Biomonitor 2-AF/-S (Biotronik)	Confirm (St. Jude Medical)	Confirm RX (St. Jude Medical)	Reveal LINQ (Medtronic)	Reveal XT (Medtronic)
Dimensions (mm, L × W × H)	88 × 15 × 6.0	56.3 × 18.5 × 8.0	49 × 9.4 × 3.1	44.8 × 7.2 × 4.0	62 × 19 × 8.0
Volume (mL)	5	6.5	1.4	1.2	9
Weight (g)	10	12	3.0	2.5	15
Electrode spacing (mm)	75	39	39.8	37.7	41
Battery life (years)	4	3	2	3	3
Sampling rate (Hz)	128	128	128	256	256
Total memory capacity (min)	>60	48	57	59	49.5
sECG storage	Up to 55 (40 s) automatically detected and 4 (7.5 min) patient-activated episodes	Up to 147 episodes	Up to 13 (4.5 min) automatically detected and 4 (15 min) patient-activated episodes	Up to 27 min automatically detected and 30 min patient-activated episodes	Up to 27 min automatically detected and 22.5 min patient-activated episodes
Remote monitoring	Biotronik Home Monitor Service Center	Transtelephonic monitoring	myMerlin App via Bluetooth-Smartphone	Medtronic Care Link Network	Medtronic Care Link Network
MRI conditional	1.5 and 3 T	1.5 T only	1.5 T only	1.5 and 3 T	1.5 and 3 T
Injectable	Yes	No	Yes	Yes	No
Accelerometer	No	No	No	Yes	Yes
Arrhythmia detection	AF, AF burden (Biomonitor 2-AF only), HVR, SVA, bradycardia, sudden rate drop and asystole	AF, tachycardia, bradycardia and asystole	AF, tachycardia, bradycardia and asystole	AT/AF, tachycardia, bradycardia and asystole	AT/AF, tachycardia, bradycardia, asystole, ventricular tachyarrhythmia

Abbreviations: AT, atrial tachycardia; H, height; HVR, high ventricular rate; L, length; sECG, subcutaneous ECG; SVA, sustained ventricular arrhythmia; W, width.

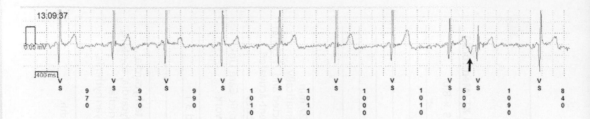

Fig. 1. Sinus rhythm in an 86-year-old patient with hypertensive cardiomyopathy. In sinus rhythm, the P-wave is not well visible and its amplitude and morphology suggests origin from the lower area of the sinus node in the presence of atrial electrical disease. Conversely, in the atrial premature contraction (second to last beat) a well evident negative P-wave (*arrow*) is present.

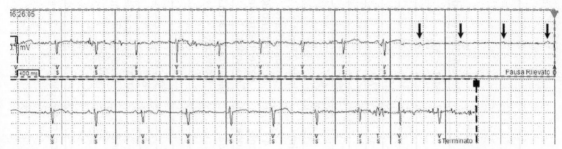

Fig. 2. Transient complete atrioventricular block in a patient with recurrent syncope. The blocked P-waves (*arrows*) can be clearly distinguished. No P-R interval or R-R interval prolongation is observed before the block, suggesting no autonomic tone influence.

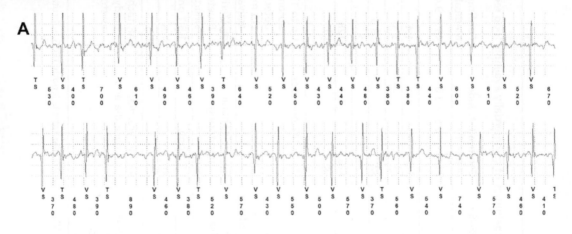

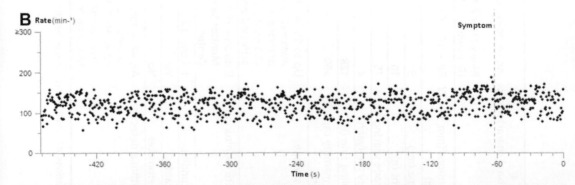

Fig. 3. (*A, B*) AF well evident in the electrocardiographic tracing of the ILR (*A*) with wide variations of the R-R cycle from 370 to 890 milliseconds. The trend of the heart rhythm variation over time is shown in (*B*). The vertical interrupted line in (*B*) indicates symptoms felt by the patient.

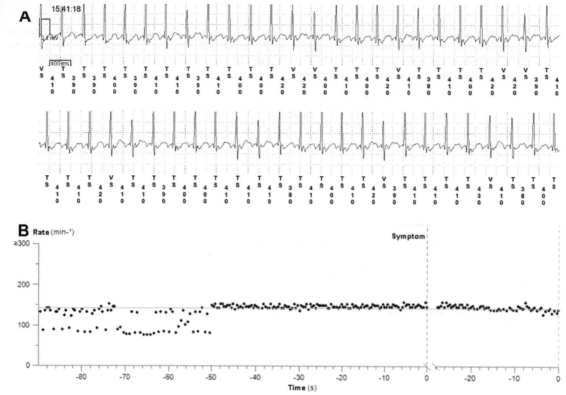

Fig. 4. (*A, B*) Same patient as in **Fig. 3**. (*A*) Organization of AF into flutter with evident F-waves and 2:1 atrioventricular conduction. As a consequence, the ventricular rate (*B*) becomes regular at 150 beats per minute. This rhythm variation is felt by the patient.

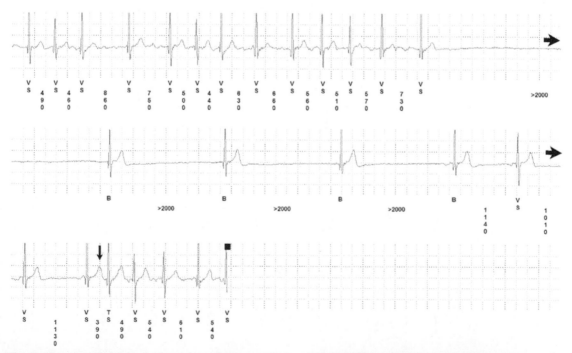

Fig. 5. Upon termination of AF, a pause of 4.3 s occurs in a patient with bradycardia-tachycardia syndrome and syncope. Subsequently, after 3 junctional beats at very low rate (<30 beats per minute), sinus rhythm restores at about 60 beats per minute, but soon after AF resumes likely with a "P-on-T phenomenon" (*vertical arrow* indicate P-wave superimposed to T-wave). *Horizontal arrows* indicate that the rhythm strips are continuous.

Fig. 4B strongly suggest the diagnosis of typical counterclockwise atrial flutter, the ultimate diagnosis can be made only on the 12-lead ECG. Finally, detection of the P-wave is also important for the correct interpretation of the rhythm emergent after atrial arrhythmia termination (Fig. 5), which can confirm the diagnosis of a bradycardia–tachycardia syndrome.[11]

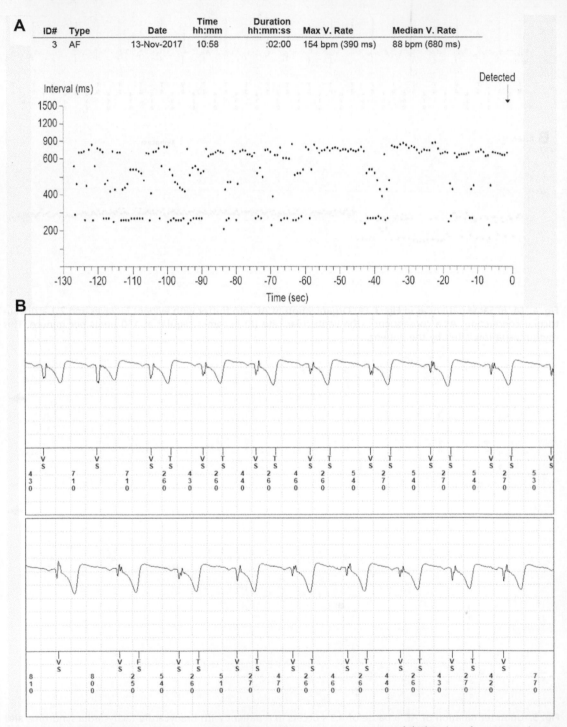

Fig. 6. (A, B) False detection of AF in a patients who received an ILR for syncope. (A) The plot of very irregular R-R intervals detected by the device and classified as AF lasting 2 minutes. (B) Two strips of tracing with normal sinus rhythm and oversensing of the T-wave interpreted as AF.

Clinical Use

As mentioned, ILRs were introduced into clinical practice to study rhythm variation in patients with syncope that remained unexplained after noninvasive and invasive testing.[1] Since then, ILRs have been used also in patients with AF and nondocumented palpitations. The recently published guidelines of the European Society of Cardiology[12] recommend with a Class I indication the implantation of an ILR in the early phase of evaluation in patients with recurrent syncope of uncertain origin, the absence of high-risk criteria, and a likelihood of syncope recurrence within the battery life. The same class of recommendation is given also for patients with high-risk criteria, in whom a comprehensive evaluation has been inconclusive and who do not have indications for implantable cardioverter-defibrillator or pacemaker implantation.[12] These recommendations are based on the evidence of a meta-analysis that included 660 patients with unexplained syncope randomized to conventional strategy (external loop recorder, tilt testing, and EPS) or prolonged monitoring with an ILR: there was a 3.7 increased probability of a diagnosis in the last group compared with the first group.[12] In studies published in recent years, the ILR yields a diagnosis in less than 2 years in a proportion of patients with syncope varying from 26% to 50%, depending on selection criteria; bradyarrhythmias, mainly owing to sick sinus node and advanced atrioventricular block, are the leading causes of symptoms.[13–16]

ILRs are being used intensively to screen for subclinical AF in high-risk patients, to define the arrhythmia burden in patients with known AF, or to assess the efficacy of a therapy, such as catheter ablation. In this field of application, the ILR represents a very powerful and useful technology, but not without limitations. In fact, the device's ability to detect AF mainly relies on the irregularity of R-R intervals and different manufacturers have developed different algorithms to implement AF detection. However, if on the one hand these algorithms have demonstrated a very high sensitivity, on the other their specificity in detecting AF may be suboptimal; in different recently published studies, a variable proportion of arrhythmia episodes were not confirmed when compared with concomitant Holter monitoring recordings.[9] These data highlight the importance of individualized device programming to minimize the burden of false-positive episodes (**Fig. 6**A, B) that represents an inappropriate overload at remote monitoring and invariably alters the correct definition of the AF burden, considering also that tracings of some episodes automatically detected by the ILR may not be available for adjudication. **Fig. 7** shows the false detection of a prolonged paused owing to undersensing in a patient who received an ILR for definition of AF burden after the first episode.

Despite these limitations, the ILR has proved very effective in demonstrating the presence of AF in the population of patients with cryptogenic stroke in which the proportion of patients with subclinical AF captured by the device varies between 16% and 30%,[17,18] depending mainly on the duration of follow-up. In one of these studies,[17] the percent of subclinical AF is significantly higher than the one detected by prolonged Holter monitoring. Moreover, ILRs proved better than 72-hour Holter monitoring for detection of

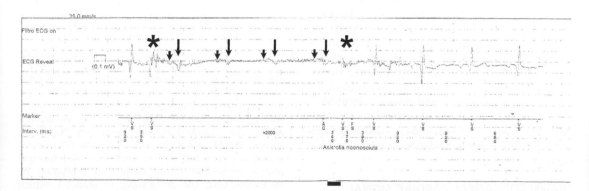

Fig. 7. Undersensing of the P- and R-waves detected by the ILR as asystole lasting 4.6 s. Actually, after the first artifact (*first asterisk*) detected as ventricular activity (VS), in the following 3 beats, both the P- and R-waves have a critically decreased amplitude probably owing to unusual body movements, which returns to normal amplitude after the second artifact (*second asterisk*), again detected as ventricular activity. The patient had no symptoms during this episode and the R-R cycles remain constant if the undersensed R-waves are considered. *Short* and *long arrows* identify the undersensed P- and R-waves, respectively.

subclinical AF also in high-risk patients (CHA_2DS_2-VASc of 3–5), in whom AF lasting >2 minutes was observed in 21% of them during prolonged follow-up.[19] Of clinical importance, any treatment in relation to the detection of subclinical atrial tachyarrhythmia by an implanted device has to be decided individually, in the light of the patient's clinical characteristics.[20] Finally, both in the past[21] and recently,[22] recurrences of AF after catheter ablation are more frequently observed if the follow-up is based on implanted devices rather than on conventional methodology, mainly based on symptoms. Interestingly, in this population recurrence may present as regular atrial tachycardia/flutter, which may be missed by the ILR, if it is programmed to detect only AF to avoid false detection of sinus tachycardia. One possible solution to this problem could be to lower the cut-off rate for arrhythmia detection and use the data of the accelerometer included in the monitoring device to exclude effort-related sinus tachycardia.[9]

Strength and Limitations

ILRs have really started a new era of electrocardiography, considering also that this technology is empowered by remote monitoring. Besides all the considerations expressed elsewhere in this article, it should be underlined how this technology opens new perspectives for speculation in cardiac rhythm disturbances. For example, self-termination of idiopathic ventricular fibrillation even after a few minutes as documented by ILRs,[23,24] a phenomenon rarely observed in the past and mainly in patients with structural heart disease, calls for further investigation aimed at clarification of its mechanism.

As with every technology, ILRs present some limitations, such as the low specificity of AF detection, which has been already discussed elsewhere in this article. Other limitations are emerging from recent reports, which describe adverse events that can occur in the follow-up. They include missensing owing to interference with transcutaneous electrical nerve stimulation[25] or device dehiscence,[26] and device migration.[27] Finally, pocket infections are possible, although rare and with consequences definitely less serious than the ones described with transvenous devices.

TRANSESOPHAGEAL CARDIAC SIGNAL RECORDING
General Considerations

Several decades ago, different catheters with variable characteristics in term of size, shape, number of electrodes, and interelectrode spacing have

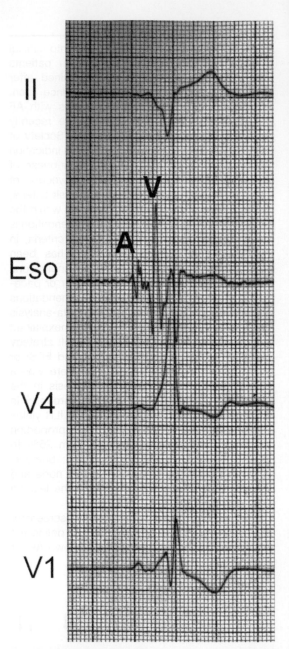

Fig. 8. Esophageal bipolar recording during sinus rhythm in a patient with Wolff-Parkinson-White syndrome with a posteromedial atrioventricular accessory pathway. Surface leads II, V1, and V4 as well as bipolar transesophageal recording (Eso) are shown. Distinct atrial (A) and ventricular (V) electrograms are recorded with a very short A-V interval and a ventricular initial deflection preceding by 40 milliseconds the delta-wave in lead V4, which suggests a strict anatomic relationship between the site of recording and the accessory pathway in this case.

been developed to record bipolar or unipolar cardiac electrical signals from the esophagus, after the catheter has been inserted, usually from the nostrils with the help of an anesthetic lubricant gel. As an alternative, pill electrodes have also been developed. These devices can be swallowed by a patient and then withdrawn from the stomach to the esophagus by pulling back the wires connected to the electrodes.[28]

Type and Quality of the Electrical Signal

Cardiac electrical signals can be recorded in the esophagus at a variable distance from the insertion site, depending on individual morphometric characteristics.[29] When recorded bipolarly, these signals are comparable with the ones recorded at EPS (**Fig. 8**). Several years ago, it was assessed that the atrial signals recorded in the esophagus originate from the posterior wall of the left atrium (**Fig. 9A–D**) for its close anatomic relationship with the esophagus.[30] When multiple esophageal bipolar atrial recordings from a multipolar catheter are analyzed and their chronology evaluated in relation to the surface P-wave, different activation patterns can be found that reflect different degrees of atrial conduction delay after electrical cardioversion in patients with persistent AF.[31] Ventricular electrograms can be recorded less easily than atrial, when the catheter is further advanced into

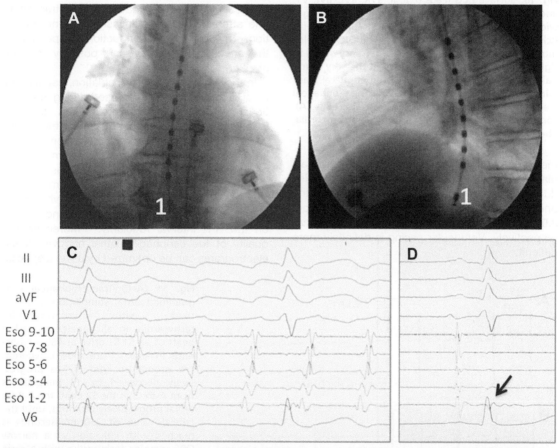

Fig. 9. (A–D) Fluoroscopic image in anteroposterior (A) and left lateral projection (B) together with surface ECG leads (II, III, aVF, V1, and V6) and bipolar recordings from a decapolar catheter positioned in the esophagus from the distal (Eso 1–2) to the proximal (Eso 9–10) electrode pair, during typical counterclockwise atrial flutter (C) and in sinus rhythm (D), restored by esophageal burst pacing. During atrial flutter, atrial activation propagates from distal to proximal, reflecting the pattern of caudocranial activation of the posterior wall of the left atrium during this arrhythmia. In sinus rhythm, the bipolar atrial esophageal recording shows simultaneous activation of the posterior left atrial wall, while their chronologic relationship with the surface P-wave and the morphology of the surface P-wave itself demonstrates the presence of delayed atrial conduction in this patient. In sinus rhythm, a ventricular signal is also evident in the distal esophageal recording (*arrow*), facilitated by the longer interelectrode spacing between the first 2 electrodes. The *small vertical lines* on top of (C) indicate 1-s intervals. The number in (A) and (B) indicates the position of the distal electrode.

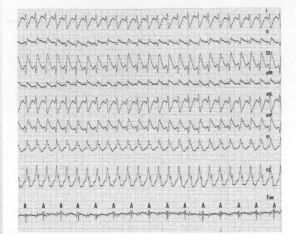

Fig. 10. Surface ECG leads (I, II, II, aVR, aVL, aVF, V1, and V2) and esophageal bipolar lead (Eso) during a wide QRS complex tachycardia in a patient with ischemic cardiomyopathy. Although the QRS complex morphology is not consistent with aberrancy owing to right bundle branch block, a notch in the very terminal part of the QRS complex in the peripheral leads mimicking a P-wave can be observed. The esophageal lead, however, shows a dissociated atrial activity (A), confirming the diagnosis of ventricular tachycardia. The paper speed is 25 mm/s.

the distal part of the esophagus, close to the cardias. Atrial pacing can be performed[32] with pulse duration and amplitude definitely higher than the ones used for intracavitary pacing, varying from 2.0 to 15.0 milliseconds and from 15 to 30 mA, respectively. Ventricular pacing is definitely more difficult.

Clinical Use

Over the years, esophageal recordings and pacing have been used to orient the diagnosis during both wide QRS complex (**Fig. 10**) and narrow QRS complex tachycardias (**Fig. 11**A, C) and to terminate cardiac arrhythmias, such as atrial flutter (see **Fig. 9**A–D) or supraventricular tachycardias (**Fig. 12**), avoiding the use of drugs or electrical cardioversion.[32–36] For its minimally invasive nature, transesophageal EPS has been used in children, especially to define the conduction properties of an accessory pathway and its ability to sustain arrhythmias.[37,38] Interestingly, the last consensus document on the management of young, asymptomatic patients with ventricular preexcitation[39] still considers the use of transesophageal EPS as an alternative to the intracavitary one after adequate noninvasive patient evaluation, to define the conduction properties of the accessory pathway and possibly indicate ablation.

In the early phases of AF ablation, esophageal atrial recordings have been used during interventional electrophysiologic procedures to help identify the site of origin of atrial premature depolarizations and, therefore, guide ablation.[40,41] For its minimally invasive nature, long-term esophageal recording is also feasible, and it has been reported to be more sensitive than Holter monitoring for the detection of atrial ectopic activity, being based on the waveform analysis and not simply on the R-R interval regularity.[42] Moreover, the quality of the esophageal atrial and ventricular electrograms can be optimized by using a specific

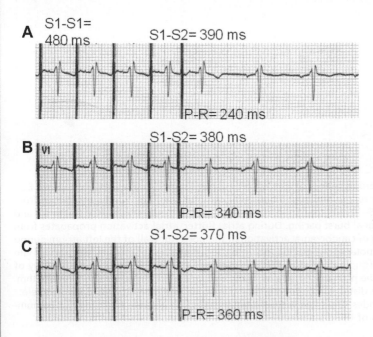

Fig. 11. (A–C) Transesophageal programmed atrial stimulation in a patient with supraventricular tachycardia. In all panels, the last 4 beats of an S1-S1 drive at 480 milliseconds in lead V1 are shown, whereas the premature beat (S2) is progressively decreased by 10 milliseconds from A to C. In the S2 beat, the P-R interval progressively prolongs, until the critical value of 360 milliseconds is reached with induction of a narrow QRS-complex tachycardia with a cycle length of 480 milliseconds. Both the modality of tachycardia induction and the absence of a clear P-wave after the QRS complex suggest atrioventricular nodal reentrant tachycardia.

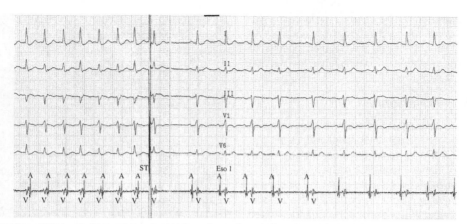

Fig. 12. Surface ECG leads (I, II, III, V1, and V6) and esophageal bipolar lead (Eso) during supraventricular tachycardia. The r′-wave in lead V1 and the very short V-A interval in the esophageal lead suggest an atrioventricular nodal reentrant tachycardia. A single premature extra stimulus delivered by the esophageal catheter (ST) advances the atrial deflection and terminates the tachycardia in the antegrade limb of the reentry circuit. The paper speed is 25 mm/s.

lead configuration, so that, in perspective, these signals can be interpreted more reliably by an automatic software during long-term esophageal monitoring.[43]

In interventional electrophysiologic procedures for the ablation of complex atrial arrhythmias in patients with congenital heart disease, the atrial esophageal bipolar recordings can be used as a reference signal for the 3-dimensional mapping system with the advantage of having a stable left atrial reference and spare an intracavitary catheter, simplifying the procedure in this particular subset of patients.[44] The recording and pacing of an atrial signal from the posterior left atrial wall, readily available with the transesophageal methodology, has been recently reported to be very useful to confirm or refute isolation of the left atrial posterior wall after catheter only or hybrid (surgical and catheter) ablation procedures in patients with persistent AF.[45] Finally, transesophageal recordings and temporary pacing of a left ventricular electrogram with a specifically

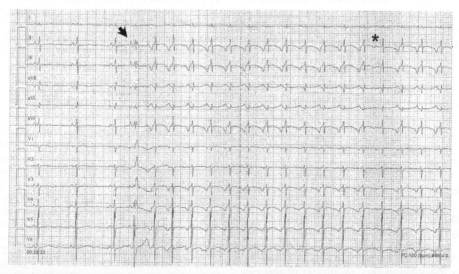

Fig. 13. Twelve-lead ECG in a patient with supraventricular tachycardia occurring during continuous monitoring the day before the ablation procedure. The tachycardia is initiated by an atrial premature beat (*arrow*) and shows a relative regular cycle length with negative P-waves in the inferior and left precordial leads. However, the beat marked with an *asterisk* occurs earlier and shows a narrower P-wave with a different morphology. Interestingly, the P-wave morphology of the fourth beat preceding this one is also slightly different from the others, suggesting a fusion beat between 2 activation wavefronts (see **Fig. 14**).

designed catheter can be used to evaluate the degree of left ventricular activation delay and the hemodynamic effect of left ventricular pacing to improve the selection of candidates for cardiac resynchronization therapy.[46]

Strength and Limitations

The major advantage of this methodology relies on its ability to record and pace atrial and ventricular electrograms with a minimally invasive approach. For this reason, new applications have been found in the recent years for specific tasks, as discussed elsewhere in this article. In contrast, the cardiac signals recorded in the esophagus provide limited information on the heart electrical activation during the broad spectrum of arrhythmias and ventricular pacing can be very difficult at tolerable pacing thresholds; evaluation of ventriculoatrial conduction during ventricular pacing is also very challenging. For these reasons, the information provided by transesophageal recordings has to be combined with a surface ECG, which configures an intermediate methodology in between an invasive electrophysiologic procedure and surface electrocardiographic monitoring. Moreover, the transesophageal EPS is a safe procedure, but a couple of considerations are important. First, severe arrhythmias can be induced during a transesophageal EPS, such as preexcited AF with fast ventricular conduction, potentially degenerating into ventricular fibrillation. Therefore, this procedure should be performed in a fully equipped laboratory, rather than in areas where a noninvasive evaluation is performed. Second, burn or esophageal injuries as a result of pacing or catheter insertion have been described,[47,48] although they have usually no consequence and can be minimized using appropriate pacing and insertion protocols.

Overall, at the present time, the transesophageal methodology should be regarded as a valuable option for specific tasks in patients with cardiac arrhythmias, but not as a substitute for an invasive electrophysiologic procedure, which remains the gold standard for the final diagnosis and the curative treatment of cardiac arrhythmias.

INTRACARDIAC SIGNAL RECORDING AND MAPPING

Sixty years have passed since the seminal works describing the intracavitary recording of the His bundle potential,[49] the use of programmed electrical stimulation for the induction and termination of clinical cardiac arrhythmias,[50] and mapping of the total excitation of the human heart.[51] Over the years, technological improvements have rendered

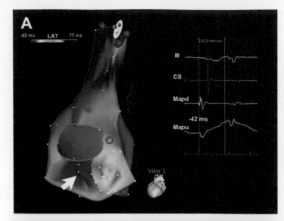

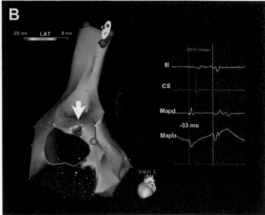

Fig. 14. (A, B) Same case as in **Fig. 13**. (A) The electroanatomic activation mapping of the right atrium during the predominant arrhythmia with a cycle length of 340 milliseconds and a negative P-wave in lead III, which is diagnosed as a focal atrial tachycardia originating from the medial lower right atrium. The *white arrow* indicates the earliest activated area during tachycardia and the inset shows the local bipolar (Mapd) and unipolar (Mapu) electrogram, which precedes the reference signal in the coronary sinus (CS) by 42 milliseconds; the unipolar atrial deflection is completely negative. This finding confirms the tachycardia origin in this site. The yellow tag identifies the His-bundle area. (B) After ablation of the first focus was performed successfully at the site of the red tag, a second focal atrial tachycardia with a cycle length of 300 milliseconds and a different P wave morphology in lead III is induced by more aggressive atrial stimulation. Remapping of the right atrium shows than now the focus is localized in the anteromedial right atrium (*white arrow*). (*Inset*) Electrograms at the site of earliest activation, where the bipolar electrogram (Mapd) precedes by 33 milliseconds the reference signal with a negative unipolar atrial deflection in Mapu. The P-wave morphology of this second tachycardia in lead III is identical to the one of the variant P-wave in the spontaneous episode, shown in **Fig. 13**.

possible refinements of these techniques, and specific pacing maneuvers have proved essential for the correct interpretation of the intracavitary electrical signals.[52–54] Currently, invasive EPS is still essential for differential diagnosis and subsequent adequate treatment with catheter ablation of cardiac arrhythmias, especially in certain wide QRS complex tachycardias, when a surface ECG could be misleading.[55]

Technological improvements have also allowed the transition from manual cardiac mapping[51] to sophisticated 3-dimensional electroanatomic mapping to understand the pathophysiology of complex atrial[44,56–58] and ventricular[59,60] arrhythmias and to guide successful ablation, also decreasing radiation exposure.[61,62]

While the technology moves ahead the frontier of knowledge and, therefore, a physician's ability to better treat a wide spectrum of cardiac arrhythmias,[63,64] the basic knowledge of electrical signal interpretation should not be neglected.[65] **Figs. 13** and **14** highlight the importance of an in-depth analysis of the surface ECG before an invasive procedure is performed. In this case, a change in the P-wave morphology on surface ECG during a clinical arrhythmia episode predicts the presence of 2 distinct atrial foci in a focal atrial tachycardia.

Finally, despite multiple options for prolonged electrocardiographic monitoring, some patients for different reasons are unable to record a surface ECG during palpitations. In a selected subgroup of these patients, an electrophysiologic interventional procedure can be used as a valuable diagnostic and therapeutic option. In our experience, over several years (from 2003 to 2015), 123 patients who complained of recurrent, nondocumented palpitations with sudden onset and termination and a heart rate of more than 120 beats per minute were considered for invasive EPS in the fasting nonsedated state. During the procedure, which included also an isoproterenol challenge, an arrhythmia responsible for the clinical symptom was induced in 74 patients (60%), with atrioventricular nodal reentrant tachycardia being the predominant arrhythmia (83%), followed by orthodromic atrioventricular reentrant tachycardia (12%) and focal atrial tachycardia (5%). The arrhythmia could be permanently cured by catheter ablation performed with no complication during the same procedure in 70 patients (95%).

REFERENCES

1. Krahn AD, Klein GJ, Yee R, et al. Final results from a pilot study with an implantable loop recorder to determine the etiology of syncope in patients with negative noninvasive and invasive testing. Am J Cardiol 1998;82:117–9.
2. Vardas PE. From the Einthoven galvanometer to the implantable loop recorder: revelations in store. Pacing Clin Electrophysiol 2000;23:1453–5.
3. Miracapillo G, Addonisio L, Breschi M, et al. Left axillary implantation of loop recorder versus the traditional left chest area: a prospective randomized study. Pacing Clin Electrophysiol 2016;39:830–6.
4. Bisignani G, De Bonis S, Bisignani A, et al. Sensing performance, safety, and patient acceptability of long-dipole cardiac monitor: an innovative axillary insertion. Pacing Clin Electrophysiol 2018;41:277–83.
5. Maines M, Zorzi A, Tomasi G, et al. Clinical impact, safety, and accuracy of the remotely monitored implantable loop recorder Medtronic Reveal LINQ™. Europace 2018;20:1050–7.
6. Ibrahim OA, Drew D, Hayes CJ, et al. Implantable loop recorders in the real world: a study of two Canadian centers. J Interv Card Electrophysiol 2017;50:179–85.
7. Roberts PR, Zachariah D, Morgan JM, et al. Monitoring of arrhythmia and sudden death in a hemodialysis population: the CRASH-ILR Study. PLoS One 2017;12:e0188713.
8. Sakhi S, Theuns DAMJ, Bhagwandien RE, et al. Value of implantable loop recorders in patients with structural or electrical heart disease. J Interv Card Electrophysiol 2018;52:203–8.
9. Lee R, Mittal S. Utility and limitations of long-term monitoring of atrial fibrillation using an implantable loop recorder. Heart Rhythm 2018;15:287–95.
10. Lacour P, Dang PL, Huemer M, et al. Performance of the new BioMonitor 2-AF insertable cardiac monitoring system: can better be worse? Pacing Clin Electrophysiol 2017;40:516–26.
11. De Ponti R, Marazzato J, Bagliani G. Sick sinus syndrome. Card Electrophysiol Clin 2018;10:183–95.
12. Brignole M, Moya A, de Lange FJ, et al. 2018 ESC Guidelines for the diagnosis and management of syncope. Eur Heart J 2018;39:1883–948.
13. Da Costa A, Defaye P, Romeyer-Bouchard C, et al. Clinical impact of the implantable loop recorder in patients with isolated syncope, bundle branch block and negative workup: a randomized multicentre prospective study. Arch Cardiovasc Dis 2013;106:146–54.
14. Maggi R, Rafanelli M, Ceccofiglio A, et al. Additional diagnostic value of implantable loop recorder in patients with initial diagnosis of real or apparent transient loss of consciousness of uncertain origin. Europace 2014;16:1226–30.
15. Podoleanu C, Da Costa A, Defaye P, et al. Early use of implantable loop recorder in syncope evaluation: a randomized study in the context of the French

healthcare system (FRESH study). Arch Cardiovasc Dis 2014;107:546–52.

16. Sulke N, Sugihara C, Hong P, et al. The benefit of remotely monitored implantable loop recorder as a first line investigation in unexplained syncope: the EaSyAS II trial. Europace 2016;18:912–8.

17. Musat DL, Milstein N, Mittal S. Implantable loop recorders for cryptogenic stroke (plus real-world atrial fibrillation detection rate with implantable loop recorders). Card Electrophysiol Clin 2018;10: 111–8.

18. Carrazco C, Golyan D, Kahen M, et al. Prevalence and risk factors for paroxysmal atrial fibrillation and flutter detection after cryptogenic ischemic stroke. J Stroke Cerebrovasc Dis 2018;27:203–9.

19. Philippsen TJ, Christensen LS, Hansen MG, et al. Detection of subclinical atrial fibrillation in high-risk patients using insertable cardiac monitor. JACC Clin Electrophysiol 2017;3:1557–64.

20. Gorenek B, Bax J, Boriani G, et al. Device-detected atrial tachyarrhythmias: definition, implications and management – an European Heart Rhythm Association (EHRA) consensus document, endorsed by the Heart Rhythm Society (HRS), Asia Pacific Heart Rhythm Society (APHRS) and Sociedad Latinoamericana de Estimulacion Cardiaca y Electrofisiologia (SOLEACE). Europace 2017;19:1556–78.

21. Israel CW, Gronefeld G, Ehrlich JR, et al. Long-term risk of recurrent atrial fibrillation as documented by an implantable monitoring device: implications for optimal patient care. J Am Coll Cardiol 2004;43: 47–52.

22. Heeger CH, Tscholl V, Salloum O, et al. What is the real recurrence rate after cryoballoon-based pulmonary vein isolation? Lessons from rhythm follow-up based on implanted cardiac devices with continuous atrial monitoring. Heart Rhythm 2018;15: 1844–50.

23. Przyżycka P, Kałowski M, Poddębska I, et al. Self-terminating ventricular fibrillation recorded by an implantable loop recorder as a cause of syncope – a case report. J Electrocardiol 2018;51:617–9.

24. Chiriac A, Mulpuru SK, McLeod CJ, et al. Almost five minutes of ventricular fibrillation and living to tell the tale (spontaneously resolved long-duration ventricular fibrillation. J Cardiovasc Electrophysiol 2018;29: 1038–9.

25. Suarez-Fuster L, Oh C, Baranchuk A. Transcutaneous electrical nerve stimulation electromagnetic interference in an implantable loop recorder. J Arrhythm 2018;34:96–7.

26. Peruzza F, Maines M, Catanzariti D, et al. A misleading prolonged asystole: a case of implantable loop recorder dehiscence. G Ital Cardiol (Rome) 2018;19:246–7 [in Italian].

27. Preminger MW, Musat DL, Sichrovsky T, et al. Migration of implantable loop recorder into the pleural space. HeartRhythm Case Rep 2017;3: 539–41.

28. Jenkins JM, Dick M, Collins S, et al. Use of the pill electrode for transesophageal atrial pacing. Pacing Clin Electrophysiol 1985;8:512–27.

29. Haeberlin A, Niederhauser T, Marisa T, et al. Optimal lead insertion depth for esophageal ECG recording with respect to the atrial signal quality. J Electrocardiol 2013;46:158–65.

30. Bagliani G, Meniconi L, Raggi F, et al. Left origin of the atrial esophageal signal as recorded in the pacing site. Pacing Clin Electrophysiol 1998;21: 18–24.

31. Bagliani G, Michelucci A, Angeli F, et al. Atrial activation analysis by surface P wave and multipolar esophageal recording after cardioversion of persistent atrial fibrillation. Pacing Clin Electrophysiol 2003;26:1178–88.

32. Gallagher JJ, Smith WM, Kerr CR, et al. Esophageal pacing: a diagnostic and therapeutic tool. Circulation 1982;65:336–41.

33. Brembilla-Perrot B, Beurrier D, Houriez O, et al. Wide QRS complex tachicardia. Rapid method of prognostic evaluation. Int J Cardiol 2004;97:83–8.

34. Tritto M, Dicandia CD, Calabrese P. Overdrive atrial stimulation during transesophageal electrophysiological study: usefulness of post-pacing VA interval analysis in differentiating supraventricular tachycardias with 1:1 atrio-ventricular relationship. Int J Cardiol 1997;62:37–45.

35. Brockmeter K, Ulmer HE, Hessling G. Termination of atrial reentrant tachycardia by using transesophageal atrial pacing. J Electrocardiol 2002;35(Suppl): 159–63.

36. Heinke M, Kuhnert H, Surber R, et al. Termination of atrial flutter by directed transesophageal atrial pacing during transesophageal echocardiography. Biomed Tech (Berl) 2007;52:180–4.

37. Hessling G, Brockmeier K, Hulmer HE. Transesophageal electrocardiography and atrial pacing in children. J Electrocardiol 2002;35(Suppl):143–9.

38. Brembilla-Perrot B, Cloez JL, Marchal C, et al. Transesophageal electrophysiologic study in non sedated children younger than 11 years with a Wolff-Parkinson-White syndrome. Ann Cardiol Angeiol 2009;58:1–6.

39. Cohen MI, Triedman JK, Cannon BC, et al. PACES/HRS expert consensus statement on the management of the asymptomatic young patient with a Wolff-Parkinson-White (WPW, ventricular preexcitation) electrocardiographic pattern: developed in partnership between the Pediatric and Congenital Electrophysiology Society (PACES) and the Heart Rhythm Society (HRS). Endorsed by the governing bodies of PACES, HRS, the American College of Cardiology Foundation (ACCF), the American Heart Association (AHA), the American Academy of

Pediatrics (AAP), and the Canadian Heart Rhythm Society (CHRS). Heart Rhythm 2012;9:1006–24.

40. Scheweikert RA, Perez Lugones A, Kanagaratnam L, et al. A simple method of mapping atrial premature depolarizations triggering atrial fibrillation. Pacing Clin Electrophysiol 2001;24:22–7.

41. Yamada T, Murakami Y, Muto M, et al. Simple and accurate catheter mapping technique to predict atrial fibrillation foci in the pulmonary veins or posterior right atrium. Heart Rhythm 2004;1:427–34.

42. Haeberlin A, Niederhauser T, Tanner H, et al. Atrial waveform analysis using esophageal long-term electrocardiography reveals atrial ectopic activity. Clin Res Cardiol 2012;101:941–2.

43. Niederhauser T, Haeberlin A, Marisa T, et al. An optimized lead system for long-term esophageal electrocardiography. Physiol Meas 2014;35:517–32.

44. Drago F, Russo MS, Marazzi R, et al. Atrial tachycardia in patients with congenital heart disease: a minimally invasive simplified approach in the use of three dimensional electroanatomic mapping. Europace 2011;13:689–95.

45. Furniss G, Panagopoulos D, Newcombe D, et al. The use of an esophageal catheter to check the results left atrial posterior wall isolation in the treatment of atrial fibrillation. Pacing Clin Electrophysiol 2018; 41:1345–55.

46. Heinke M, Ismer B, Kuhnert H, et al. Transesophageal left ventricular electrogram-recording and temporary pacing to improve patient selection for cardiac resynchronization. Med Biol Eng Comput 2011;49:851–8.

47. Arzbaecher R, Jenkins JM. A review of the theoretical and experimental bases of transesophageal atrial pacing. J Electrocardiol 2002;35(Suppl): 137–41.

48. Kohler H, Zink S, Scharf J, et al. Severe esophageal burn after transesophageal pacing. Endoscopy 2007;39(Suppl 1):e300.

49. Scherlag BJ, Lau SH, Helfant RH, et al. Catheter technique for recording His bundle activity in man. Circulation 1969;39:13–8.

50. Durrer D, Schoop L, Schuilenburg RM, et al. The role of premature beats in the initiation and the termination of supraventricular tachycardia in the Wolff-Parkinson-White syndrome. Circulation 1967;36: 644–62.

51. Durrer D, van Dam RT, Freud GE, et al. Total excitation of the isolated human heart. Circulation 1970;41: 899–912.

52. Waldo AL. From bedside to bench: entrainment and other stories. Heart Rhythm 2004;1:94–106.

53. Veenhuyzen GD, Quinn FR, Wilton SB, et al. Diagnostic pacing maneuvers for supraventricular tachycardia: part 1. Pacing Clin Electrophysiol 2011;34:767–82.

54. Veenhuyzen GD, Quinn FR, Wilton SB, et al. Diagnostic pacing maneuvers for supraventricular tachycardia: part 2. Pacing Clin Electrophysiol 2012;35: 757–69.

55. De Ponti R, Marazzato J, Bagliani G, et al. Peculiar electrocardiographic aspects of wide QRS complex tachicardia: when differential diagnosis is difficult. Card Electrophysiol Clin 2018;10:317–32.

56. De Ponti R, Tritto M, Lanzotti ME, et al. Computerized high-density mapping of the pulmonary veins: new insights into their electrical activation in patients with atrial fibrillation. Europace 2004;6:97–108.

57. De Ponti R, Verlato R, Bertaglia E, et al. Treatment of macro-re-entrant atrial tachicardia based on electro-anatomic mapping: identification and ablation of the mid-diastolic isthmus. Europace 2007;9:449–57.

58. De Ponti R, Marazzi R, Zoli L, et al. Electroanatomic mapping and ablation of macroreentrant atrial tachycardia: comparison between successfully and unsuccessfully treated cases. J Cardiovasc Electrophysiol 2010;21:155–62.

59. Gokoglan Y, Mohanty S, Gianni C, et al. Scar homogenization versus limited-substrate ablation in patients with non-ischemic cardiomyopathy and ventricular tachycardia. J Am Coll Cardiol 2016;68: 1990–8.

60. Briceno DF, Romero J, Gianni C, et al. Substrate ablation of ventricular tachycardia: late potentials, scar dechanneling, local abnormal ventricular activities, core isolation, and homogenization. Card Electrophysiol Clin 2017;9:81–91.

61. Stabile G, Scaglione M, Del Greco M, et al. Reduced fluoroscopy exposure during ablation of atrial fibrillation using a novel electroanatomical navigation system: a multicentre experience. Europace 2012;14: 60–5.

62. De Ponti R. Reduction of radiation exposure in catheter ablation of atrial fibrillation: lesson learned. World J Cardiol 2015;7:442–8.

63. Stabile G, Solimene F, Calò L, et al. Catheter-tissue contact force values do not impact mid-term clinical outcome following pulmonary vein isolation in patients with paroxysmal atrial fibrillation. J Interv Card Electrophysiol 2015;42:21–6.

64. Takigawa M, Derval N, Frontera A, et al. Revisiting anatomic macroreentrant tachycardia after atrial fibrillation ablation using ultrahigh-resolution mapping: implications for ablation. Heart Rhythm 2018; 15:326–33.

65. Josephson ME. Electrophysiology at a crossroads. Heart Rhythm 2007;4:658–61.

The Value of Baseline and Arrhythmic ECG in the Interpretation of Arrhythmic Mechanisms

Qiong Chen, MD[a,b,1], Alessio Gasperetti, MD[a,1],
Domenico G. Della Rocca, MD[a,*],
Sanghamitra Mohanty, MD[a], Omer Gedikli, MD[a],
Chintan Trivedi, MD[a], Alfredo Chauca-Tapia, MD[a],
Luigi Di Biase, MD, PhD[a,c,d,e,f], Andrea Natale, MD[a,c,d,g,h,i]

KEYWORDS

- Electrocardiogram • Cardiac arrhythmias • Baseline electrocardiogram • Tachycardia
- Atrial-ventricular conduction

KEY POINTS

- ECG is important in the diagnosis of arrhythmia, and baseline ECG also plays an important role before arrhythmia occurrence.
- The baseline ECG from P wave, PR interval, QRS wave, J wave, ST-T, and QT interval are analyzed systematically, and the role of baseline ECG in the diagnosis of arrhythmia discussed.

INTRODUCTION

Owing to the rapid development of new electrophysiologic techniques, our understanding of arrhythmias and their underlying mechanisms has reached unprecedented levels. Nonetheless, the surface 12-lead electrocardiograph (ECG) still represents an important tool in the armory of the physician studying rhythm disorders, allowing a first-line, noninvasive, rapid, and inexpensive evaluation. In most cases the pathogenesis of clinical arrhythmias is due to electrophysiologic abnormalities. These abnormalities are often mirrored by baseline ECG alterations, sometimes even in an obvious manner; the skilled clinician must spot and recognize them before the arrhythmia develops, to start appropriate therapies for prevention of arrhythmic events or to stratify the risk according to patients' outcomes. A systematic revision of baseline ECG alterations, following the normal ECG waves and interval succession order, is presented here.

[a] Texas Cardiac Arrhythmia Institute, St David's Medical Center, 3000 N. IH-35, Suite 720, Austin, TX 78705, USA; [b] Henan Provincial People's Hospital, No. 7 Weiwu, Zhengzhou, Henan Province, China; [c] Department of Internal Medicine, Dell Medical School, University of Texas, 1501 Red River Street, Austin, TX 78712, USA; [d] Department of Biomedical Engineering, Cockrell School of Engineering, University of Texas, 301 East Dean Keeton Street, Austin, TX 78712, USA; [e] Arrhythmia Services, Department of Medicine, Montefiore Medical Center, Albert Einstein College of Medicine, 111 East 210th Street, Bronx, NY 10467, USA; [f] Department of Clinical and Experimental Medicine, University of Foggia, Via A. Gramsci 09/91, Apulia, Foggia 71122, Italy; [g] Interventional Electrophysiology, Scripps Clinic, 9898 Genessee Avenue, La Jolla, CA 92037, USA; [h] Department of Cardiology, Metro Health Medical Center, Case Western Reserve University School of Medicine, 2109 Adelbert Road, Cleveland, OH 44106, USA; [i] Division of Cardiology, Stanford University, 870 Quarry Road, Stanford, CA 94305, USA
[1] These authors contributed equally to this work.
* Corresponding author.
E-mail address: domenicodellarocca@hotmail.it

Card Electrophysiol Clin 11 (2019) 219–238
https://doi.org/10.1016/j.ccep.2019.02.007

P-WAVE ABNORMALITIES

The P wave represents the whole process of atrial depolarization. Depolarization starts from the sinus node and it is transmitted along the Bachman bundle (BB) and the internodal tracts to the myocardium of both atria and to the atrioventricular (AV) node. The P wave is usually characterized according to its morphology, duration, and amplitude. A normal P wave is positive in I, II, aVF, and V4 to V6, and negative in aVR; positive P waves are generally blunt but slight incision can be sometimes observed. Atrial depolarization time, including P-wave duration, should be less than 120 ms, with an electrical vector moving from downward and leftward. Normal P-wave amplitude ranges between 0.05 and 0.25 mV, depending on the patient's constitution and heart position. P-wave alterations normally mirror atrial morphologic abnormalities. The most common abnormal P waves are the "P mitrale" and "P pulmonale"; in addition to these, an intra-atrial block (IAB) may be identified on the ECG.

P Mitrale

At ECG evaluation, a P mitrale appears to be broad (>120 ms), significantly notched, and bifid, with an interpeak interval >40 ms in the limb leads (especially in the inferior leads). In V1, the terminal negative deflection of the P wave appears wider

(>40 ms) and deeper (>1 mm) than normal, with larger area than the initial P-wave-positive deflection (**Fig. 1**). The P mitrale is associated with left atrial (LA) dilatation, most commonly caused by valvular heart diseases (eg, mitral stenosis, mitral regurgitation, and aortic stenosis), systemic hypertension, and hypertrophic or postischemic cardiomyopathies.

P Pulmonale

The P pulmonale appears as a tall, upright, and relatively narrow P wave greater than 2.5 mm in lead II with a prominent initial positive deflection (>1.5 mm) in V1 (**Fig. 2**). A P pulmonale is usually associated with right atrium (RA) dilation and fibrosis: the activation of the RA being delayed results in a simultaneous depolarization of both atria, forming a P wave of increased amplitude. It is generally caused by primary or secondary advanced pulmonary hypertension.

Intra-atrial Block

An IAB is an interatrial conduction delay characterized by a P-wave duration greater than 120 ms, with a notched or biphasic morphology in the inferior leads and/or in V1 or V2. This electrocardiographic change is due to a collagen deposition between atrial cells, causing a partial or complete BB block. IAB leads to a delayed

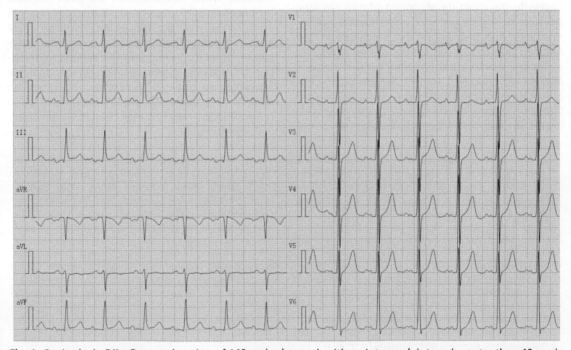

Fig. 1. P mitrale: in DII a P-wave duration of 140 ms is observed, with an interpeak interval greater than 40 ms; in V1 there is a biphasic P wave, with a wider and deeper terminal negative deflection.

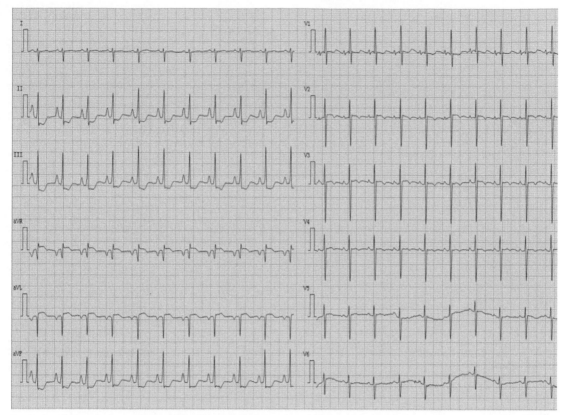

Fig. 2. P pulmonare in a 76-year-old man with chronic obstructive pulmonary disease. In the inferior leads a tall, upright, and relatively narrow P wave greater than 2.5 mm can be identified. A rightward axis deviation and ECG criteria for right ventricle hypertrophy are also present.

and asynchronous activation of the atrial syncytium: the impulse needs to find an alternative way to the BB to propagate. It initially propagates through the inferior RA, penetrates into the septum, then enters the LA, the coronary sinus (CS), and inferior LA before finally depolarizing the posterior LA roof (**Fig. 3**).

Absence of P Wave

In some clinical scenarios, no P wave can be found. Three potential options should then be considered:

- Atrial activity subduction: the P wave is present but is covered by QRS or T-wave signal; it can be unveiled in case of a sudden change in heart rate or the other situation (eg, wide complex tachycardia, atrial tachycardia)
- Hidden atrium activity: in atrial fibrillation (AF) or atrial flutter (AFL), the P wave is not visible on the surface ECG, but the atrial activity is still there and can be visualized by an intracardiac ECG or transesophageal ECG

- No atrial activity: no atrial activity can be recorded. Examples can be sinus and atrial arrest in hyperkalemia (**Fig. 4**).

Predictive Value of P-Wave Abnormalities

The P-wave analysis can be used by the electrophysiologist as an a priori parameter for atrial arrhythmia development risk; recent studies in paroxysmal and persistent AF patients revealed that a prolonged P-wave duration (PWD) recorded during sinus rhythm was associated with higher rates of postpulmonary vein antrum isolation recurrences and of progression from paroxysmal to persistent AF.[1–4] In addition, atrial enlargement, atrial fibrosis, and IAB might predispose to formation of electrical re-entry circuits in the atrium, which may increase the risk of AF, a risk factor that may lead to AF, AFL, or atrial tachycardia.[5–7]

Besides PWD, other independent predictive markers of arrhythmia recurrence are a wide P-wave dispersion (such as the difference between the widest and narrowest P waves), an abnormal P-wave axis, and the presence of premature atrial contractions (PACs).[8] Specifically,

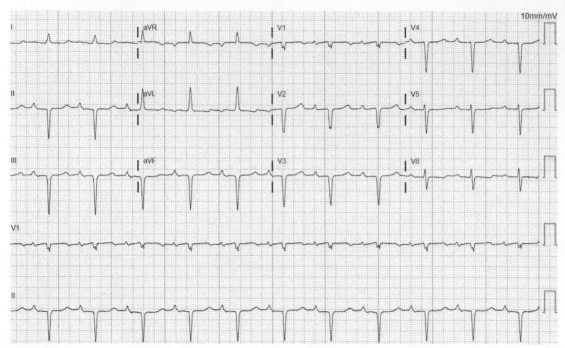

Fig. 3. A 73-year-old man with intra-atrial block; P-wave duration is 160 ms with a biphasic morphology in V1 and inferior leads.

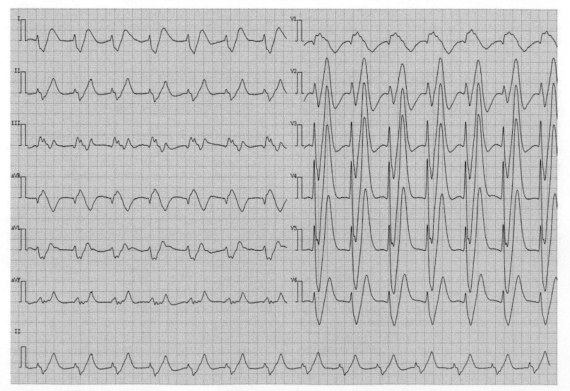

Fig. 4. A 58-year-old man with acute renal failure related hyperkalemia (K^+ >8.0 mmol/L) with sinus arrest. P-wave disappearance, nonspecific intraventricular functional block with QRS widening, and high T waves with a narrow base.

frequent PACs have been identified in recent meta-analyses as strong predictors for AF, both at baseline and during exercise.[9–11]

PR INTERVAL ALTERATIONS

The PR interval is defined as the interval from the beginning of atrial depolarization to the beginning of ventricular depolarization; it is composed of the P wave and the PR segment, which represent the impulse going through the AV node. Normally in adults it ranges from 120 to 200 ms; conduction abnormalities may prolong, shorten, or vary the normal PR duration. The most common reasons for PR interval prolongation are AV blocks (AVB), dual AV node pathway (DAVNP), and the presence of an IAB. Conversely, reasons for PR interval shortening include ventricular pre-excitation enhanced AV nodal conduction, which occurs when unfiltered atrial impulses reach the lower AV junction and the ventricles, and interfering AV dissociation. Four of these PR interval alterations hold high arrhythmic relevance and therefore need to be addressed.

Dual Atrioventricular Node Pathway

This condition is due to the presence of 2 separate conduction pathways in the compact part of the AV node, called the "fast" pathway, with a longer refractory period, and the "slow" pathway, with a shorter refractory period.[12] The slow pathway (usually the target for catheter ablation) is located inferiorly and slightly posteriorly to the AV node, following the anterior margin of the CS, whereas the fast pathway is located superiorly to the AV node.

A definitive diagnosis of DAVNP is obtained on the demonstration of a discontinuous anterograde AV nodal conduction in response to a programmed atrial stimulation protocol in the electrophysiology laboratory. The diagnostic sign of a DAVNP is the presence of the so-called jump, a sudden conduction delay that causes an increase greater than 50 ms in the PR interval during programmed atrial stimulation (**Fig. 5**).

Given the duality of the conduction pathways, several situations have to be considered. If one of the pathways is capable of retrograde conduction, an electrical re-entry may form and an atrioventricular node re-entry tachycardia (AVNRT) may develop. The usual trigger of this arrhythmia is a PAC or a sudden change in the atrial rate: the premature depolarization will reach the AV node, and 2 different mechanisms of arrhythmia may follow depending on the refractory status of the pathways.

- Typical AVNRT: the depolarization reaches a still refractory fast pathway but an already repolarized slow pathway; therefore, the slow pathway conducts the electrical impulse to the ventricles. If sufficient time has passed to allow complete repolarization of the fast pathway, the electrical activity before leaving the lower part of the AV node can also be retro-conducted by the fast pathway, closing the re-entry. This generates an AV nodal "echo" beat and, if this pattern is perpetuated, a "typical" AVNRT (**Fig. 6**). The surface ECG is characterized by a P wave with a short RP interval and a sudden increase in ventricular frequency.
- Atypical AVNRT: the anterograde depolarization is conducted by the fast pathway, while the retrograde conduction happens along the slow pathway before the electrical activity leaves the AV node, closing the re-entry. An AV nodal echo beat will arise as well but the P wave generating on the surface ECG will be followed by a long RP interval.

If instead the retrograde capacity of the 2 pathways is scarce, the impulse will be conducted to the ventricles alternating by the fast or the slow pathway and 2 stable different PR intervals can be record in the same individual, with a difference in length greater than 50 ms. No arrhythmia can arise given the fact that no re-entry is present.

In rare cases, if the 2 pathways have such a difference in conduction velocity and refractory periods when electrical activity is transmitted via the slow pathway that the fast one is already out of the refractory period, a normal sinus beat will result in a ventricular activation along both pathways. On the surface ECG a P wave followed by 2 narrow QRS will be recorded ("double firing"). This may evolve into a dual AV nodal non-re-entrant tachycardia[13] (**Fig. 7**).

Finding at the baseline ECG analysis more than one stable PR interval with a jump greater than 50 ms should always lead to the suspicion of a dual AV pathway and, if this finding is corroborated by clinical symptoms, an arrhythmologic consultation should be required to eventually assess and diagnose the patient with an electrophysiologic study.

Ventricular Pre-excitation

Ventricular pre-excitation is defined as an earlier activation of the ventricular myocardium via an impulse originating from the atrium that is not normally conducted along the AV node pathway. The following pathways can be involved in

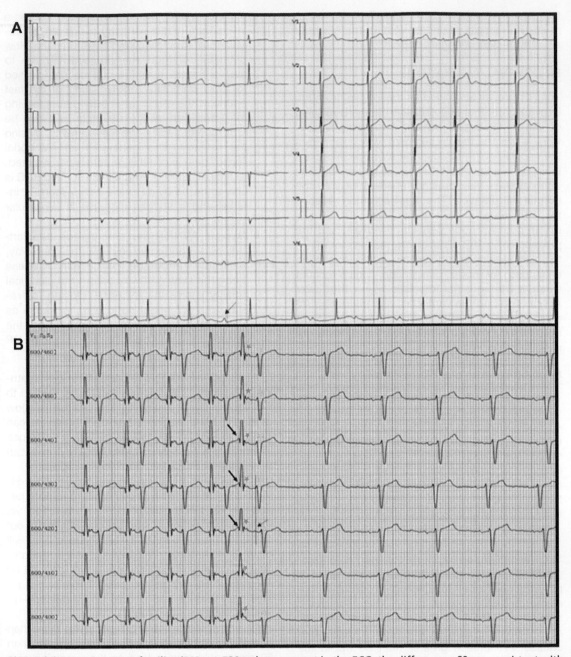

Fig. 5. (*A*) Two PR pattern families (240 ms, 520 ms) are present in the ECG, the difference >60 ms, consistent with DAVNP. (*B*) S1-S2 programmed stimulation; the stimulus-QRS interval jumped 70 ms at 600/420 ms, suggesting DAVNP. Red arrow, jump; black arrow, stimulus; green star, P wave; yellow star, QRS. DAVNP, dual AV node pathway.

pre-excitation[14]: (1) accessory AV muscle bundles; (2) accessory nodoventricular muscle bundles; (3) atriofascicular bypass fibers; (4) fasciculoventricular accessory connections; (5) intranodal bypass fibers; and (6) nodal malformations.[15] The term "ventricular pre-excitation syndrome" is used when a ventricular pre-excitation is combined with a clinically symptomatic tachycardia.[16]

Wolff-Parkinson-White syndrome

An AV bypass tract (Kent bundle) is present. On the ECG, a manifest ventricular pre-excitation is characterized by a PR interval less than 120 ms,

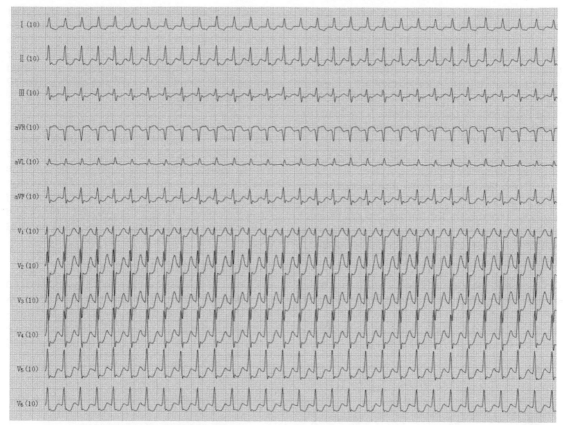

Fig. 6. Narrow complex tachycardia at 200 beats/min. P wave is not found in the RR' interval but as an incision in the terminal deflection of the QRS in the inferior leads. RP' interval is less than PR interval and the RP' interval less than 70 ms. These findings are diagnostic for AV node re-entrant tachycardia.

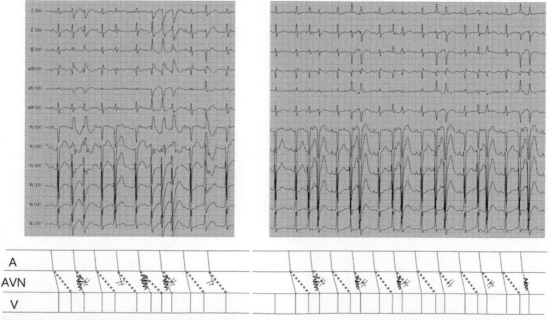

Fig. 7. "Double firing." DAVNP, with some P waves followed by 2 supraventricular QRS caused by consecutive antegrade conduction via fast and slow pathways can be observed for the entire registration. Blue dotted line, slow pathway; whirly line, conduction delay; double line, conduction blocked.

and a delta wave (a slurred upstroke or downstroke at the beginning of the QRS complex) incision in a QRS, whose width exceeds 120 ms. The PJ interval is normal and secondary ST changes may be found. The delta wave in V1 may be positive (type A pre-excitation) if the Kent bundle connects the LA and the left ventricle, or negative (type B pre-excitation) if instead the bundle connects the right chambers (**Fig. 8**). The pattern may be concealed as well, with no clearly identifiable delta wave but a short PR and a wide or upper-normal limit QRS.

Kent bundles always have both anterograde and retrograde conduction abilities, therefore meeting the basic conditions for forming an AV re-entry, such as the presence of 2 pathways, slow conduction, and one-way block. This condition can lead to the insurgence of the following.

Orthodromic atrioventricular re-entrant tachycardia The impulse is conducted from the atria to the ventricles through the AV node and then from the ventricles again back to the atria through the Kent bundle. This tachycardia is characterized by an RP interval greater than 70 ms and shorter than the PR interval, with a narrow QRS (unless a functional intraventricular block occurs). If the pathway is left sided the RP interval in V6 is shorter than the RP interval in V1, whereas in a right-sided pathway the RP interval in V6 is longer than the RP interval in V1 (**Fig. 9**).

Antidromic atrioventricular re-entrant tachycardia The impulse is conducted from the atria to the ventricles through the Kent bundle and the re-entry is closed by a retro-conduction through the AV node. This tachycardia is characterized by an RP interval longer than the PR interval and a PR interval less than 120 ms, with a wide QRS (**Fig. 10**).

Lown-Ganong-Levine syndrome
On the ECG, LGL syndrome is characterized by a PR interval <120 ms and a normal QRS complex (**Fig. 11**).[17] In this situation, an appropriate premature stimulus may induce AVRT. The pathophysiology of this syndrome has not as yet been fully

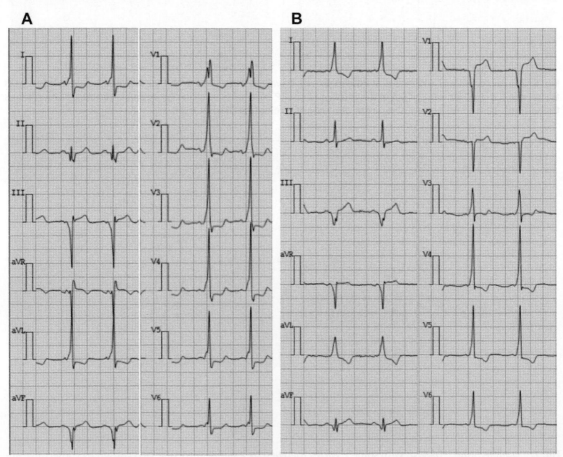

Fig. 8. Wolff-Parkinson-White syndrome ECG pattern: PR interval less than 120 ms with delta wave in the initial upstroke (*A*, left pathway; type A) or downstroke (*B*, right pathway; type B) of the QRS in V1.

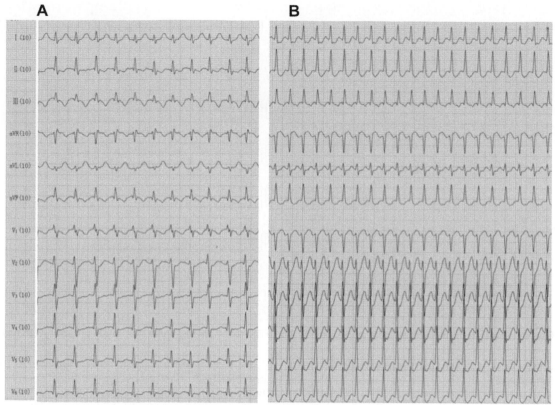

Fig. 9. Narrow QRS tachycardia with an RP′ less than PR and RP′ greater than 70 ms; diagnostic for orthodromic AV re-entrant tachycardia. (*A*) Right-side pathway (RP′ V1 < RP′ V6), heart rate (HR) 167 beats/min; (*B*) Left-side pathway (RP′ V1 > RP′ V6), HR 214 beats/min.

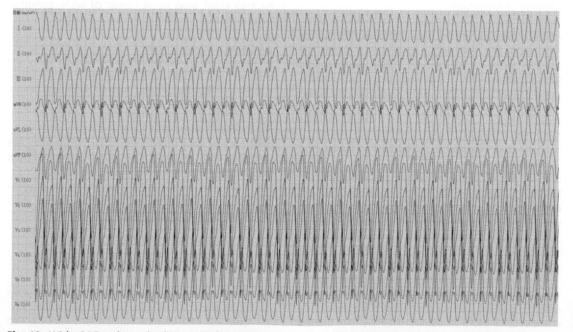

Fig. 10. Wide QRS tachycardia (HR ~250 beats/min) consistent with antidromic AV re-entrant tachycardia.

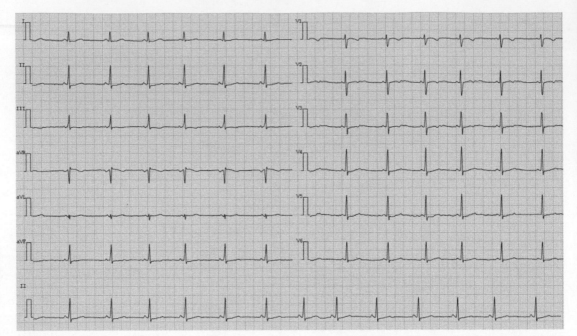

Fig. 11. Short PR, normal QRS syndrome. ECG shows short PR interval (90 ms) and a normal QRS duration (85 ms).

understood, and various hypotheses have been formulated.

Accessory pathway hypothesis The James fibers have been proposed, but never fully confirmed, as the culprit additional pathway bypassing the AV node to justify the short PR and supraventricular tachycardia development but with a narrow QRS due to the normal AV-His-Purkinje system impulse propagation.

Atrioventricular node abnormalities Alterations regarding the AV node have been proposed as the basis of this theory, both morphologic (hypoplasia of the node) and functional (abnormally fast transmitting channels accelerating conduction)

Mahaim
Mahaim fiber is a special AV bypass with slow and decreasing conduction. This type of bypass has only AV and no ventricular arrhythmia (VA) conduct function. Mahaim fiber connections are located between the RA or the AV node and the right ventricle in or close to the right bundle branch. They can be atriofascicular, AV, nodofascicular, nodoventricular, and so forth, depending on their variable proximal and distal insertions[18] (**Fig. 12**).

On the electrocardiogram, during sinus rhythm the PR interval is normal or longer than normal, and the pre-excited wave is visible. It can induce a wide QRS tachycardia with left bundle branch block (LBBB) morphology (**Fig. 13**).

Ventricular pre-excitation adds another level of complexity in most tachycardias: wide complex tachycardias require a rapid differential diagnosis between ventricular tachycardia (VT) and supraventricular arrhythmias conducted with aberrances, an eventual pre-excitation in AF also representing a contraindication to most antiarrhythmic drugs.[19] Looking for a pre-excitation pattern in a previous baseline ECG is an important step in all cases of wide complex tachycardia.

Atrioventricular Block

AVB is an abnormal conduction between the atria and the ventricles. Three types of AVB are usually described (**see Fig. 13**).

First-degree atrioventricualar block
Each atrial activation is transmitted to the ventricle with an AV conduction delay. On the ECG, every P wave is followed by a QRS complex (P-QRS ratio 1:1) but the PR interval is >200 ms (>180 ms in children younger than 14 years of age) (**Fig. 14**A).

Second-degree atrioventricualar block
It is a more severe AV conduction delay. This condition can be further classified into

- Type 1 (Mobitz I, Luciani-Wenckebach phenomenon): there is a progressive prolongation of PR interval in several conducted beats, then a P wave is not conducted; the

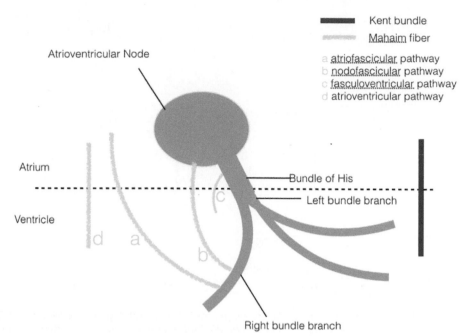

Kent bundle

Mahaim fiber

a atriofascicular pathway
b nodofascicular pathway
c fasculoventricular pathway
d atrioventricular pathway

Fig. 12. Red line, Kent bundle; blue line, Mahaim fibers. a, atriofascicular pathway; b, nodofascicular pathway; c, fasculoventricular pathway; d, atrioventricular pathway.

nonconduction cycle repeats, more or less regularly; the first beat after the nonconducted one has a shorter PR interval than the last conducted one (**Fig. 14**B).

- Type 2 (Mobitz II): the PR interval can be normal or longer and remains unchanged in all beats before a P wave, which suddenly

fails to be conducted to the ventricles (**Fig. 14**C).

High-grade atrioventricular block
If there are 2 or more nonconducted successive P waves this would be called high-grade AV block, represented by a P/QRS ratio of 3:1 or

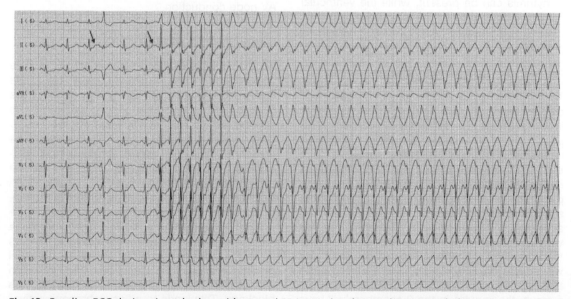

Fig. 13. Baseline ECG during sinus rhythm with normal PR interval and normal QRS morphology in a patient with a premature atrial contraction followed by rapid atrial pacing initiated a Mahaim fiber tachycardia with left bundle branch block morphology.

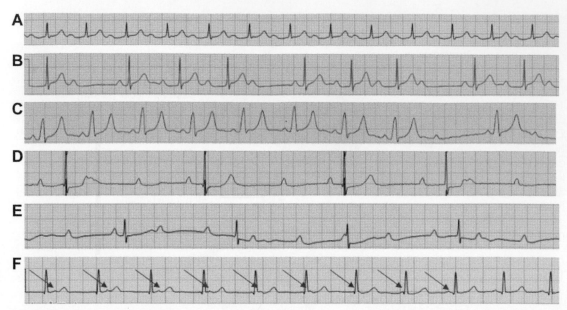

Fig. 14. AVB and interference phenomenon. (*A*) First-degree AVB; (*B*) second-degree AVB Mobitz 1; (*C*) second-degree AVB Mobitz 2; (*D*) high-grade second-degree AVB; (*E*) third-degree AVB; (*F*) AV interference dissociation. AVB, AV block.

higher and extremely slow ventricular rate, but with AV conduction still present (**Fig. 14**D).

Third-degree atrioventricualar block

This is the most severe form of AVB, with complete dissociation between atrial and ventricular electrical activity. P waves and QRS complexes are present with 2 independent rhythms. The atrial rhythm can be sinus, but any kind of atrial arrhythmia can be present, while the ventricular activity is frequently a junctional escape rhythm (normal QRS morphology, 40–60 beats/min) (**Fig. 14**E).

Interference Atrioventricular Dissociation

The interference phenomenon is defined as a different origin of atrial and ventricular activation in the absence of a third-degree AV block. This phenomenon refers to a series of continuous interference (≥3 beats) between the atrium and the ventricle. In a condition of normal sinus rhythm, the sinoatrial (SA) node is the physiologic pacemaker and all the lower ectopic rhythms are suppressed; when there is a slow SA activity or an acceleration in an ectopic subnodal rhythm, the ventricular heart rate can be equal to or higher than the atrial rate. Thus, the ectopic heart rate will be the one depolarizing the ventricle while the sinus impulse will depolarize the atrium. As a result, the impulse in the 2 chambers will have a different origin. On the ECG, the interference AV dissociation appears as a dissociation of P

waves and QRS complexes (**Fig. 14**F). The 2 rhythms should be described at the same time and the P-P and R-R intervals assessed and compared. This rhythm may resemble a third-degree AV block, but the pathogenesis is different: in the interference AV dissociation the AV conduction is normal and the dissociation is due to 2 different origins of the atrial impulse, whereas in the third-degree AV block there is no AV node conduction.

QRS COMPLEX ALTERATIONS

Ventricle depolarization, which normally occurs along the His-Purkinje system, gives rise to the QRS complex on the ECG. Its normal width ranges between 60 and 100 ms. QRS abnormalities bearing arrhythmic significance include mainly fascicular and bundle branch blocks; these are common in patients with a structural heart disease, but are often found also in patients without any known heart disease.

When a conduction block along one of the fascicles or the His bundle is present, there will be an area of delayed ventricular activation. As a rule of thumb, activation of that area occurs when the impulse conducted by the contralateral branch reaches the area via the common myocardial fibers, therefore bypassing the blockage. This leads to an asynchronous activation of the 2 ventricles, resulting in a wide QRS complex on the surface ECG. Those conduction blocks can be classified anatomically on the basis of the affected branch:

Left Bundle Branch Anomalies

Left anterior fascicular block
This condition is the result of a conduction anomaly in the anterior fascicle of the left bundle. On the ECG, a left axis deviation (QRS axis usually between −45° and −90°) can be found. The QRS complexes have a normal or slightly widened length (80–110 ms); qR complexes in leads I and aVL and rS complexes in II, III, and aVF can be found: diagnosis can be made in the presence of an S wave in DIII deeper than the S wave in DII (**Fig. 15A**).

Left posterior fascicular block
This condition occurs instead when the conduction delay affects the posterior fascicle of the left bundle branch. On the ECG there is a right axis deviation (QRS axis > +90°). The QRS complexes have a normal or slightly widened length (80–110 ms), with rS complexes in leads I and aVL, and qS in leads II, III, and aVF. This is a rare condition and it is usually a diagnosis of exclusion; all other causes of right axis deviation should be excluded (eg, right ventricle hypertrophy, arm lead switch, and dextrocardia).

LBBB
LBBB is characterized by a significant slowing or block of conduction through the left bundle. According to the QRS length, it can be defined as either incomplete (QRS 100–120 ms) or complete (QRS >120 ms). A prominent S wave can be seen in V1, with broad monophasic R waves in

lateral leads (I, aVL, V5-V6). The QRS axis is frequently shifted leftward. ST segment and T-wave alterations are usually present because of abnormal ventricular activation: they go in the opposite direction to the main vector of the QRS complex (appropriate discordance—eg, a negative T wave in a lead with a strongly positive QRS vector) (**Fig. 15B**).

Right Bundle Branch Anomalies

Right bundle branch block (RBBB) is a conduction defect caused by slowing or delay of conduction through the right bundle. Just like the LBBB, according to the QRS length it can be classified as incomplete (100–120 ms) or complete (>120 ms). It is not usually associated with a rightward axis deviation, owing to the smaller right ventricle myocardial mass. In leads V1 to V3 the "rabbit ear pattern" is usually found (there is a terminal R wave in those leads, usually denoted as an RsR′ complex), with wide and deep S waves in leads I, aVL, V5, and V6 (**Fig. 15C**).

Bilateral Anomalies

A bilateral anomaly (BLA) always appears as alternating bundle branch block: it is a rare condition whereby there is a high degree of blockage to both bundle branches. The ECG pattern presents an LBBB/RBBB alternating QRS morphology; it is highly associated with advanced heart block with a poor prognosis without adequate intervention. These ventricular conduction abnormalities may be associated with ischemic problems. As an example, the development of an LBBB pattern on a recent ECG may be secondary to ischemia

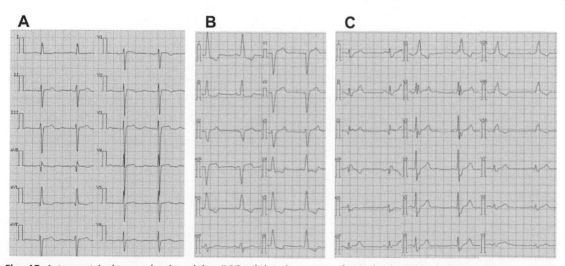

Fig. 15. Intraventricular conduction delay ECGs. (A) Left anterior fascicular hemiblock (QRS axis 61°); (B) left bundle branch block; (C) right bundle branch block (peripheral-standard precordial-right and posterior leads).

and may also suggest the presence of a large area of myocardial necrosis, with an increased risk (especially in the first hours of the event) of developing sustained VAs.[20,21]

Epsilon Wave

A particular alteration of the QRS complex that should always be searched for and ruled out in a first ECG evaluation is the epsilon wave. It a small post QRS wave, frequently described as a wave with a "grassy knoll" appearance, usually present in leads V1 and V2; it represents one of the major ECG criteria for arrhythmogenic right ventricular dysplasia/cardiomyopathy (ARVD/C) diagnosis, being specific for that disease.[22] (**Fig. 16**). This electrical signal is due to fragmentation of the normal impulse conduction caused by the presence of a fibro-fatty infiltrate with different electrical capacity replacing myocardial tissue in the ventricles.

ARVD/C is a subtle disease, highly underdiagnosed given the lack of symptoms for a long period of time. This ECG alteration should never go undetected, especially in asymptomatic patients, as they are prone to developing VA. A complete and invasive arrhythmic evaluation should be performed and an implantable cardioverter-defibrillator discussed, sudden cardiac death (SCD) caused by electrical alteration often being the first clinical manifestation of this disease.

ST SEGMENT ABNORMALITIES

The ST segment is the segment between the end of the S wave (called the J point) and the beginning of the T wave. It represents the interval of time between ventricular depolarization and repolarization. Usually it is flat and isoelectric. Most commonly, ST alterations are associated with ischemic events, but there are some arrhythmic syndromes, gathered under the umbrella of "J-wave syndrome" definition, that can cause them.[23] The J-wave syndrome is a clinical syndrome, first proposed in 2004,[24] whose hallmark is the presence of an early repolarization.

Classically, it can be divided into

- Hereditary J-wave syndrome: Brugada syndrome (BrS), idiopathic ventricular fibrillation (IVF), and early repolarization syndrome (ERS)
- Acquired J-wave syndrome: hypothermic J wave (HTJW) and acute ischemic J wave (AIJW)

Being acquired or genetically inherited, J-wave presence is due to an amplification of the transient outward potassium current (I_{TO}) that can cause electrical instability: all of these syndromes in fact present an increased risk of initiating a ventricular fibrillation (VF).

BrS

BrS is a genetically inherited channelopathy whose causative genetic abnormality is a

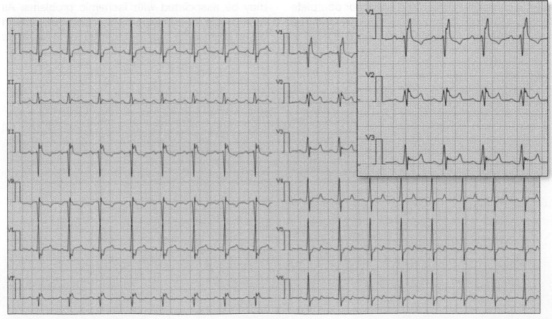

Fig. 16. Right bundle branch block with an epsilon wave in V1 to V3 in an arrhythmogenic right ventricular dysplasia/cardiomyopathy.

missense mutation in the sodium channel gene.[25] This syndrome may present with 3 different ECG patterns:

- Type 1 pattern: a coved ST elevation greater than 2 mm in at least one of the leads V1 to V3, followed by a negative T wave with no iso-electric separation (**Fig. 17**).
- Type 2 pattern: a "saddle-back" ST segment elevation ≥2 mm in leads V1 to V3 and a positive or biphasic T wave.
- Type 3 pattern: presents with a type 2 pattern but with an ST elevation less than 1 mm.

These ECG changes may be transient or always present at baseline; the same patient may present with different patterns at different times. Multiple factors may unmask or augment these patterns: fever, drugs (eg, sodium channel blockers, calcium channel blockers, cocaine), and electrolyte disturbances are the most common.

To diagnose the syndrome, the clinical criteria must be associated with a type 1 Brugada-like ECG pattern (types 2 and 3 are not diagnostic). Clinical criteria are presence of ventricular sustained arrhythmias or SCD, family history of SCD or type 1 ECG pattern in other family members, and VT inducibility with programmed ventricular stimulation.

Early Repolarization Syndrome

ERS was previously considered as a benign physiologic variant, but Haissaguerre and colleagues[26] first described the relationship between ERS and IVF/SCD in 2008. The ERS is defined as the presence of an early repolarization ECG pattern associated with symptomatic VAs. The 2015 consensus paper defined the following ECG criteria[27] for ERS (**Fig. 18**):

a. Presence of an end-QRS notch or slur on the downslope of an R wave
b. J peak greater than 0.1 mV in 2 or more contiguous leads, excluding V1 to V3
c. QRS width less than 120 ms
d. ST segment elevation may be present: if it is upward and followed by an upright T wave, the pattern is defined as early repolarization with ascending ST segment; if the ST segment is horizontal or downward sloping, the pattern is defined as early repolarization with descending or horizontal ST segment.

ERS can be divided into 3 subtypes, according to the characteristics of ECG, epidemiology, and clinical manifestations[28]:

- Type 1: the early repolarization pattern can be found in the lateral precordial leads (V2 to V5).

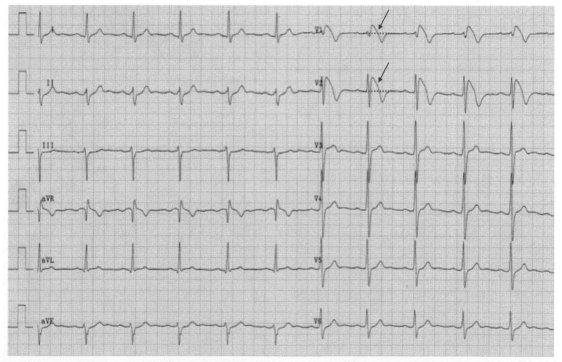

Fig. 17. Brugada type 1 "coved-like" pattern. EGC shows an ST elevation greater than 2 mm in V1 and V2 (*red arrow*), ST segment gradually descending, followed by a negative T wave under isoelectric line (*red dotted line*).

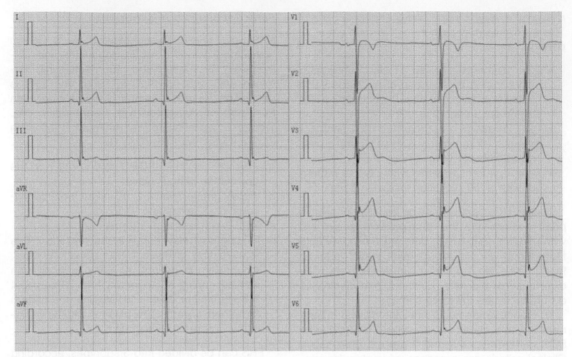

Fig. 18. Early repolarization syndrome. ECG shows a J wave in V3 to V6, inferior leads, and DI, with a normal-width QRS (100 ms), and an ST elevation >1 mm in V3 to V5.

This form is common among healthy male athletes but rarely seen in VF survivors

- Type 2: the early repolarization pattern is mainly found in the inferior or inferolateral leads and the risk of VA is higher than in type 1
- Type 3: the early repolarization pattern can be observed in the inferior, lateral, and right precordial leads. This form carries the highest risk of malignant VA

The following risk factors and ECG abnormalities are associated with an increased risk of IVF[28–31]:

a. Multiple leads with early repolarization ("global early repolarization")
b. The inferior leads are the ones where an early repolarization pattern has been more strongly associated with arrhythmia insurgence
c. J-wave amplitude greater than 0.2 mV, with J-wave/ST segment dynamic changes
d. ST segment with horizontal or downward slope
e. A short coupling interval, accompanied by an "R-on-T" phenomenon
f. A concomitant corrected QT interval alteration (<340 ms or >450 ms).

QT INTERVAL ABNORMALITIES

The QT interval reflects the duration of the cellular action potential and is a marker of depolarization

and repolarization. Its length is affected by age, gender, drugs, and hormonal imbalance. Given the dependence of QT duration on heart rate, its value is analyzed as corrected QT (QTc) to improve the accuracy of this measurement for detection of patients at increased risk of VA. Several formulas have been proposed for QT correction, the most used being the Bazett formula:

- Bazett: $QTcB = QT/RR^{1/2}$
- Fridericia: $QTcFri = QT/RR^{1/3}$
- Framingham: $QTcFra = QT + 0.154\,(1 - RR)$
- Hodges: $QTcH = QT + 0.00175\,([60/RR] - 60)$
- Rautaharju: $QTcR = QT - 0.185\,(RR - 1) + k$ ($k = +0.006$ seconds for men and $+0$ seconds for women)

The Framingham and Hodges formulas perform better at higher heart rates (>100/min). Normal values for QTc are ≤450 ms for men and ≤460 ms for women. The QTc should be always measured and monitored because the arrhythmic risk increases at both extreme ranges of normality. Many drugs (class Ia and class III antiarrhythmic drugs, many antidepressants and antipsychotics, fluoroquinolones, antifungal drugs) and electrolyte imbalances (eg, hypokalemia, hypercalcemia) can influence the QT interval (**Fig. 19**), generally by prolonging it, but there are 2 genetically inherited conditions that should

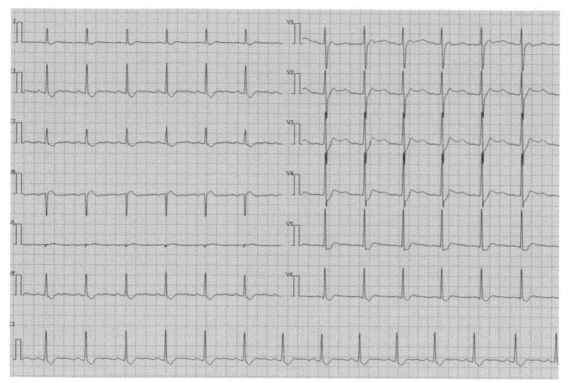

Fig. 19. Short QT interval (QT = 280 ms) caused by hypercalcemia (serum Ca^{2+} = 3.4 mmol/L) in an 8-year-old boy.

not be overlooked when performing a QT interval evaluation.[32]

Long QT Syndrome

Long QT syndrome is a clinically and genetically heterogeneous syndrome characterized by a lengthening of the QT interval and a propensity to develop severe VA such as torsades de pointes and VF, leading to syncope and sudden death. On the surface ECG, this syndrome is characterized by an abnormally long QT interval ($\geq$450 ms) often accompanied by T-wave/U-wave abnormality **(Fig. 20)**.

LQTS is caused by a decrease in repolarizing currents or an increase in depolarizing currents because of genetic mutations in many proteins (mostly ion channels): 13 genetic LQTS subtypes have been identified so far, whose hereditary patterns can be autosomal dominant or recessive. Mutations in LQT1, LQT2, and LQT3 loci are responsible for about 90% to 95% of all LQTS.

Different mutations present with different ECG manifestations, with the common hallmark of an increased QTc[33]:

- LQT1: broad-based early-onset monophasic T waves
- LQT2: low-amplitude late T waves, usually notched

These syndromes are caused by an anomaly in potassium channels for a loss-of-function mutation (α-subunit of the I_{KS} channel for LQT1 and I_{KR} for LQT2) and usually trigger VA under physical or emotional stress.

- LQT3: long isoelectric ST segment, followed by a narrow-based T wave

LQT3 is instead caused by a mutation with gain of function in α subunit sodium channel and is associated with the development of slow heart rate and arrhythmias during sleep and rest. As usual, the presence of the ECG pattern is not sufficient to address it as LQTS; clinical symptoms are required. Any sort of VA can be developed, but torsades de pointes is still the most common and life-threatening one.

Two phenomena should always be addressed for a rule-out analysis in every LQTS suspect:

a. R-on-T: an ectopic QRS firing on a T wave. This firing can induce malignant VA (torsades, polymorphic VT or VF) when the transmural dispersion of repolarization is increased; it is particularly important in patients with an LQTS because this phenomenon often represents the trigger for many VAs[34] **(Fig. 21)**.

b. T-wave alternation: a phenomenon of beat-to-beat variability in the repolarization phase of

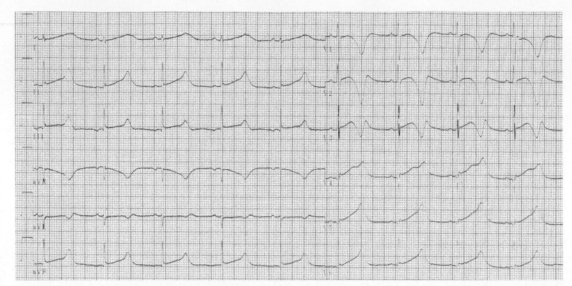

Fig. 20. Long QT syndrome (QT/QTc 592/586 ms) in an 8-year-old girl, HR 59 beats/min, with a history of syncope.

the ventricles that has been closely associated with an increased risk of ventricular tachyarrhythmia events and SCD. It refers to regular changes in the shape, amplitude, and polarity of every other T wave; it is a nonspecific LQTS finding and can be used as an indicator of higher risk of ventricular arrhythmias and SCD.[35]

Lastly, it is of a paramount importance not only to recognize the presence of an LQTS but also to characterize its subtype, given the fact that different drugs have been proved protective in different subtypes.

Short QT Interval Syndrome

Short QT syndrome is an uncommon channelopathy, characterized by a shortening of the effective refractory period of the atria and ventricles, increasing in transmural dispersion of repolarization.[32,36] At the ECG, an abnormally short QT interval (<350 ms) will be visible, with high T-wave symmetry in the chest leads.

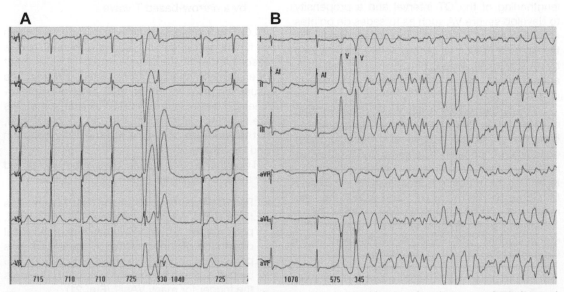

Fig. 21. R-on-T phenomenon; (A) Two PVCs with a short coupling interval but in a baseline normal QTc interval. No sustained VA arises. (B) A PVC on a T wave triggers VF in a patient with a long QTc interval. PVC, premature ventricular contraction; VA, ventricular arrhythmia; VF, ventricular fibrillation.

Mutations in 6 causative genes have been reported so far, 3 genes encoding for K$^+$ cardiac channels (*KCNQ1*, *KCNJ2*, and *KCNH2*) and 3 encoding for L-type calcium channels (*CACNA1C*, *CACNB2*, and *CACNA2D1*), with some overlapping with the mutations causing LQTS and BrS: a loss of function of these genes cause LQTS, whereas a gain of function causes SQTS.

In 2003, Gaita and colleagues[37] first reported that short QT interval is associated with a familial form of SCD. Schimpf and colleagues[38] reviewed the clinical characteristics of short QT syndrome in 2008 and reported that the short QT syndrome is associated with AF, syncope, and SCD. Short QT interval and reduced ventricular refractory period together with an increased dispersion of repolarization constitute the potential substrate for re-entry and life-threatening ventricular tachyarrhythmia. SQTS predisposes affected individuals to an increased risk of ventricular and atrial arrhythmias, in particular VF, being an important cause of recurrent episodes of syncope and SCD.

SUMMARY

Surface 12-lead ECG represents an important tool in the armory of the physician studying rhythm disorders, allowing a first-line, noninvasive, rapid, and inexpensive evaluation of arrhythmia risk. It is of pivotal importance to spot and recognize baseline ECG abnormalities before the arrhythmia develops, so as to initiate appropriate therapies for prevention of arrhythmic events or to stratify the risk according to patients' outcomes.

REFERENCES

1. Steinberg JS, Altman RK. Don't neglect the electrocardiogram: P-wave proves a potent predictor. JACC Clin Electrophysiol 2018;4(4):544–6.
2. Jadidi A, Müller-Edenborn B, Chen J, et al. The duration of the amplified sinus-P-wave identifies presence of left atrial low voltage substrate and predicts outcome after pulmonary vein isolation in patients with persistent atrial fibrillation. JACC Clin Electrophysiol 2018;4(4):531–43.
3. Dilaveris PE, Gialafos EJ, Andrikopoulos GK, et al. Clinical and electrocardiographic predictors of recurrent atrial fibrillation. Pacing Clin Electrophysiol 2000;23(3):352–8.
4. Conte G, Luca A, Yazdani S, et al. Usefulness of P-wave duration and morphologic variability to identify patients prone to paroxysmal atrial fibrillation. Am J Cardiol 2017;119(2):275–9.
5. Johner N, Namdar M, Shah DC. Intra- and interatrial conduction abnormalities: hemodynamic and arrhythmic significance. J Interv Card Electrophysiol 2018;52(3):293–302.
6. Tse G, Wong CW, Gong M, et al. Predictive value of inter-atrial block for new onset or recurrent atrial fibrillation: a systematic review and meta-analysis. Int J Cardiol 2018;250:152–6.
7. Aizawa Y, Sato M. P-pulmonale and new-onset atrial fibrillation. Circ J 2014;78(2):309–10.
8. Wang YS, Chen GY, Li XH, et al. Prolonged P-wave duration is associated with atrial fibrillation recurrence after radiofrequency catheter ablation: a systematic review and meta-analysis. Int J Cardiol 2017;227:355–9.
9. Prasitlumkum N, Rattanawong P, Limpruttidham N, et al. Frequent premature atrial complexes as a predictor of atrial fibrillation: systematic review and meta-analysis. J Electrocardiol 2018;51(5):760–7.
10. Hwang JK, Gwag HB, Park SJ, et al. Frequent atrial premature complexes during exercise: a potent predictor of atrial fibrillation. Clin Cardiol 2018;41(4):458–64.
11. Della Rocca DG, Santini L, Forleo GB, et al. Novel perspectives on arrhythmia-induced cardiomyopathy: pathophysiology, clinical manifestations and an update on invasive management strategies. Cardiol Rev 2015;23(3):135–41.
12. Mani BC, Pavri BB. Dual atrioventricular nodal pathways physiology: a review of relevant anatomy, electrophysiology, and electrocardiographic manifestations. Indian Pacing Electrophysiol J 2014; 14(1):12–25.
13. Peiker C, Pott C, Eckardt L, et al. Dual atrioventricular nodal non-re-entrant tachycardia. Europace 2016;18(3):332–9.
14. Basso C, Corrado D, Rossi L, et al. Ventricular preexcitation in children and young adults: atrial myocarditis as a possible trigger of sudden death. Circulation 2001;103(2):269–75.
15. Anderson RH, Becker AE, Brechenmacher C, et al. Ventricular preexcitation. A proposed nomenclature for its substrates. Eur J Cardiol 1975;3(1):27–36.
16. Bhatia A, Sra J, Akhtar M. Preexcitation syndromes. Curr Probl Cardiol 2016;41(3):99–137.
17. Benditt DG, Pritchett ELC, Smith WM, et al. Characteristics of atrioventricular conduction and the spectrum of arrhythmias in Lown-Ganong-Levine syndrome. Circulation 1978;57(3):454–65.
18. Katritsis DG, Wellens HJ, Josephson ME. Mahaim accessory pathways. Arrhythm Electrophysiol Rev 2017;6(1):29–32.
19. Wellens HJ, Durrer D. Wolff-Parkinson-White syndrome and atrial fibrillation. Relation between refractory period of accessory pathway and ventricular rate during atrial fibrillation. Am J Cardiol 1974; 34(7):777–82.
20. Bhar-Amato J, Davies W, Agarwal S. Ventricular arrhythmia after acute myocardial infarction: 'the

perfect storm.'. Arrhythm Electrophysiol Rev 2017; 6(3):134–9.

21. Gorenek B, Lundqvist CB, Terradellas JB, et al. Cardiac arrhythmias in acute coronary syndromes: position paper from the joint EHRA, ACCA, and EAPCI task force. Eur Heart J Acute Cardiovasc Care 2015;4(4):386.

22. Marcus FI, McKenna WJ, Sherrill D, et al. Diagnosis of arrhythmogenic right ventricular cardiomyopathy/dysplasia: proposed modification of the task force criteria. Circulation 2010;121(13):1533–41.

23. Antzelevitch C, Yan GX, Ackerman MJ, et al. J-wave syndromes expert consensus conference report: emerging concepts and gaps in knowledge. J Arrhythm 2016;32(5):315–39.

24. Priori SG, Napolitano C. J-wave syndromes: electrocardiographic and clinical aspects. Card Electrophysiol Clin 2018;10(2):355–69.

25. Brugada R, Campuzano O, Sarquella-Brugada G, et al. Brugada syndrome. Methodist Debakey Cardiovasc J 2014;10(1):25–8.

26. Haissaguerre M, Derval N, Sacher F, et al. Sudden cardiac arrest associated with early repolarization. N Engl J Med 2008;358(19):2016–23.

27. MacFarlane PW, Antzelevitch C, Haissaguerre M, et al. The early repolarization pattern: a consensus paper. J Am Coll Cardiol 2015;66(4):470–7.

28. Rezus C, Floria M, Moga VD, et al. Early repolarization syndrome: electrocardiographic signs and clinical implications. Ann Noninvasive Electrocardiol 2014;19(1):15–22.

29. Viskin S, Havakuk O, Antzelevitch C, et al. Malignant early repolarization: it's the T-wave, stupid…. Heart Rhythm 2016;13(4):903–4.

30. Mazzanti A, Underwood K, Nevelev D, et al. The new kids on the block of arrhythmogenic disorders: short QT syndrome and early repolarization. J Cardiovasc Electrophysiol 2017;28(10):1226–36.

31. Hasegawa K, Watanabe H, Hisamatsu T, et al. Early repolarization and risk of arrhythmia events in long QT syndrome. Int J Cardiol 2016;223:540–2.

32. Tse G, Chan YW, Keung W, et al. Electrophysiological mechanisms of long and short QT syndromes. Int J Cardiol Heart Vasc 2016;14:8–13.

33. Tester DJ, Ackerman MJ. Genetics of long QT syndrome. Methodist Debakey Cardiovasc J 2014; 10(1):29–33.

34. Oksuz F, Sensoy B, Sahan E, et al. The classical "R-on-T" phenomenon. Indian Heart J 2015;67(4): 392–4.

35. Pandey M, Dutta R, Kothari SS. Massive biventricular rhabdomyoma in a neonate. Ann Pediatr Cardiol 2017;10(2):218–9.

36. Bjerregaard P. Diagnosis and management of short QT syndrome. Heart Rhythm 2018;15(8):1261–7.

37. Gaita F, Giustetto C, Bianchi F. Short QT syndrome: a familial cause of sudden death. Circulation 2003; 108(8):965–70.

38. Schimpf R, Borggrefe M, Wolpert C. Clinical and molecular genetics of the short QT syndrome. Curr Opin Cardiol 2008;23(3):192–8.

Electrocardiographic Approach to Complex Arrhythmias
P, QRS, and Their Relationships

Fabio M. Leonelli, MD[a],*, Roberto De Ponti, MD, FHRS[b],
Giuseppe Bagliani, MD[c,d]

KEYWORDS

- Electrocardiography • Complex arrhythmias • Interpretation method • Laddergram
- Precision electrocardiology

KEY POINTS

- A systematic approach to bradycardias and tachycardias is presented based on known electrophysiologic behavior of sinus node, atria, ventricles, and the conduction system.
- From an initial illustration of the basic atrioventricular relationship during bradycardias and tachycardias, increasingly more complex arrhythmias are discussed, using basic principles as building blocks.
- Laddergrams are used extensively to clarify the relationship between atria and ventricles in simple and complex tachycardias.
- This is an attempt to present a method leading to precise electrocardiology interpretation of complex arrhythmias.

A METHOD OF ELECTROCARDIOGRAPHIC ANALYSIS

A detailed electrocardiographic (ECG) analysis of an ongoing tachycardia is only possible in a clinically stable patient. Any hemodynamically unstable arrhythmia needs to be quickly dealt with leaving no time for immediate detailed ECG analysis and its tracings reviewed at a later stage. A systematic approach to interpretation of ECG in arrhythmias is important to rapidly reach a correct diagnosis.

Short of suggesting another decision tree based on the presence or absence of some ECG features, we propose a stepwise approach to the ECG interpretation of arrhythmias in a clinically

stable patient, offering the reason behind each choice. The analysis is based on gathering observations. Depending on their degree of certainty the observations can be considered:

Diagnostic: Phenomena owing to unique features of one specific arrhythmia (fusion in ventricular tachycardia [VT])

Highly suggestive: ECG findings not specific of a single tachycardia, but often useful to narrow down the differential diagnosis (QRS width).

Ancillary: Relevant observation useful to start establishing a differential diagnosis or to better define some aspects of an arrhythmia component (ie, P wave morphology to identify atrial tachycardia origin).

Disclosure statement: The authors disclose no conflicts.
[a] Cardiology Department, James A. Haley Veterans' Hospital, University South Florida, 13000 Bruce B. Downs Boulevard, Tampa, FL 33612, USA; [b] Cardiology Department, University of Insubria, Varese, Italy; [c] Foligno General Hospital, Cardiology Department, Arrhythmology Unit, Foligno, Italy; [d] Cardiovascular Diseases Department, University of Perugia, Perugia, Italy
* Corresponding author.
E-mail address: Fabio.Leonelli@va.gov

Card Electrophysiol Clin 11 (2019) 239–260
https://doi.org/10.1016/j.ccep.2019.02.001
1877-9182/19/© 2019 Elsevier Inc. All rights reserved.

The initial observations are based on the recognition of an ECG event (Pw, QRS) and their morphology (inverted Pw, wide QRS etc). This initial set of data will lead to a number of logically derived deductions regarding some aspect of the arrhythmia mechanism (ie, direction of wavefront propagation, atrioventricular [AV] conduction, etc). Other important informations are based on the recognition of dominant patterns during the arrhythmia (regularity or irregularity of events, QRS morphology and variations, etc).

These observations are based on a knowledge of anatomy, cellular physiology, and the electrophysiologic properties of cardiac tissue. The more comprehensive this knowledge, the more extensive and correct the interpretation of the gathered information will be. These findings by themselves or linked together will lead, by deduction, to a number of different diagnoses of variable likelihood. As the analysis proceeds, the clinician will begin to search for other observations, leading to a final diagnosis.

A diagnosis should always be stated in terms of probability because exceptions to the rules are frequent and most observations may have more than one acceptable explanation. The most probable diagnosis is the one with the most congruent number of observations.

Pathologic arrhythmias are characterized by abnormalities in impulse formation, rate, or propagation. These abnormalities can occur in isolation or combined and the goal of ECG interpretation is to define each one of these problems.

The first observation is based on the 2 most obvious abnormalities: the R-R interval and the QRS width. A bradycardia defined by an R-R interval of less than 60 bpm introduces the question of impulse formation and conduction.

BRADYCARDIAS (R-R INTERVAL <60 BPM)
Failure of Impulse Generation or Conduction

The first observations to identify the cause of the bradycardia are:

1. Identify each P wave and establish the P-P interval.
2. Clarify the P and QRS relationship.

Bradycardias may not be pathologic because they may represent a normally functioning sinus node (SN) with intrinsically slower discharge rates or side effect of medications. It is difficult to distinguish between sinus bradycardia owing to an early SN dysfunction and a physiologic bradycardia. Symptoms, circadian variation of heart rate, or response to exercise will usually distinguish physiologic from pathologic SN rates.

Sinus arrest, a typical manifestation of SN dysfunction, can be due to a failure to generate or deliver to the atria 1 or more sinus depolarizations and its ECG manifestation is the absence of expected P waves; this pattern can occur randomly, regularly, or as a consequence of periods of fast atrial stimulation (SN suppression). ECG analysis of the P-P relationship can help in differentiating between an inability to generate a sinus impulse or block by the surrounding tissue of a normal sinus pulse. The hallmark of this latter condition are normal P-P intervals interspersed by longer P-P pauses, which are multiples of the basic P-P interval.

In pure SN dysfunction, each Pw is followed by a QRS demonstrating a normal AV conduction.

In contrast, pathologic AV conduction, the other cause of bradycardia, manifests with a normal P-P rate that is faster than the accompanying R-R rate. In this case, SN function is normal and some form of conduction block is causing the slowing of the R-R rate. Conduction abnormalities progress from a simple delay of conduction (first-degree AV block [AVB]) to an episodic block of conduction, either progressive or sudden (second-degree Wenckebach and Mobitz variants) to prolonged periods of conduction block either partial (2:1 AVB) or total (third-degree or complete heart block; **Fig. 1**)

The majority of AVBs are benign and do not cause bradycardia. Only profound alterations of AV conduction result in bradycardia and those are:

2:1 AVB
Paroxysmal AVB
Complete heart block

These conditions often represent progressive stages of conduction system's pathology. ECG recognition of these types of AVB is fairly straightforward; it is nevertheless important, in deciding the appropriate therapy, to determine the level of block (AV node [AVN] vs the His Purkinje system [HPS]) and whether the block is a reversible phenomenon or it represents a permanent damage likely to progress. HPS disease will progress and any evidence of advanced pathology at this level requires pacing therapy. AVN disease is often reversible and usually slowly progressive; thus, therapy is often dictated by the patient's symptomatology.

2:1 atrioventricular block
A 2:1 AVB is easily diagnosed; having identified every P, the R-R rate is exactly one-half of the sinus rate, but it is not specific for either AVN or HPS block because it is observed in both conditions. Ancillary observations pointing to AVN block

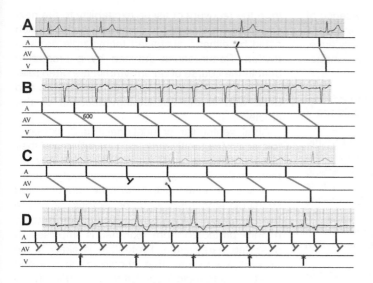

Fig. 1. Common bradycardia ECG patterns. (*A*) Sinus arrest. Two sinus beats are followed by a 3.8-ms pause without evidence of P waves. The period of sinus arrest is terminated by an atrial escape beat, see different P wave morphology and shorter PR, before sinus rhythm resumes at a slower rate. This last observation is in keeping with a period of hypervagotonia possibly causing the sinus arrest. (*B–D*) AVBs. (*B*) First-degree AVB. Prolonged AV conduction. The ECG manifestation of this block is a PR in excess of 200 ms. The normal morphology of the QRS and the degree of PR prolongation (600 ms) strongly suggest AVN as the site of delay. (*C*) Second-degree AVB. A single, nonconducted sinus P wave. In this case, a regular sinus rhythm shows a progressive AV conduction delay culminating in a nonconducted P (Wenckebach type). The following beat is a junctional escape (*asterisk*) occurring at the same time as the sinus P. Conduction resumes with a PR shorter (400 ms) than the last conducted (520 ms). This sequence regularly repeated, group beating, is the hallmark of abnormal AV node decremental conduction. Second-degree AVB can also occur in the HPS with different manifestations (see text). (*D*) Complete heart block. Two different dissociated rhythms are present: sinus rhythm at a rate of 680 ms and a wide complex bradycardia at rate of 1720 ms. The slower rhythm is due to a subsidiary pace maker most likely situated in one of the HPS bundles. The absolute regularity of the escape rhythm is diagnostic of complete AVB.

include evidence of Wenckebach periodicity, minimal P-R increments preceding the nonconducted P, or a 2:1 block during hypervagotonia demonstrated by a slowing of sinus rate. Baseline ECG with evidence of a bundle branch block (BBB) does not automatically localize a 2:1 block to HPS because, in up of 20% of patients with wide QRS, the block is in the AVN. A 2:1 AVB occurring during exercise is always localized to the HPS regardless of the QRS duration because the catecholaminergic response during physical effort will improve AVN conduction while decreasing the recovery period of the His bundle.

Paroxysmal atrioventricular block

Paroxysmal AVB is characterized by 2 or more nonconducted P waves and it is seen during tachycardia or may be initiated by an atrial or ventricular ectopic beat. Both presentations are usually due to abnormal electrophysiologic properties of diseased HPS fibers becoming less responsive to subsequent impulses (Ref a). Conduction will be blocked until a critically timed premature beat resets the abnormally elevated transmembrane potential.[1,2]

As with less advanced AVBs, profound hypervagotonia is usually associated with clear triggers, such as cough, micturition, or vasovagal stimulation, and can cause periods of paroxysmal AVB

at times lasting several seconds. Manifestations of increased vagal tone preceding the block that can be observed are:

A gradual slowing of the heart rate, PR prolongation, or Wenckebach periodicity
P-P prolongation during the period of ventricular asystole and longer P-R on resumption.

Vagally induced block reliably localizes it at the AVN level. This type of block is functional and nonprogressive and requires pacing therapy only in case of severe repetitive symptoms.

Complete heart block

The most advanced AV conduction block is a complete hart block (CHB), which is characterized by the presence of 2 completely dissociated rhythms. One is usually sinus rhythm because the SN function remains unperturbed; the sinus intrinsic rate is usually the fastest of the two and it is easily identified by observing P morphology and rate. The second rhythm represents a subsidiary pacemaker. CHB is only one of the causes of AV dissociation; other situations where atrial and ventricular activity is independent include:

The presence of 2 rhythms with very similar rates emerge from different cardiac structures (atria, AV junction, or HPS)

A VT not affecting SN function with evidence of episodic ventriculoatrial (VA) dissociation; VT is not always a dissociated rhythm because, not infrequently, fixed or episodic VA conduction can be observed.

The emergence of subsidiary pacemakers is common to any form of bradycardia should the V rate decrease to rates compromising organ perfusion. Cardiac cells with physiologic automatic properties are distributed widely within the atria and conduction system. They will start discharging when the higher rate of another pacemaker falls below their intrinsic rate. A narrow QRS localizes the subsidiary pacemaker to an area above the HPS bifurcation; a wide QRS, not present in a baseline ECG, is diagnostic of an escape rhythm from the HPS or the ventricular muscle.

Subsidiary pacemakers need to be differentiated from automatic ectopic foci firing at rates of less than 100 bpm and competing with sinus rhythm (idioventricular and junctional rhythms). With automatic foci, AV conduction is preserved; therefore, these 2 rhythms can interfere with each other with episodic occurrences of atrial and ventricular fusion, resetting, retrograde capture, and so on.

Both in case of escape and automatic ectopic rhythms, plotting P-P versus R-R in a ladder diagram (see **Fig. 1**) will establish the capture of each focus and their reciprocal interactions.

Absence of antegrade capture in CHB is manifested by the persistent regularity of both rhythms at different rates. Retrograde conduction may at times be present in CHB possibly due to electrotonic dissociation within the conduction axis (AVN and HPS).

By definition, the 2 rhythms present in CHB are regular because are unaffected by each other. Some degree of irregularity may be due phasic variations induced by respirations or more sporadically by the effects on SN of retrograde atrial capture from junctional or ventricular subsidiary pacemakers.

Supraventricular capture will be promptly identified as a variation in the R-R interval with advancement of a single R and should lead to reconsideration of the diagnosis of CHB.

ATRIAL AND VENTRICULAR EXTRASYSTOLES

Atrial or ventricular extrasystole are depolarizations generated by an ectopic focus occurring prematurely respect to a dominant rhythm (**Fig. 2**).

An ectopic beat, to become ECG manifest, requires that the surrounding tissue is excitable; this situation will occur during a time window from the recovery of tissue excitability to the next spontaneous beat of the dominant rhythm, which could be either a sustained tachycardia or sinus rhythm. Perturbations induced by a premature beat in the course of an arrhythmia are often relevant in the understanding of its mechanism and dealt with in the subsequent sections of this article.

Atrial, ventricular, or junctional (**Fig. 3**) extrasystole occur frequently during sinus rhythm and their clinical relevance depends on their frequency, effects on the SN, and the conduction system function and its relationship with other documented sustained arrythmias. At times, ectopic beats are the expression of an automatic regular ectopic rhythm protected from extraneous impulses, a so-called parasystole. Protection is likely to be present if impulses that should discharge and reset the automatic focus fail to do so (**Fig. 4**).

The majority of ectopy observed in clinical practice occurs randomly.

Sporadic premature beats, in SR, can be highly symptomatic but are, in general, of little hemodynamic consequence, although, as their frequency increases, they can severely interfere with normal cardiac function.[3] A more in-depth ECG evaluation of these beats and the response of SN and conduction system to premature stimulations can provide information on the status of these structures as well as ectopy's arrhythmic mechanism and site of origin.

The identification of a premature atrial contraction can be difficult when it occurs inside a QRS or a T wave; a comparison of the preceding waveforms is necessary to ascertain its presence and morphology. When identified, the chamber of origin can be predicted[4] and, if identical to tachycardia P wave, a similar origin and a probable automatic mechanism can be deduced.

Premature stimulation induced by a premature atrial contraction can, if correctly timed, penetrate into the SN and prematurely depolarize it. An atrial premature contraction (APC) after a sinus P interval will, in this case, be very close to a normal P-P interval because the SN, after the premature depolarization, will resume its normal spontaneous rate. A shift to a different SN exit site is at times observed, leading to minor variations in the sinus P morphology.

A dysfunctional SN, as in SN disease, when prematurely depolarized, can require a much longer period of recovery of its function or be totally suppressed; this abnormality will be manifested by long APC-P intervals, at times accompanied by the emergence of a subsidiary pacemaker.

If an earlier APC is unable to discharge the SN because it is blocked by refractoriness of the

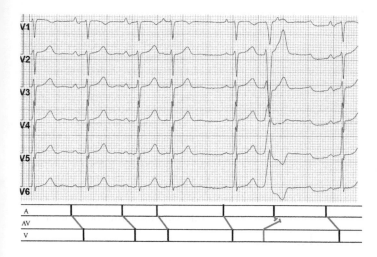

Fig. 2. Premature beats, QRS morphology, and P wave relationship. A supraventricular and a ventricular extrasystole. The first is preceded by an atrial ectopic beat with a P different from sinus P and a narrow QRS similar to a QRS in SR. The second extrasystole is ventricular because of its wide with left bundle branch morphology, there is no preceding P, ruling out aberrant conduction. SN function continues unperturbed as the VPC is followed by a sinus P with blocked conduction owing to ventricular premature contraction penetrance in the AVN-HPS system.

tissue surrounding this structure, the SN rate will remain unchanged and the P-P interval encompassing the APC will be unaltered.

A premature beat, not preceded by P, with QRS morphology identical to the baseline QRS originates from the junction above the HPS bifurcation (junctional premature beat). This beat can at times retrogradely depolarize the atria (see **Fig. 3**) with, at times, subsequent antegrade conduction to the ventricles using a different AVN pathway, therefore, demonstrating the presence of dual AVN pathways.

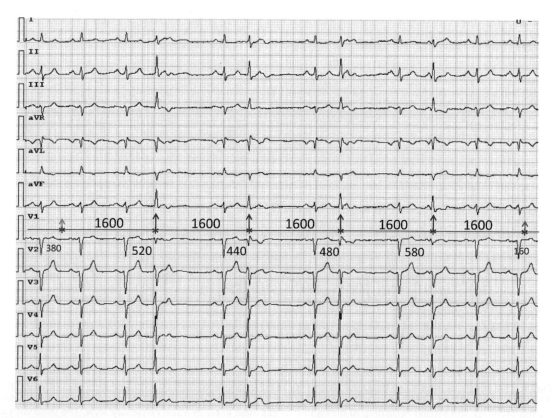

Fig. 3. Parasystole. Four junctional ectopic beats with minimal aberrancy during SR cl 680 to 720 ms. The relationship with preceding sinus P is variable but the interectopic interval is fixed at 1600 ms. This finding suggests the presence of an automatic focus, which is not influenced by the previous sinus beat (entrance block) in keeping with a parasystolic focus.

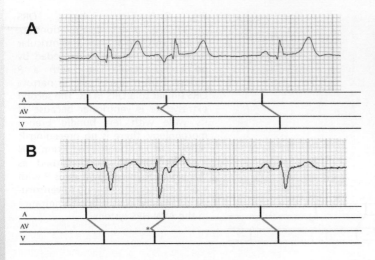

Fig. 4. Premature beats, QRS morphology, and P wave relationship. Both extrasystole have a morphology similar to the normally conducted preceding beats and, therefore, are junctional premature beats. In A, the extrasystole is preceded by a an inverted P, which could be due to a coronary sinus premature beat with a short PR owing to its vicinity to the AVN-HPS conducting system. The other possibility is a retrograde P from a junctional extrasystole conducting with some anterograde delay. In B, an inverted P follows a junctional premature beat with more usual retrograde timing.

Any premature supraventricular beat, regardless of their site of origin, will engage the AVN–HPS. Conduction to the V will be determined by recovery of excitability of each constituents of the conduction system leading to a number of possible scenarios including (**Fig. 5**):

- Antegrade block in the AVN-HPS manifested by a nonconducted ectopic P.
- Prolongation of physiologic AVN conduction with a long P-R.
- Block of fast AVN pathway and conduction via a slow AVN pathway manifested by a much

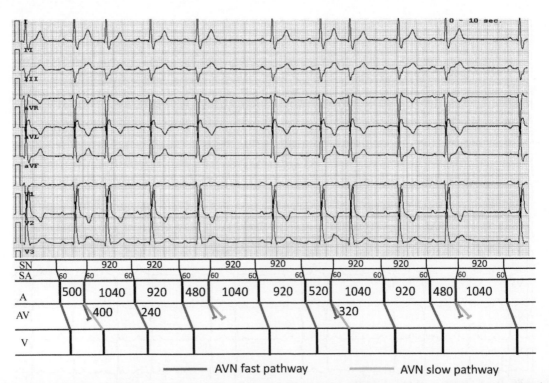

——— AVN fast pathway   ——— AVN slow pathway

Fig. 5. The effects of premature beats on SN and AV conduction. Sinus rhythm with first-degree AVB and right BBB; SV ectopy with variable degree of prematurity; first APC with a couple of 500 ms, conducts with PR prolongation (400 ms), the second occurring 20 ms earlier, blocks most likely in a still refractory AVN. The third with a couple of 520 ms conducts with a PR of 320 ms; the fourth at with a couple of 480 ms blocks again in the AVN. Every premature beat resets the SN because the postectopic sinus beat occurs with an interval of 1040 ms compared with a sinus cl of 920 ms. The difference between these 2 intervals (120 ms) is due to the time needed to reach the SN form the ectopic focus (approximately 60 ms) and from the SN to the atria (equal interval of 60 ms).

longer P-R than normally observed during sinus rhythm.

- A block in one of the HPS subdivisions and conduction with fascicular, R or left BBB (LBBB) morphology (**Figs. 6** and **7**)

In the presence of an AP, either with concealed or antegrade conduction, a premature atrial beat can have multiple consequences depending on the dominant rhythm and the effective refractory period of AVN and AP (**Fig. 8**).

Although these behaviors are, in general, physiologic, a number of abnormal responses are also possible, manifesting themselves with alternating BBB, variable conduction along a normal conduction axis, and an accessory pathway (AP) or induction of a reentrant tachycardia. These responses will be discussed in detail in Giuseppe Bagliani and colleagues' article, "QRS Variations During Arrhythmias: Mechanisms and Substrates. Toward a Precision Electrocardiology," in this issue.

Retrograde conduction after a ventricular premature contraction (VPC) is possible if the HPS-AVN is engaged after these anatomic structures have recovered excitability. The same combinations described for APCs are possible, including retrograde engagement of 1 of the 2 AVN pathways and antegrade conduction along the other (**Figs. 9–11**)

TACHYCARDIAS (R-R INTERVAL MORE THAN 100 BPM)
First Look: Narrow or Wide, Regular or Irregular

The ECG analysis of tachycardia is focused on determining the arrhythmia mechanism and the propagation of the abnormally generated electrical impulse. Although the information gathered is the same as in bradycardias, the principles used in the analysis are different. QRS width and the R-R interval are the first observations at the beginning of the study, as we are dealing with an impulse characterized by an abnormal origin and an excessive rate.

At first look, it is obvious to group the tachycardias in narrow complex tachycardias (NCT) versus wide complex tachycardias (WCTs), depending on a QRS duration width of more or less than 110 ms. The second step is an attentive analysis of R-R, which contains a great deal of subtle information. The presence of a regular R-R (variations of approximately 30 ms) indicates a stable arrhythmia circuit and next step in the analysis will focus on the mechanism of the tachycardia.

Irregularly Irregular R-R

An irregular R-R interval is due, save for some rare arrythmias, to a variable AV conduction response to a fast supraventricular rhythm. When exposed to a fast regular stimulation the AVN will adapt to the rate and develop a pattern of conduction which is either fixed (2:1, 3:1, etc) or demonstrates predictable variations (typical or atypical Wenckebach) in a regularly irregular pattern.

When the stimulation is very fast and random, the effects of concealed conduction will alter the orderly AVN response and the impulses will be conducted to the V in a completely haphazard pattern (irregularly irregular). Many sustained supraventricular rhythms will produce regularly irregular R-R intervals, but only atrial fibrillation (AF) and multifocal atrial tachycardia produce an irregularly irregular R-R.

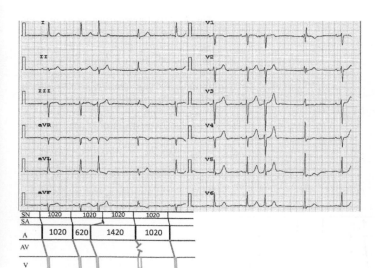

Fig. 6. Ectopy and SN resetting. Two supraventricular extrasystole during SR, cl 1020 occurring at similar P-P interval; they are followed by the emergence of an SN beat 1420 ms later, occurring at the same time of an escape beat conducted with some degree of aberrancy, probably owing to phase 4 aberrancy or a fascicular escape. The APC does not reset the node because the sinus P-P timing encompassing the APC is equal to 2 spontaneous sinus cycles (compensatory pause).

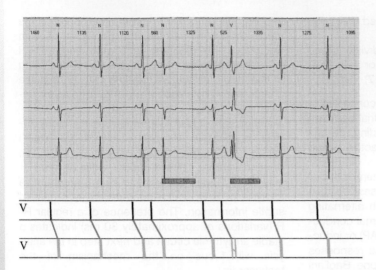

Fig. 7. APCs inducing BBB. The first APC conducts with a normal QRS; the second induces right BBB. The P-APC interval is shorter in the second beat (480 ms vs 600 ms) and because the AVN conduction remains the same in both beats (PR of approximately 220 ms), the R-R interval of the second beat is shorter encroaching in the RB effective refractory period (Ashman's phenomenon).

The next step is to determine the nature of the SV rhythm leading to this type of V response. AF is diagnosed in the absence of a morphologically reproducible Pw in more than 1 lead.

Frequent APCs or multifocal atrial tachycardia are not uncommonly confused with AF, if the P waves are not well-visualized. Close observation of the tracing may be necessary to identify Ps and observe how their morphology is variable and distinct from the sinus P.

One situation where R-R analysis is particularly useful occurs when evaluating an irregular R-R in the absence of a visible P. In the majority of these cases, the knee jerk diagnosis is AF based on superficial observations. The presence of variable but reproducible R-R patterns (regularly irregular response) over a period of observations strongly suggests the presence of a regular SV rhythm with a small P wave. Atypical or typical atrial flutter (AFL) in the presence of severely scarred atria are often the arrhythmias producing these ECGs (see **Fig. 7; Figs. 12** and **13**).

In AF, observing the QRS morphology may be very relevant for a patient's management. A wide QRS is normally due to preexisting BBB or newly developed aberrancy (see Giuseppe Bagliani and colleagues' article, "QRS Variations During Arrhythmias: Mechanisms and Substrates. Toward a Precision Electrocardiology," in this issue); it is necessary to keep in mind the uncommon situation of AF in the presence of a fast, antegradely conducting

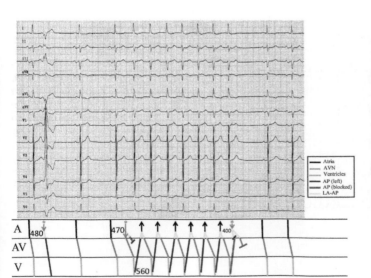

Fig. 8. Atrial premature beats in WPW syndrome. During SR, a first ectopic beat (*asterisk*) (P-ACP 480 ms) blocks in the AVN and conducts with a short PR using a previously concealed left later AP. The second APC with a marginally shorter delay (470 ms) conducts using a slow AVN pathway and triggers an orthodromic AV reentrant tachycardia with a PR of 320 ms and RP of 240 ms. A third APC during SVT at an interectopic interval of 400 ms blocks antegradely in the slow AVN pathway terminating the tachycardia.

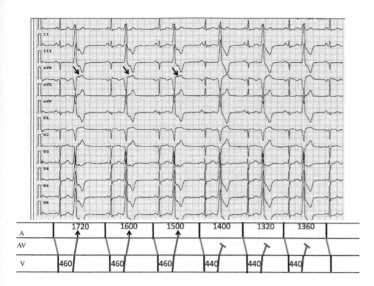

Fig. 9. Premature ventricular contractions and retrograde conduction. A bigeminal rhythm with fixed coupled VPCs. The first 3 PVC with an R-R interval of 480 ms conduct retrogradely to the atria. The other 3 coming 20 ms earlier block in the HPS-AVN system and there is no retrograde P wave after the beats. The retrograde P does not reset the SN as manifested by a variable P-P unrelated to P retroconduction.

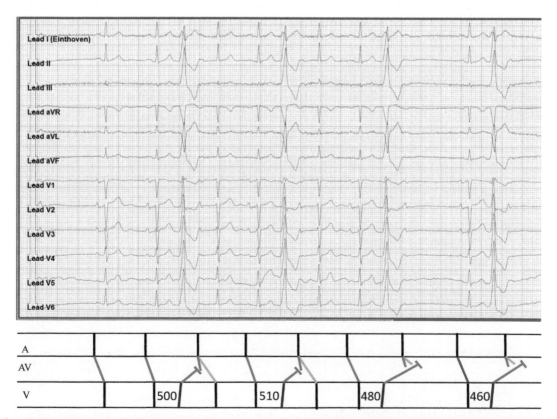

Fig. 10. Premature ventricular contractions uncovering dual AVN physiology. Four PVCs are recorded during SR with slight variations in the R-R′ interval. The P-R following the first and the second VPC is 180 ms longer than the P-R in SR. This finding is in keeping with an AVN fast pathway block owing to AVN penetration by VPC retrogradely and sinus beat antegradely; the following sinus beat will conduct to the ventricles using the slow pathway and prolonging the PR. Third and fourth VPC occur at a shorter coupling interval (480–460 ms) penetrate in the AVN and render both fast and slow AVN pathway refractory. The subsequent sinus P will be unable to conduct to the ventricles.

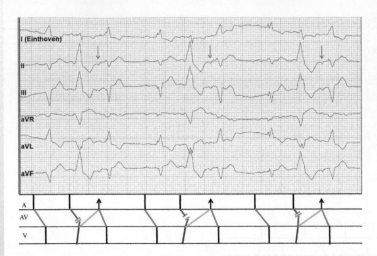

Fig. 11. Premature ventricular contractions and reciprocation. Sinus rhythm with 3 VPCs at variable R-R interval. Each of the VPCs is followed by a retrograde P (*arrows*) with a QRS-P interval of 500 ms and antegrade conduction with PR of 180 ms (reciprocation). To explain these findings, we need to suppose a retrograde conduction along the slow AVN pathway (*green line*) and anterograde conduction along the fast pathway of the AVN (*blue line*).

AP. A baseline ECG should, in the most cases, demonstrate a Wolff-Parkinson-White (WPW) pattern, clarifying the situation. The width of a delta wave is dynamic and related to the amount of V activated by the wavefront traveling in the AP compared with the V depolarized carried by the AVN-HPS. AVN and AP refractoriness will be the major determinant of delta wave's presence and magnitude (see **Fig. 8**). The longer the AP refractory period, the less obvious and constant the delta wave will be; on the contrary, the shorter the R-R causing increased AVN delay or block, the more manifest will be the delta wave. The shorter preexcited R-R is related to the shortest refractory

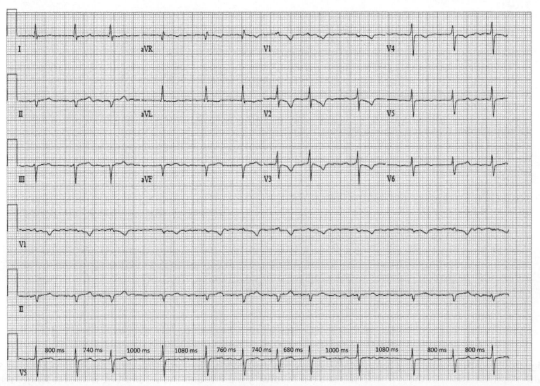

Fig. 12. AF? The importance of measurements. A narrow complex irregular rhythm without reproducible P waves. AF seems to be an easy diagnosis. Measuring R-R intervals demonstrates a regularly irregular pattern with predominantly around 1000 and 740 ms. An enlargement of an event monitor strip reveals a regular reproducible slow voltage flutter waves. This is more in keeping with concealed AVN conduction as response to a regular rhythm. An EPS demonstrated a scar-related left atrial flutter.

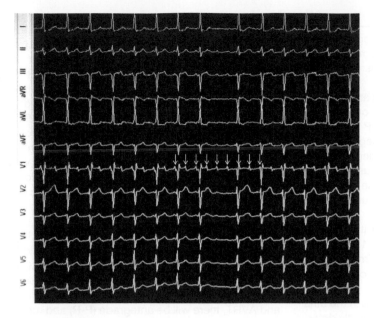

Fig. 13. P-QRS relationships: obvious diagnostic clues. NCT with a clearly visible P wave: the first 3 beats of the tachycardia suggest a 1:1 conduction with a long PR. This interval prolongs and a second P of same morphology becomes evident (beat 4–8). AVN conduction slows further and 3 P are not conducted (9–11). The tachycardia resumes with an apparent 1:1 conduction followed by a progressive PR prolongation. Differential diagnosis is confined to AT or atypical AFL. Arrhythmia CL, P wave morphology, and long baseline between P-P intervals are suggestive of AT.

period of the AP and, if less than 220 ms, is associated with an increased likelihood of ventricular fibrillation induction and sudden cardiac death.

Regular narrow complex tachycardias

Let's now observe NCT (QRSd < 110 ms) with a regular R-R response. These arrhythmias are obviously supraventricular in origin, because the V are activated through the normal AVN-HPS axis; having established that the AV-HPS is involved in the arrhythmia, the only diagnostic goal is to determine whether this structure is an integral part of the arrhythmia or just a bystander activated by an independent atrial focus. For this purpose, we need to identify and carefully evaluate the P and its relationship with QRS.

Finding and Observing the P Wave

Identification of the P wave is the initial task at times rendered difficult by intrinsic low voltage of this waveform or by its relationship with QRS or T. The determinant of P voltage are:

- Amount of tissue activated,
- Degree of organization of the depolarizing waveform, and
- The relationship between direction of main propagating vector and the axis of the exploring lead.

Wavelets in AF depolarize a small amount of tissue in a disorganized and inscribe no recognizable atrial activity. On the contrary, a P wave generated by a regular rhythm depolarizing the atria in an organized fashion will generate a large wavefront

moving in a constant, predictable direction. The resultant vector, will inscribe a well-defined P with a morphology informing us on its origin, direction, and to some extent sequence of atrial depolarization. Atria activated sequentially, as in isthmus-dependent flutter, will often inscribe characteristic P wave with morphologies reflecting both atria's contributions.

Anatomic localization of distinct P origin is possible and very important in the understanding of the arrhythmia mechanism.[4] In particular, a wavefront originating inferiorly at the level of interatrial septum will depolarize the atria in a retrograde direction (inferosuperior) inscribing a negative deflexions in leads II, III, and aVF, positive in aVR and aVL, and positive, tall narrow, and peaked wave in V1. Anatomically, this area corresponds with the triangle of Koch, where the AVN is located; any arrhythmia incorporating the AVN in its mechanism or any impulse traveling retrogradely in the HPS will emerge in this region, generating a retrograde P wave.

Furthermore, APs located in this area (so-called septal and paraseptal APs) will feature a P with similar characteristics. These features localize the atrial site of the tachycardia, but in general do not diagnose the arrythmia mechanism.

One exception to the rule is typical isthmus dependent flutter, a macro reentry depolarizing the atria in a predictable fashion pattern generating a sawtooth P of constant morphology with a dominant retrograde vector. The morphology of the flutter wave, so typical to be diagnostic in the majority of cases,[5] is in fact multicomponent with a negative part being the most recognizable.

P and QRS Relationship

When 2 consecutive P are clearly recognized, the cycle length (CL) of a regular SV arrhythmia is known and identification of every P is now aided by this measurements.

If one is unclear on how many Ps are present, long ECG recordings of arrhythmia can identify changes in the relationship between P and QRST and fully demonstrate the atrial depolarization (**Figs. 14** and **15**). Maneuvers delaying the AVN conduction time, such as carotid sinus massage or vagomomimetic drugs, will increase R-R intervals, allowing the emergence of an P undisturbed by QRS or ST-T waveforms.

When Ps have been clearly identified, it is possible to assess if P and QRS are associated in 1:1 or higher ratio. A 2:1 P-QRS ratio or a regularly irregular R-R (described elsewhere in this article) is observed in atrial tachycardias, such as AT or AFL where the arrhythmia mechanism is fully contained in the atria (see **Fig. 13**) with conduction to the V mostly determined by AVN decremental conduction.

ECG differentiation between AT and AFL based on P morphology and rate is not always possible. Distinct P waves separated by a clear isoelectric line tend to suggest focal AT, but this criterium is not foolproof because postablation flutters often share the same feature.[5]

NCT with a 1:1 P-QRS relation can be due to ATs with rates allowing full adaptation of AVN conduction or AV nodal reentrant tachycardia (AVNRT) and AV reentrant tachycardia (AVRT), where the AVN is integral part of the reentrant circuit. Differentiation between these 3 possibilities is based on P morphology and an observation of long recordings to identify the specific behaviors of these arrhythmias.

The atrial arm of the AVNRT or AVRT reentrant circuit emerges in the inferior side of the right or left atrium. The P generated by this wavefront is a retrograde P as previously described; the identification of a high antegrade P (positive in I and II and negative in aVF) rules out AVNRT or AVRT. Identification of a retrograde P is helpful but nondiagnostic because an atrial tachycardia originating in the vicinity of the coronary sinus os will have the same morphology. The P-QRS relationship, on the other hand, contains the diagnostic information necessary to differentiate these 3 arrhythmias.

Depending on the mechanism of the tachycardia, there may be only antegrade conduction, as in ATs, in which case the AVN is just a bystander, or in the case of reentrant rhythm using AVN as part of the reentrant circuit such as AVNRT and AVRT, there will be antegrade (P-R) and retrograde (R-P) conduction.

P-R versus R-P: Is the Atrioventricular Node a Bystander or a Part of the Arrhythmia Circuit?

Observing an NCT implies that antegrade conduction occurs along the normal AVN-HPS axis. A bystander AVN presupposes a supraventricular rhythm disassociated from V, where the AVN is used only to conduct the impulse to V (see **Fig. 13**). Antegrade or retrograde conduction are not necessary to maintain the arrhythmia. Therefore, there will be a variable P-R and R-P relationship during the arrhythmia with P-R interval determining, with an inverse

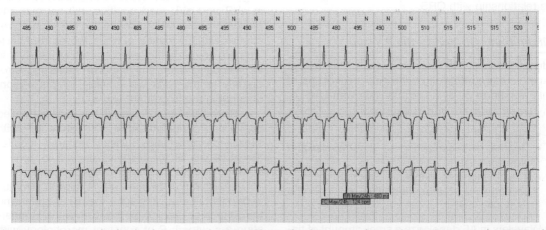

Fig. 14. PR and RP: who leads whom? NCT cl 440 to 460 ms. The diagnostic observation in this case is the PR-RP relationship: at first this relationship is not fixed and, as the RP prolongs, the PR shortens. Second, these interval variations are preceded by small variations in the PP interval so that, as the PP prolongs, the PR shortens and the RP prolongs. These observations are diagnostic of an AT with variable cl and variable antegrade AVN conduction; the RP is directly related to the PR and moves in the opposite direction (shortening of PR prolongs the RP and vice versa).

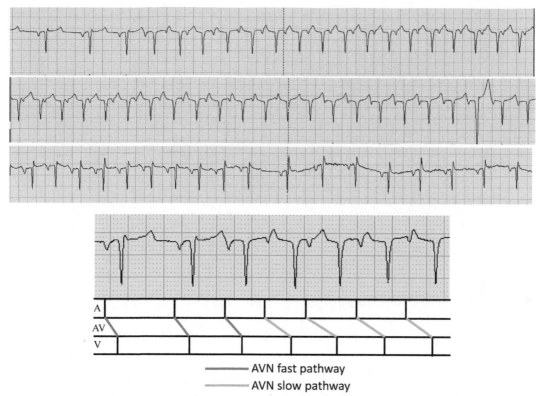

AVN fast pathway
AVN slow pathway

Fig. 15. PR and RP: confirmation of diagnosis. Initiation of AT of **Fig. 14**, after 2 sinus beats and termination of the same arrhythmia with a QRS. Note the different morphology of the atrial tachycardia P wave and PR similar to SR. The AT ends with a QRS ruling out AVNRT and AVRT.

relationship, the following R-P (see **Figs. 14** and **15**). In general, in AT, the P-R measurements tend to be close to the one in sinus rhythm and in the majority of ATs the P-R will be shorter than R-P (see **Fig. 10**).

The 2 reentrant rhythm using the AVN-HPS as part of the reentry are, as mentioned, AVNRT and AVRT. In both arrhythmias, there is an antegrade and a retrograde arm of the circuit, which, in the case of AVNRT, are both located in the region of AVN body. In AVRT, presenting as an NCT, antegrade propagation travels through the AVN-HPS and retrograde conduction uses an AP situated somewhere across the tricuspid or mitral valve ring. The diagnosis of these 2 arrhythmias requires a demonstration of both arms of the reentrant circuit. When these 2 reentrant rhythms have become stable, their A-V and V-A relationship has minimal variations in view of the electrophysiologic properties of the linking arms. In an NCT, the study of antegrade and retrograde conduction is deduced by observing the P-R and R-P duration, and the stability and changes at the beginning, the end of the arrhythmia burst, and during perturbations induced by external stimuli.

P-R and R-P interval analysis is a fundamental step in understanding the role of the AVN in the arrhythmia and, therefore, in the differential diagnosis of tachycardias.

Any A-V conduction block during a stable NCT strongly suggests a bystander role of the AVN, excludes AVRT, makes AVNRT extremely unlikely, and basically confirms the presence of an independent atrial rhythm. A ventricular ectopic beat can terminate both AVNRT and AVRT (**Fig. 16**), but the phenomenon is extremely rare with atrial tachycardias. Given the relative size of AVRT reentrant circuit, a VPC is much more likely than in AVNRT to penetrate this circuit and by blocking retrogradely in the AVN-HPS terminated the tachycardia. A VPC that terminates an NCT without reaching the atria (no retrograde P wave present) excludes AT as the mechanism of the arrhythmia and is diagnostic of AVN-HPS participation in the circuit.

Observations of the P-R interval made at the onset of tachycardia can provide important clues to its mechanism. A demonstration of the initiation of tachycardia by APC associated with a critical degree of P-R prolongation is diagnostic of reentry

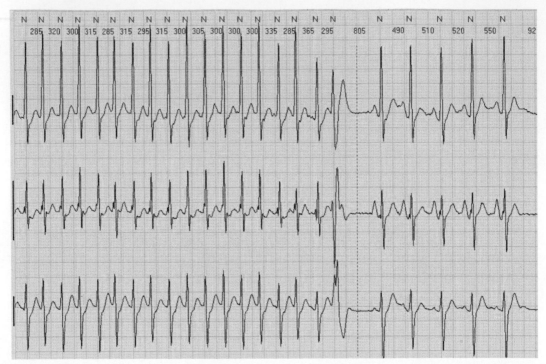

Fig. 16. Rhythm disturbances during stable arrhythmia: fundamental observations. Holter recording of an NCT cl 300 ms. The arrhythmia terminates with a VPC. From the tracing a retrograde P is identifiable when comparing SVT and SR tracing with a possible VA interval of 60 to 80 ms. The mode of the arrhythmia's termination makes AVRT most likely because the VPC is unlikely to penetrate the AVNRT reentry circuit owing to its narrow gap; the VPC has terminated this NCT without reaching the atria, because no retrograde P is visible following the ectopic beat, and this rules out AT.

involving AVN because site this is the site of the conduction delay. This finding suggests that the mechanism of the tachycardia is either A-V nodal reentry or A-V reentry involving a concealed bypass tract. If the first P following an APC does not conduct to V, this rules out reentry using a concealed bypass tract and makes AVNRT extremely unlikely.

In these arrhythmias, the V-A interval represents retrograde conduction and its analysis during stable tachycardias is far more informative than evaluation of antegrade conduction.

Retrograde conduction can occur in NCTs either via a pathway in the paranodal tissue surrounding the AVN (AVNRT) or via an AP located along left or right AV rings.

V-A conduction is demonstrated, in a stable tachycardia, when linking[a] between ventricular and subsequent A depolarization is consistently observed. This almost fixed relationship between the V and A interval, during stable NCT, is because

retrograde pathways of typical AVNRT (fast pathway) and AVRT (AP) show minimal or no decremental properties. Therefore, any V depolarization during reentry is conducted to the A within a very narrow time window.

VA conduction time (from the beginning of QRS to the beginning of documented retrograde P) has diagnostic implications. The V-A conduction time using either the normal conduction system, as observed during VT, or AP, as in AVRT, is always longer than 60 ms and allows the inscription of a retrograde P close but distinct from the QRS (**Fig. 17**). A retrograde P generated by a reentrant circuit within the AVN region (AVNRT or junctional tachycardia) travels a shorter distance and, therefore, will emerge in the atria in less than 50 ms. This P is, therefore, recorded within the QRS, leaving no traces of its presence or subtly altering its morphology by inscribing at the beginning of QRS small q or pseudo-S inferiorly or at the end an R′ in V1 not present in SR (**Fig. 18**). The V-A

---

[a]Linking is here used to describe a fixed relationship between A and V depolarizations linked by interposed anatomic structures (ie, slow and fast AV pathways or AP and AVN).

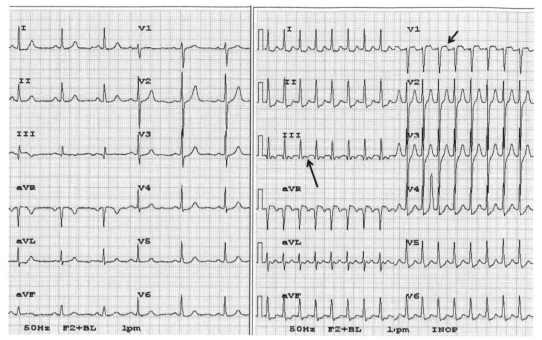

Fig. 17. P-QRS relationships: the search for diagnostic clues. NCT cl 360 ms. Search for P leads us to the small deflection on the ST upslope by comparing this interval in SR and during the arrhythmia. The P (*arrows*) is fully identified following the QRS with an RP of 160 ms. These observations strongly suggest an AVRT using a concealed by pass or, less likely, AVNRT using an atypical reentrant circuit.

interval can, therefore, be used to distinguish between typical AVNRT and AVRT.

Exceptions to the shorter V-A time in typical AVNRT are not infrequent and slower retrograde conduction with longer R-P is not so rare in atypical AVNRTs combining faster antegrade and slower retrograde conduction (**Fig. 19**) or even more uncommonly a slow–slow combination.[6,7]

An AP is a small muscular strand embedded in the mitral or tricuspid ring connecting the homolateral A and V. The electrical impulse will enter the AP retrogradely after having traveled through the ipsilateral His Purkinje System (HPS) bundle explaining the longer VA timing. A functional block in this bundle will result in delayed engagement of the AP by the reentrant activation wavefront prolonging the tachycardia CL.

The other major diagnostic concept is that the AVNRT reentrant circuit is fully contained within the region of the AVN and does not need atria or ventricles to be maintained. It is, therefore, possible to dissociate one chamber from the other without interfering with the arrhythmia CL (**Fig. 20**). Premature atrial and ventricular contractions can capture the respective chambers of origin without affecting the arrhythmia continuing unaltered in the other chambers.

In AVRT, the atria and ventricles are integrant part of the tachycardia circuit and any perturbation induced in one chamber will affect the other and, even for one beat, the cl of the tachycardia.

In both arrhythmias, antegrade conduction is the weak link of the circuit and the spontaneous termination of either arrhythmias occurs more commonly owing to antegrade conduction block and therefor a retrograde A is the last recorded wave (**Fig. 21**). This will never occur in AT, where the arrhythmia terminates because of spontaneous termination of the atrial focus; this arrhythmia will, therefore, end with a QRS (see **Fig. 15**).

It is necessary, when analyzing these types of NCTs, to distinguish between diagnostic and suggestive observations. Evidence of participation of AVN in the mechanism of the arrhythmia is the key observation that excludes AT and leaves only AVNRT and AVRT in the differential diagnosis. The different behavior of the reentrant circuits will distinguish between these 2 arrhythmias.

Wide Complex Tachycardias

As initially mentioned, the analysis of the QRS is, in most cases, the first observation made when confronted with ECG tracing of an arrhythmia. Although a narrow QRS is diagnostic of SVT, both VT and an aberrantly conducted SVT will result in a wide QRS. Numerous criteria have been elaborated based on clinical observations

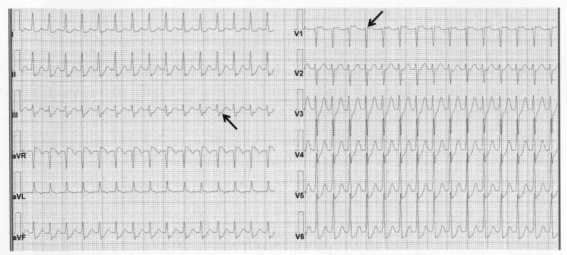

Fig. 18. P-QRS relationships: the search for diagnostic clues. NCT cl 350 ms. No P wave is obvious but a small deflection deforming the ST upslope in fixed relationship with QRS (fixed QRS-P interval) is highly suggestive of a retrograde P (*arrows*). Unchanged PR and RP intervals and the occurrence of part of the P during QRS (see V1) are findings highly suggestive of AVNRT.

that allow, in the great majority of cases, to distinguish between aberrancy and VT.[6]

Saltatory or Aberrant Conduction?

The ECG criteria usually used in the differential diagnosis of WCT are based on:

1. Differences in location of arrythmia breakthrough and Ventricular propagation between SVT with aberrancy and VT and
2. Coexistence of a dissociated SR during VT.

A widening of the QRS is due, in both situations, to a slow muscle–muscle conduction (saltatory conduction) that is present during WCTs, during the greatest part of ventricular depolarization.

SVT with aberrancy represents a pure BBB, which is a combination of an initial wavefront of normal depolarization of the ventricle activated by a functional bundle and a slow muscle to muscle conduction in the portion of ventricle supplied by the blocked branch.

In VT, the wavefront of activation emerges in the ventricular muscle and progresses with saltatory conduction until it may encounter HPS terminal arborizations and reenter this fast conducting system.

Many of the criteria differentiating the mechanism of WCT are, therefore, based on QRS features predicting the timing and degree of HPS engagement. Because altered propagation induced by a BBB is well understood and generate predictable ECG findings, the electrocardiographic manifestations of aberrancy will reproduce a R or LBBB pattern with an early fast

conduction followed by a slow wave of propagation.

In VT, wavefront propagation is highly unpredictable and depends, among other factors, on muscle to muscle connections, the presence of scars, the size of the ventricles, and the degree of retrograde engagement of the HPS. Retrograde invasion of the peripheral ramifications of the conduction, when it occurs, will allow the propagating wavefront to be distributed to parts of the ventricle in a fast and organized fashion. Electrocardiographically, this change in propagation is manifested by a late narrowing of the QRS because the speed of transmission increases during HPS conduction.

The closer the origin of VT to the denser septal ramifications of HPS, the larger the amount of ventricle activated using the normal conduction system. This will lead to a narrower QRS duration especially during VT using HPS fascicles as reentrant paths (fascicular VTs; **Figs. 22–24**). Accordingly, the sensitivity of conventional ECG criteria used to differentiate VT from aberrancy is reduced in patients with these types of VT, also defined as idiopathic VT.[8] This is most obvious in VT originating from septal sites, particularly Purkinje sites and the septal outflow tract regions.

Impulse penetration in the HPS can vary owing to alternating conduction delay or block in some portion of the conduction system or at the interface with ventricular muscle, leading to an alternating pattern of electrical activation(electrical alternans).

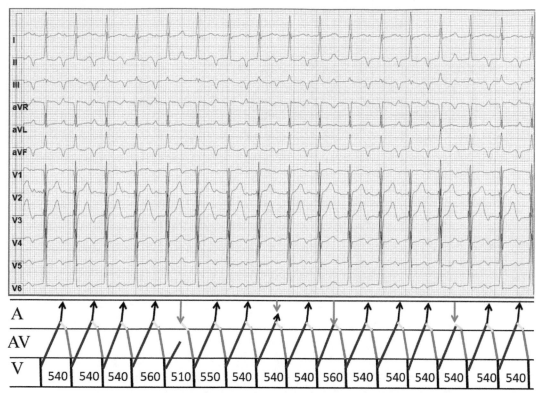

Fig. 19. An unusual case requiring close scrutiny. Not infrequently, we are challenged by tracings that are of very high complexity, either because the different waveforms are difficult to discern or because a rare electrophysiologic behavior is present in a rare tachycardia. This tracing is an example of this situation: A NCT cl 540 ms with a clear retrograde P with a long RP of 260 ms and a similar PR. of 320 ms. The fixed RP and PR intervals, as a first observation, are highly suggestive of a reentrant circuit incorporating the AVN. The cl of the tachycardia and the long almost symmetric RP and PR tell us that this is a rare mechanism such as a slow–slow AVNRT or one of the AVRTs using a slowly conducting retrograde pathway. Another puzzling observation is a drastic changes of P morphology occurring at beats 6, 11, and 15 and a subtle change at beat 11. The drastic change consists of P becoming predominantly positive in the inferior leads in keeping with an antegrade depolarization wavefront and sinus origin. In beat 11, the negativity is decreased in keeping with a fusion beat. Furthermore, the RR interval of beat 6 is 50 ms shorter than the rest of the tachycardia, in keeping with penetration of that sinus beat in the tachycardia reentrant circuit and resetting. Because the sinus PP is not constant, the retrograde activation form the SVT most likely resets the SN. In summary, there is evidence of an NCT with a fixed prolonged RP and PR, and evidence of persisting SN depolarization with atrial capture, fusion, and resetting. The type of RP and PR association and the observation that the cl of the tachycardia is advanced, despite full atrial capture, only once by a sinus beat makes an AT unlikely. The unusual form of AVNRT or a rare tachycardia using an embryonic remnant of the AVN, so called paroxysmal junctional tachycardia or Coumel tachycardia, would fit these requirements.

Together with the widening of the QRS, in VT, there is also evidence of abnormal propagation vectors generated by the anomalous location of tachycardia origin.

The vector associated with aberrant SVT is determined by the presence of left anterior fascicular block or left posterior fascicular block and, therefore, within −30 and +110°. In VT, the axis is often unphysiologically abnormal because the ventricular breakthrough point of this arrhythmia can be localized anywhere, most commonly in the left ventricle.

Because SR, unless suppressed by retrograde conduction, continues unaffected during VT, ECG manifestations of 2 independent rhythms during WCT can be considered diagnostic of VT. Direct evidence of this phenomenon is identification of dissociate P wave (see **Fig. 23**); indirect evidence of this dissociation is the observation of fusion when a critically timed sinus beats captures a part of the ventricles with a wavefront fusing with the VT propagating activation front (see **Fig. 24**). The resultant QRS is somewhat premature, with a resultant morphology with initial characteristics

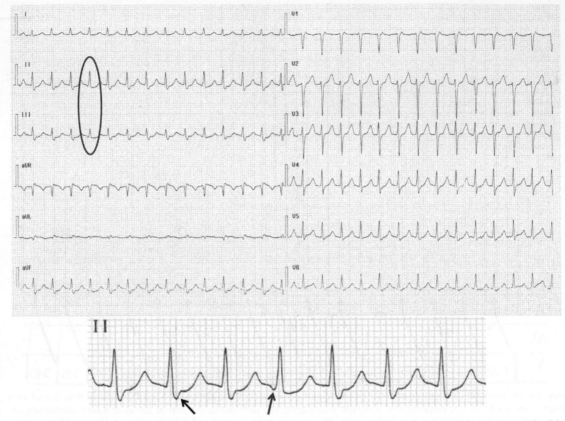

Fig. 20. Attention to details makes the diagnosis. NCT cl 380 ms. The same observations as in **Fig. 18** are applicable in the analysis of this SVT. Furthermore, beat 4 is morphologically different from the rest because it has lost the deflection immediately after QRS; close observation suggests that the retrograde P is now occurring earlier and is visible at the beginning of the QRS. A possible shift in conduction velocity of the fast pathway may have caused this. Because R-R continues at the same rate, we can deduce that the atria are not integral part of the tachycardia. This line of deductions leads to the diagnosis of AVNRT (or far less likely automatic junctional tachycardia).

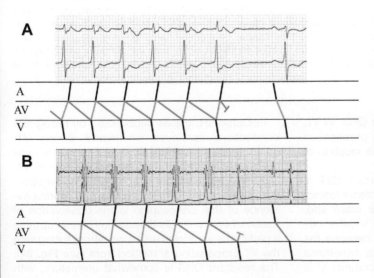

Fig. 21. The importance of observing SVT termination. (*A*) An ECG recording and laddergram of NCT spontaneous termination. Tachycardia termination occurs on the slow pathway leaving a P as the last ECG waveform. This finding rules out an atrial tachycardia, but cannot in itself differentiate between AVNRT/AVRT. Regular NCT morphology and a VA interval of 60 ms make AVNRT highly likely. (*B*) Esophageal recording, ECG, and laddergram of NCT spontaneous termination. Tachycardia termination occurs on the fast pathway leaving a QRS as the last ECG waveform. This finding is not helpful because it does not help us in differentiating between AT, AVNRT, and AVRT. Regular NCT morphology and a constant VA interval of 45 ms make AVNRT highly likely.

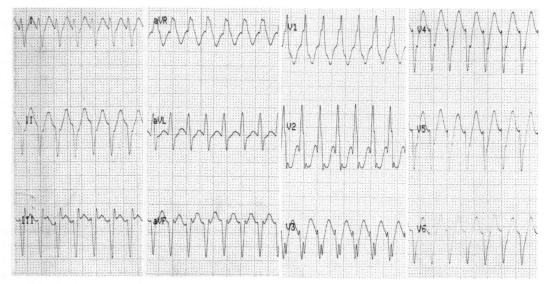

Fig. 22. How to resolve diagnostic uncertainties. We may face a problem of interpretation when we are faced with findings strongly suggesting a different diagnosis. In this case, a regular tachycardia with a QRS width of 130 ms and a retrograde P (lead aVF) seems to have a right BBB morphology with a rapid initial upstroke (see lead V3-V6) consistent with SVT with aberrancy, yet a clearly abnormal axis with an NE direction (R in aVR) suggests VT. Reaching a diagnosis is also made more difficult by low-resolution recordings (see **Fig. 23**).

of SN capture and later QRS portions resembling VT QRS. AV dissociation and fusion, considered some of the most specific diagnostic criteria of VT, have a low sensitivity because they can be documented in approximately 20% of patients.

Conversely, a retrograde P during a wide QRS tachycardia could represent either SVT with a fixed or functional bundle branch block or a VT with retrograde atrial conduction. In general, retrograde activation can be demonstrated in more than 50% of normal individuals and in up to 30% of patients during VT using electrophysiology study.

This discrepancy is probably due to a conduction block of the retrograde activation within the HPS/AVN system when exposed to the fast rates

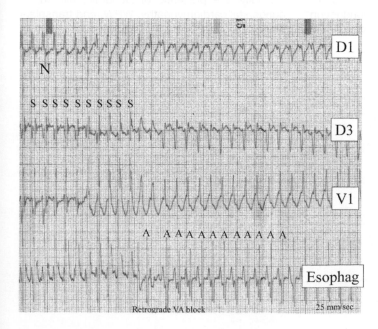

Fig. 23. How to resolve diagnostic uncertainties. The same case as in **Fig. 22**. Using an esophageal lead, rapid atrial pacing was initiated and induces the tachycardia as demonstrated by the change in QRS morphology. The esophageal recording shows the loss of atrial depolarization during the arrhythmia. This behavior could still be consistent with an aberrantly conducted AVNRT (see **Fig. 24**).

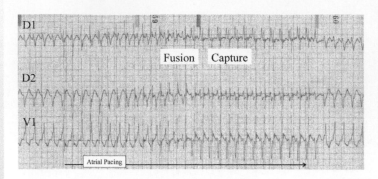

Fusion   Capture

Atrial Pacing

Fig. 24. How to resolve diagnostic uncertainties. The same case as in Figs. 22 and 23. Atrial pacing during the arrhythmia induced in Fig. 23 is diagnostic. During this maneuver, there is evidence of progressive fusion and normalization of the QRS at rates faster than the clinical arrhythmia, which continues as soon pacing is interrupted. These findings are all diagnostic of VT, most likely using a fascicular reentrant circuit.

associated with VT and the difficulty of confirming, on ECG recordings, a retrograde P often hidden in the abnormal ST-T tract.

The V-A interval during VT is often longer than P-R in sinus rhythm and can, rarely, mimic V-A in AVNRT or AVRT both in duration and fixed relationship but, more frequently, shows evidence of nondecremental block or retrograde Wenckebach.

Correct precordial lead placement is a fundamental prerequisite to a correct diagnosis. Some of the criteria to differentiate WCT are based on voltage of specific QRS components or ratio between them from observations in lead V1-V2 and V6. Subtle changes suggesting variation in septal depolarization during electrical alternans are identified in leads V2 and V3, possibly owing to greater amplitude of the QRS in these leads. A lead placed in the wrong location, by altering the QRS morphology, will not uncommonly make a WCT differential diagnosis much more difficult.

Muscle saltatory conduction characterizing VTs can be mimicked by drugs or electrolyte abnormalities affecting the velocity of conduction by directly blocking Na channels or prolonging

Na channels recovery therefore extending repolarization.

The morphology of the QRS depends both on the degree of channel blockade and on the rate-related aberrancy induced in the conduction system. At slow stimulation rates and/or moderate channel impairment, the resultant QRS closely resembles a wider resting QRS. As the block increases and the arrhythmia CL decreases, the resultant QRS becomes increasingly bizarre and it may be so excessively prolonged to assume a sinusoidal morphology.

Distinguishing true VT from SVT altered by the effect of drugs or electrolytes imbalances is difficult and often requires knowledge of the patient's clinical background. In reality, a knowledge of the baseline ECG and the presence and nature of cardiac pathologies, as well as medications and basic metabolic status, should serve as a background to any ECG interpretation of WCTs.

Finally, the presence of ischemic, dilated, or congenital cardiomyopathy, WPW, and transplant status can all render the interpretation of a WCT

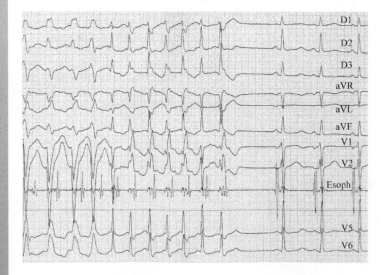

D1
D2
D3
aVR
aVL
aVF
V1
V2
Esoph
V5
V6

Fig. 25. When the VA interval is diagnostic. A tachycardia with variable QRS morphology and cl 260 to 340 ms.

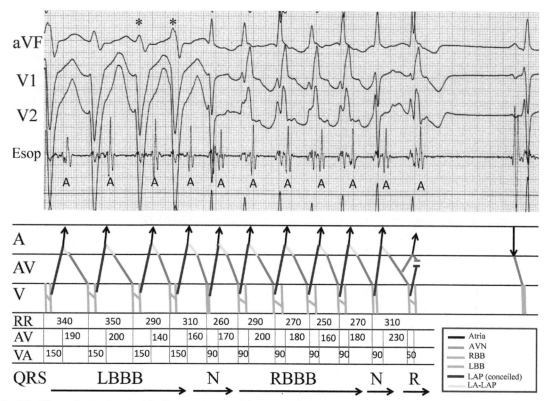

Fig. 26. When the VA interval is diagnostic. A Laddergram of **Fig. 25**. The first 3 beats with an LBBB morphology have an R-R of 340 and 380 ms; a retrograde A is visible on esophageal recording with a fixed VA of 150 ms. The fourth beat is premature, with a slightly different morphology occurring 110 ms earlier than previous R-R and anticipates the retrograde A by the same interval. The fifth beat narrows, the VA shortens to 90 ms and the tachycardia cl shortens by 60 ms. The last beat is delayed with right BBB with a cl of 280 ms and a VA interval of 50 ms. The laddergram clearly explains these observations. There is a variable antegrade conduction 140 to 230 ms explaining the cl variations. This also explains the prematurity of the different beat. Normalization of the following beat is due to a reverse Ashman phenomenon, where the shortening of the RR (*asterisk*) induces shortening of the effective refractory period in both branches. The following RR is longer due to AVN delay and allows normalization of LB conduction; hence, the normal QRS. The tachycardia terminates with an A with antegrade block. These observations point to an AP, which will require a longer time to be engaged retrogradely in the presence of a homolateral BBB. VA is the measure of this time duration and the fact that is longer in LBBB than in normal conduction or right BBB diagnoses a left side AP participating in the reentry. The cl also depends on VA duration because this is the retrograde arm of the orthodromic reentry. The final beat with right BBB morphology is more difficult to explain: we hypothesize that there is a variable antegrade conduction (see changing AV intervals) and last beat finds a slow AVN pathway able to conduct antegradely and generates a single AVNR beat. This finding explains the short VA of 50 ms and the right BBB preceded by longer R-R because the changed input in the AVN modifies HPS access finding RB refractory.

very difficult unless clinical information regarding patient's history and baseline ECG are known.

Comparing a baseline ECG in SR with the arrhythmia tracing is, in fact, a fundamental initial step in the analysis of any arrhythmia, but is especially relevant when confronted with wide QRS tachycardias. Preexisting BBBs will be faithfully reproduced in supraventricular arrhythmias, allowing a rapid and secure diagnosis.

Antidromic tachycardias sustained by antegradely conducting APs are extremely rare in clinical practice, but an irregular WCT, during AF in WPW, can be, as discussed, very difficult to interpret unless the baseline ECG showing preexcitation is first reviewed.

The observation of a longer V-A interval and a prolongation of the arrhythmia CL during periods of functional BBB is diagnostic of AP localized on the same side of the block (**Figs. 25** and **26**).

REFERENCES

1. Lee S, Wellens HJJ, Josephson ME. Paroxysmal atrioventricular block. Heart Rhythm 2009;6:1229.

2. El-Sherif N, Jalife J. Paroxysmal atrioventricular block: are phase 3 and phase 4 block mechanisms or misnomers? Heart Rhythm 2009;6(10):1514.

3. Chugh S, Shen WK, Luria DM, et al. First evidence of premature ventricular complex-induced cardiomyopathy: a potentially reversible cause of heart failure. J Cardiovasc Electrophysiol 2000;11:328.

4. Bagliani G, Leonelli F, Padeletti L. P wave and substrate of arrhythmias originating in the atria. Normal electrophysiology substrates and the electrocardiographic diagnosis of cardiac arrhythmias: part I. Card Electrophysiol Clin 2017;9:365. Elsevier publisher.

5. Leonelli F, Bagliani G, Boriani G, et al. Arrhythmias originating in the atria diagnosis of cardiac arrhythmias: part I. Card Electrophysiol Clin 2017;9: 383. Elsevier publisher.

6. Bagliani G, Leonelli FM, De Ponti R, et al. Advanced concepts of AtrioVentricular nodal electrophysiology: observations on the mechanisms of AtrioVentricular Nodal reciprocating tachycardias. Card Electrophysiol Clin 2018;10(2):277–97. Elsevier Publisher.

7. De Ponti R, Bagliani G, Boriani G, et al. General approach to a wide QRS complex part I. Card Electrophysiol Clin 2017;9:461. Elsevier publisher.

8. Yadav AY, Nazer B, Drew BJ, et al. Utility of conventional electrocardiographic criteria in patients with idiopathic ventricular tachycardia. JACC Clin Electrophysiol 2017;3:669–77.

Challenges in Bradicardias Interpretation

Fabio M. Leonelli, MD[a],*, Roberto De Ponti, MD, FHRS[b], Giuseppe Bagliani, MD[c,d]

KEYWORDS

- Bradycardia • Sinus node dysfunction • Atrioventricular node dysfunction
- His-Purkinje dysfunction • Atrioventricular blocks • Bundle branch block • Bundle branch delay

KEY POINTS

- Bradycardia is a manifestation of abnormal impulse generation or impulse conduction.
- The cause of the pathologies leading to bradycardia is varied and often progressive.
- Understanding of the anatomy and physiology of sinus node (SN), atrioventricular node (AVN), and His-Purkinje system is fundamental for a correct interpretation of bradycardia's electrocardiographic manifestations.
- The electrocardiographic changes may be obvious and easy to diagnose when the pathologies affecting SN or any part of the conduction system are fully developed.
- Before SN disease of AV blocks become manifest, several subtle electrocardiogram (ECG) findings may occur in some specific situations leading to an early diagnosis of impending severe dysfunction of impulse generation or conduction.

INTRODUCTION

Bradycardia's analysis is conceptually different from tachycardia, because the latter is the evaluation of a new pathologic impulse generation, whereas bradycardia is failure of physiologic mechanisms of generation or impulse conduction.

Failure is rarely instantaneous but in most cases is progressive and of increasing severity. Often the clinical presentation is sporadic and nonspecific; clues to the nature of the problems may be present but they are often not so obvious and subtle telltale observations may require analysis of multiple recordings and knowledge of normal and abnormal sinus node (SN) and conduction system electrophysiological properties.

The end result of the failure is the same: insufficient ventricular contractions. Because critical reduction of cardiac output is incompatible with life, evolution has created a compensatory mechanism to counteract the effects of bradycardia: subsidiary pacemakers.

Evaluation of bradycardia should therefore include the following steps:

1. Clinical consequences of bradycardia
2. Cause of bradycardia: impulse generation or conduction deficit
3. Evaluation of obvious abnormalities
4. Presence of effective subsidiary pacemakers
5. Assessment of pathology's progression and severity
6. Clinical therapy

CLINICAL CONSEQUENCES OF BRADYCARDIA

Symptoms are correlated to the severity and duration of periods of decreased cardiac output. From syncope to periodic weakness and shortness of breath one or the entire gamut of nonspecific

Disclosure Statement: F. Leonelli: Any disclosure.
a Cardiology Department, James A. Haley Veterans' Hospital, University South Florida, 13000 Bruce B. Downs Boulevard, Tampa, FL 33612, USA; b Cardiology Department, University of Insubria, Varese, Italy; c Cardiology Department, Arrhythmology Unit, Foligno General Hospital, Foligno, Italy; d Cardiovascular Diseases Department, University of Perugia, Perugia, Italy
* Corresponding author.
E-mail address: fabio.leonelli@va.gov

Card Electrophysiol Clin 11 (2019) 261–281
https://doi.org/10.1016/j.ccep.2019.02.002
1877-9182/19/© 2019 Elsevier Inc. All rights reserved.

complaints may be reported by the same patient. Baseline electrocardiogram (ECG) may be completely normal and show some nonsignificant alterations or abnormalities that may be related to the presentation. Identifying bradycardia as the culprit of the symptoms requires either demonstrating an association between symptoms and abnormality or, at least, evidence of SN or coronary sinus (CS) pathology that could, in its most severe manifestations, become symptomatic in the future.

Either of these 2 conditions need to be fulfilled before implanting a pacemaker, the most common therapy for bradycardia.

CAUSE OF BRADYCARDIA

A defective impulse generation or an intermittent or complete block of atrioventricular (AV) conduction causes bradycardia. SN, AV node (AVN), and His-Purkinje System (HPS) are complex cardiovascular structures allowing limited direct functional evaluation due to difficulties in recording their electrical activity; our understanding of their physiology is based on a large number of animal studies, detailing their electrophysiological properties and an immense quantity of clinical observations.

The ECG faithfully records fixed or dynamic abnormalities of the SN and CS during stable sinus rhythm or during episodic perturbances of their electrophysiologic status quo; these findings need to be observed, confirmed with other evidence of the same abnormality, their specificity and sensitivity evaluated, and the clinical severity assessed.

The dominant role that the autonomic nervous system plays in SN and AVN function complicates the interpretation of bradycardia electrocardiographic findings. Assessment of its tone, particularly vagal tone, is an integral part of the evaluation of finding's clinical relevance.

In the study of bradycardias or tachycardias, the authors use the same principles of electrocardiographic analysis but in the former observations to be collected are often subtler and the deductive logic used to reach a diagnosis more complex.

Impulse Generation

Sinus node anatomy
The SN and the sinoatrial (SA) tissue that surrounds it are arranged in an intricate anatomic structure with complex dynamic properties. Intrinsic automaticity is the fundamental SN property, whereas the surrounding cells with intermediate atrionodal properties serve the purposes of functioning as subsidiary pacemaker, directing

the impulse along predetermined pathways and filtering the outside impulses coming from the atria. Each one of these features can be abnormal with clinical consequences of varying severity.

Sinus node automaticity
Automaticity, the spontaneous cyclical attainment of threshold depolarization, is the key physiologic feature of SN cells. The rate of discharges varies along the entire body of the SN, with higher rates in the upper portion of this structure decreasing as lower SN cells are engaged. Shifting of the intrinsic SN activity is dictated mostly by the vegetative system tone. The spontaneous variations of rates observed during a normal 24-hour period are termed circadian variations of rates and is a fundamental feature of a normal SN.

The SN and the SA tissue that surrounds it are arranged in an intricate anatomic structure with complex dynamic properties. SN surrounding cells have intermediate atrionodal properties and serve the purposes of functioning as subsidiary pacemaker, directing the impulse along predetermined pathways and filtering the outside impulses coming from the atria. Each one of these features can exhibit pathologic features with clinical consequences of varying severity.

When discharged from an outside stimulus, the SN cells will undergo a new depolarizing cycle at their intrinsic rate discharging at an interval similar to the baseline sinus rate (resetting). A dysfunctional SN will require a longer repolarizing period at times lasting a few minutes (SN suppression) or allowing the emergence of another group of SN generating a slightly different P wave.

Impulse Conduction

Conduction system anatomy
The normal conduction axis is constituted by a closely connected system encompassing the AVN and the HPS. This complex structure serves multiple purposes; being the only AV connection allows a full control of the timing between atrial and ventricular depolarization, optimizing filling and contraction of the 4 cardiac chambers. Atrioventricular conduction, or PR interval in the ECG, is a dynamic interval strongly influenced by autonomic tone; it will shorten during sympathetic drive, as during exercise, and increase during vagal stimulation, as during sleep.

Atrioventricular node
AVN with its decremental properties is the site exerting a fundamental delaying action, which is normally manifested with progressive slowing of conduction to the point of AV block of a single beat. These properties, the mechanism of which

is still not completely understood, serve also as protection barrier during pathologically fast atrial stimulation, as in AF, preventing excessive ventricular stimulation potentially inducing ventricular arrhythmias.

His-Purkinje system

HPS with its subdivisions ending in an intricate arborization is constituted by highly specialized fast conducting cells distributing electrical stimulation in an orderly sequential fashion to both ventricles. The pattern of depolarization of these chambers is organized to allow a highly efficient torsionlike contraction by successively engaging muscular fibers in an apicobasal sequence.

Impulse propagation along HPS occurs in an "all-or-none" modality determined by refractoriness and conduction velocity that differ among the system's subdivisions.

EVALUATION OF OBVIOUS ABNORMALITIES

In the case of complete failure of impulse generation or conduction the ECG is a very valuable diagnostic instrument. **Box 1** illustrates the ECG criteria for bradycardias classification. Trying to sort out the mechanism and the failing anatomic structure may be more difficult.

Absence of impulse generation is manifested by absent P waves, sporadically or permanently.

Fibrosis, ischemia, exposure to toxins, or electrolytes abnormalities can prevent formation of a spontaneous sinus impulse; subtler pathologies of the SA junction may block a normally generated sinus impulse (SA block). P waves are absent in the ECG of both conditions, making the distinction between these 2 pathologies very difficult (**Figs. 1** and **2**).

Equally, complete heart block (CHB) with complete AV electrical disconnection is an easy ECG diagnosis, but the level of block may be not so obvious.

CHB can manifest itself abruptly most often as the result of ischemia, drugs, severe electrolytes imbalance, or anatomic malformations, but it is usually the end result of progressive dysfunction of conduction system. Progression is neither predictable nor uniform, and the initial stages of this progression are clinically silent with subtle and often sporadic changes. Finding these changes in tracings antedating the appearance of CHB can be very valuable in determining where in the Conduction System the block occurs.

SUBSIDIARY PACEMAKERS

Failure of a dominant pacemaker requires emergence of a subsidiary pacemaker to prevent circulatory collapse. The importance of this

---

> **Box 1**
> **ECG patterns of bradycardia**
>
> 1. Pathologies of Impulse Generation
>   1.1. Sinus arrest: absent P wave (see **Fig. 1**)
>   1.2. Sinoatrial block: absent P wave (see **Fig. 2**)
> 2. Pathologies of Impulse Conduction
>   2.1. First-degree AVB: fixed prolongation of PR interval (see **Fig. 9**)
>   2.2. Second-degree AVB: single nonconducted P
>   2.2.1. Type I (Wenckebach phenomenon): single nonconducted P preceded by progressive PR prolongation and shortest PR after the block (see **Fig. 10**)
>   2.2.2. Type II (Mobitz phenomenon): single nonconducted P, unchanged PR interval before and after the block (see **Fig. 11**).
>   2.2.3. Fixed 2:1 artioventricular block (AVB): conducted P followed by nonconducted P in 2:1 ratio (see **Fig. 12**)
>   2.3. Advanced AVB
>   2.3.1. Paroxysmal AVB: cluster of 2 or more nonconducted P (see **Fig. 13**)
>   2.4. Complete AVB
>   2.4.1. Third-degree AVB (complete AVB): no AV conduction is present; P and QRS are dissociated (see **Figs. 3** and **4**)

---

function underlies the vast distribution of cells with automatic properties that, in normal circumstance, can take over a failing pacemaker function.

Subsidiary Pacemaker Origin

Most common site of origin of a subsidiary pacemaker is the AVN junction (**Fig. 3**) characterized electrocardiographically by a narrow QRS originating above His bifurcation (unless a BBB was previously present). If junctional rhythm captures the atria, a retrograde P wave (negative in the inferior leads) will be apparent. Presence of a slower sinus rhythm may create some difficulties in assessing the level of AV block because of competing ventricular capture. Retrograde P can reset the SN interfering with its functional assessment. Response to sympathetic stimulation is

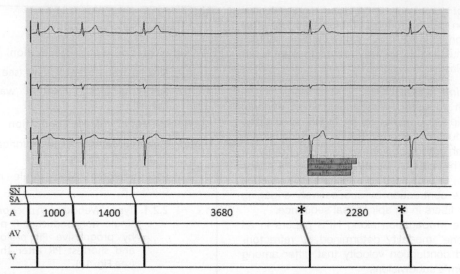

SN SA							
A	1000	1400	3680	*	2280	*
AV						
V						

Fig. 1. Sinus arrest. The figure shows sinus rhythm with a variable PP interval progressively increasing leading to a pause of 3.68 sec. The pause is terminated by emergence of an escape atrial rhythm (*asterisk*) with different P wave morphology and PP interval of 2.28 sec. Progressive slowing of sinus rate with a period of sinus arrest followed by emergence of a slower sinus rhythm highly suggests vagally mediated sinus arrest.

frequently observed in junctional pacemaker with rate increase well above their usual spontaneous rate of 55 to 65 bpm.

More rarely fascicles or distal HPS can also become source of subsidiary pacemakers (**Fig. 4**). In this case, the QRS is wide and the intrinsic rate slower and unresponsive to atropine or sympathetic stimulation. Wide QRS escape

rhythms can be due to distal HPS foci or junctional escape rhythms with preexisting BBB as noted in 20% to 50% of patients. In general, more proximal subsidiary pacemakers tend to be more reliable and have a more physiologic behavior. The more distal sites are less sensitive to autonomic system stimuli and are more unstable, as they are more easily suppressed.

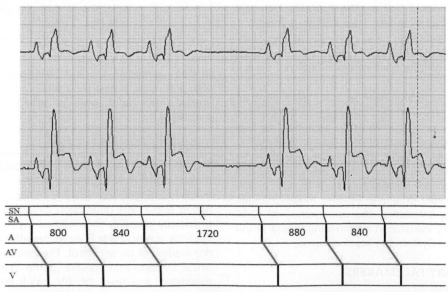

SN SA						
A	800	840	1720	880	840	
AV						
V						

Fig. 2. SA block. Recording from a Holter monitor shows a dominant sinus rhythm with some PP variations and a bundle branch block. Following the third beat there is a spontaneous pause of 1720 msec, twice the mean basic sinus PP interval (860 msec).

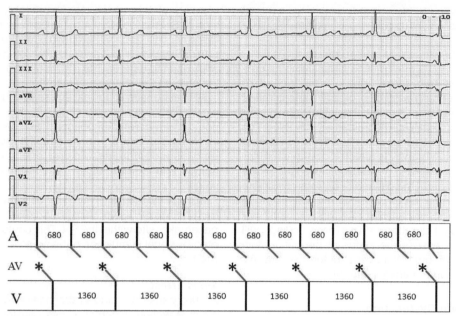

Fig. 3. CHB with junctional escape. Sinus rhythm with regular PP interval at a rate that is initially difficult to identify unless the observers scan the entire ECG strip. Some of the P waves are initially buried in the T wave and progressively emerge to demonstrate complete dissociation from a narrow regular QRS rhythm. Sinus cycle length (CL) of 680 msec and junctional CL of 1360 msec are unchanged all throughout the strip confirming the diagnosis of CHB.

ASSESSMENT OF PATHOLOGY'S PROGRESSION AND SEVERITY

In many cases, before reaching the fully developed picture of sinus arrest or CHB, there are multiple clues allowing a precise diagnosis of the defective anatomic structure involved and the likelihood of its progression to total failure of conduction.

Often, to reach a satisfactory diagnosis, 12 lead ECGs have to be supplemented by long-term

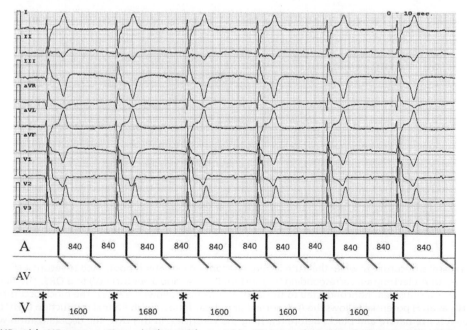

Fig. 4. CHB with HP escape. Sinus rhythm with a stable PP interval at 840 msec and wide QRS with RBBB morphology. As in **Fig. 3**, PP and RR CL are stable but different at 840 and 1600 msec, respectively. This again confirms CHB with an escape rhythm probably originating in the left common bundle before its bifurcation in view of an RBBB with a normal axis morphology.

electrocardiographic recordings using external Holter and event monitors or implantable loop recorders.[1]

ECG and Intracardiac Recordings: the advantage of the ECG over routine intracardiac recordings is that the former gives a full picture of activation of both ventricles, clearly demonstrating the effects of even a minimal delay of branch conduction. Intracardiac recordings usually inform us on the overall delay within the HPS, unable to specify which branch is affected and to what degree. Observing QRS morphologic changes allows us to understand the difference between complete and functional block induced by interplays of refractoriness, stimulation rate, and dynamic action potential duration (APD). These findings will allow us to assess the status of the conduction system and often intervene before severe AV blocks become manifest (**Fig. 5**).

Sinus Node Dysfunction

Heart rate variability

Heart rate variations with activity and sleep wake cycle are an essential feature of SN function; blunting of this parameter is probably the first sign of SN dysfunction. Most automatic recording systems can accurately quantify circadian heart rate (HR) variation but no clear physiologic boundaries exist to differentiate a normal from abnormal behavior in the absence of symptoms.

HR responses to formal stress test have been extensively studied; lower HR at max exercise and reduced rate of changes as the exercise level increases are a more specific indicator of sick sinus syndrome but the effect of drugs, aging, and comorbidities reduce their clinical value.

Abrupt slowing of sinus rate accompanied by morphologic P wave changes suggest a shift of pacemaker site within the SN. This could be mediated by vagal stimulation or being an early sign of SND.

Sinus arrest

A sinus pause is a sudden absence of an expected sinus P without external events causing it. Sinus pause can be due to SN failure to depolarize (see **Fig. 2**) or block of a normally generated impulse in the SA tissue.

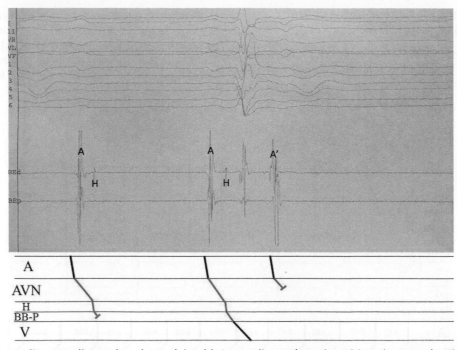

Fig. 5. Intracardiac recordings: when the truth is told. A recording catheter is positioned to record a His potential, marked as H, an A electrogram corresponding to a surface P wave, and a ventricle (V) to a QRS. The first A probably represents a sinus beat nonconducted to the ventricles (A not followed by a V). The block occurs below the common His as an H potential follows the A. A normal sinus beat follows with normal conduction (AHV complex). The last beat is premature and blocks before reaching the ventricles. In this case, the depolarization wavefront does not reach the bundle of missing H, because it blocks in the AVN. AVN conduction corresponds to A-H timing. Although such a precise information on level of conduction block are not directly available from surface ECG, several observations during analysis of an ECG recording can provide an equally detailed knowledge of the status of the AVN-HPS axis.

To analyze the cause of sinus pauses it is important to chart the events occurring in the SN from generation of the impulse to travel through SA tissue and emergence in the atria to inscribe a P. By reconstructing all these intervals in a laddergram it is possible to work out any relationship existing between duration of the pause, spontaneous SN depolarization rate, and SA conduction time. This can occur randomly for a single beat (see **Fig. 1**) or more than one P wave may be missing; a PP interval encompassing the pause, which is a multiple of the basic sinus rate, is in keeping with SA block of a few, normally generated sinus impulses (see **Fig. 2**). Sinus pauses not explainable by simple mechanisms may be due to more complex patterns at times closely resembling Wenckebach phenomenon (**Fig. 6**).

In rare cases SN ectopy can reset the SN but be blocked in the perinodal tissue. The end result is a sinus pause without obvious indication of its cause (**Fig. 7**) and requires a laddergram of the event to correctly diagnose the cause of the pause.

These findings need to be interpreted in the contest of patient's symptoms, his/her medical therapy as well as a conjecture on the patient's vagal influence at the time; in particular, rest versus activity, sleep versus wake, and situations inducing hypervagotonia, such as straining or sleep apnea, need to be fully evaluated by an in-depth clinical history.

Subtle evidence of sinus node dysfunction

Subtler evidence of SN dysfunction can be documented by its response to atrial premature contractions (APC) occurring spontaneously during asymptomatic electrocardiographic recordings.

These abnormalities tend to be more independent from vagal tone and therefore indicate SND.

To penetrate the SN and discharge it, an APC needs to be timed during a narrow time window when the SN and the tissue surrounding are fully repolarized. The effect of premature stimulation will vary depending on whether APC does or does not depolarize the SN.[2]

Observing P-APC interval and the following P will elucidate SN response to APCS or periods of supraventricular tachycardia (**Fig. 8**); identification of every P and correct timing of events is fundamental for this analysis. Evidence of SN dysfunction is suspected when the interval between APC and first postectopic sinus beat is particularly long, particularly if a subsidiary pacemaker emerges to maintain ventricular rate during a particularly long pause.

Progression of SND is unpredictable; probably begins with sinus bradycardia at rest, loss of circadian variation of HR, and blunted response to exercise. During this period, which may span many years, symptoms of fatigue and effort intolerance may emerge accompanied by episodes of sinus arrest asymptomatic or syncope or presyncope.

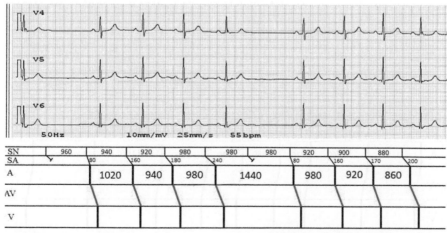

Fig. 6. Variable PP interval: the hidden events. SA Wenckebach: the figure shows sinus beats with variable PP intervals and pauses at the beginning of the strip and following the first 4 beats. To correctly identify the problem a laddergram is necessary. On this graph we see that the PP interval (AA in the laddergram) is the result of 2 different intervals: SN CL, which varies probably due to sinus arrhythmia, and sinoatrial (SA) time, which progressively lengthens. Although the SA conduction is gradually prolonged, the increment of the delay is decreasing reproducing a Wenckebach periodicity. This pattern of decreasing increments results in a gradual foreshortening of the PP interval, best seen in the last 3 beats. The following pause is due to a sinus beat blocked within the SA tissue before it could reach and depolarize the atria.

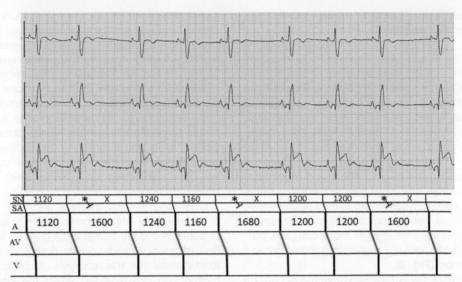

SN	1120		*	X	1240	1160		*	X	1200	1200		*	X	
SA															
A	1120	1600			1240	1160	1680			1200	1200	1600			
AV															
V															

Fig. 7. Variable PP interval: the hidden events. Blocked perisinus node ectopy with SN resetting. Sinus rhythm with RBBB CL 1120 to 1260 msec. Three longer P-P intervals are present lasting between 1600 and 1680 msec. No atrial premature contractions (APC) resetting the SN is visible and yet the SN seems to be reset. The most likely explanation is the occurrence of perisinusal ectopies (*asterisk*) blocked in the SA tissue and resetting SN depolarization (X).

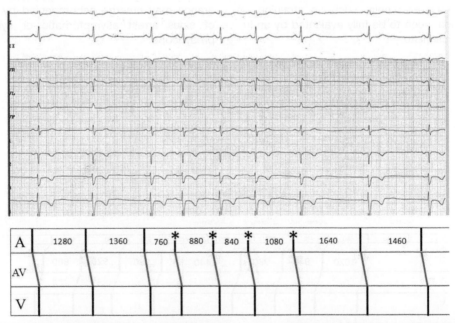

A	1280	1360	760 *	880 *	840 *	1080 *	1640	1460
AV								
V								

Fig. 8. P wave morphology and PP interval. Perisinus node ectopy and SN resetting. In this tracing there are irregular PP intervals; first 3 Ps coming at a steady interval are followed by 4 Ps with variable inter-beat interval; the strip ends with 2 more Ps with the same interval as the initial one. Puzzling is the fact that the P wave morphology is the same in every beat regardless of their intrinsic rate. We can assume that first and last beat originate in the SN with an intrinsic rate between 1280 and 1460 msec; the highly variable PP of the following waves excludes SN as their origin. Given their morphology their origin is in the perinodal region; we must conclude that the strip represents sinus beats and a burst of premature atrial contractions from the perinodal region. The SN has been reset by the last ectopic P and resumes with an interval (1640 msec) longer than the intrinsic sinus rate.

Conduction System Abnormalities

The conduction system is composed of 2 connected components: AVN and HPS, with profound differences in physiologic function, electrophysiological properties, and manifestations of functional failure.

Their anatomic closeness and yet their electrophysiologic diversity create a functional interdependence where the timing of antegrade (AVN to HPS) or retrograde (HPS to AVN) depolarizations will dictate how these structures will respond. Impulse delay, total or partial block of AVN pathways, or one or more of HPS subdivisions can be observed. These responses depend on the frequency of stimulation (heart rate) and encroachment of the impulse on the action potential phase of each conduction system component. To be able to interpret these findings and assess whether they are physiologic or abnormal is a complex endeavor.

Atrioventricular nodal blocks

From an electrocardiographic point of view, AV blocks, representing an abnormal P-QRS relationship, can be schematically summarized as follows:

First-degree AVB: fixed prolongation of PR interval (**Fig. 9**)

Second-degree AVB: single nonconducted P
- Type I (Wenckebach phenomenon): single nonconducted P preceded by progressive PR prolongation (**Fig. 10**)
- Type II (Mobitz phenomenon): single nonconducted P preceded by unchanged PR interval (**Fig. 11**)

Fixed 2:1 A/V block: conducted P followed by nonconducted P in 2:1 ratio (**Fig. 12**)

Paroxysmal AVB: cluster of 2 or more nonconducted P (**Fig. 13**)

Third-degree AVB (complete AVB): no AV conduction is present; P and QRS are dissociated

AVN is constituted by a network of cells with different electrophysiologic characteristics designed to respond to increasingly higher stimulation by decrementing conduction. This feature is physiologically present in the heart only in the AVN.

Alterations within its cellular network will accentuate these characteristics with evidence of progressive slowing even during normal heart rates (see **Fig. 10**).

Progressive slowing to block and its periodicity (Wenckebach block) localizes this abnormality to AVN (see **Fig. 10**). Given its high degree of redundancy, and the profound effect of vegetative system, these changes are episodic, frequently clinically silent, and it is often difficult to separate normal responses from pathologic ones. In view of AVN large functional reserve it is the patient's clinical response to these functional deficits that will dictate therapy.

Progression can be ideally plotted as first-degree AVB, Wenckebach at slower rates, 2:1

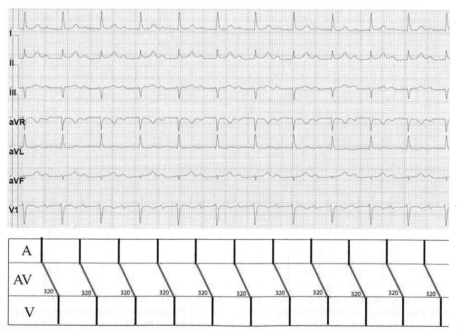

Fig. 9. First-degree atrioventricular block. Sinus rhythm CL with normal QRS and PR of 320 msec. This is a typical first-degree AVB due to conduction delay within the AVN.

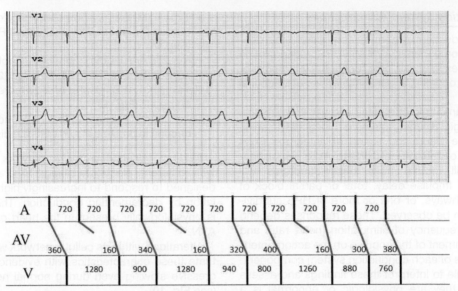

A	720	720	720	720	720	720	720	720	720	720	720
AV	360	160	340	160	320	400	160		300	380	
V		1280	900	1280	940	800	1260		880	760	

Fig. 10. Second-degree AVB type I. Sinus rhythm with stable PP interval of 720 msec. Variable P-QRS relationship is present with 1:1 and 2:1 ratio. The laddergram clearly shows the regular PP interval, the progressive P-QRS delay ending with a nonconducted P. At the same time the RR interval shortens. The PR interval after the block is the shortest of the series. All these findings are the diagnostic features of second-degree type I AVB block due to abnormal AVN conduction.

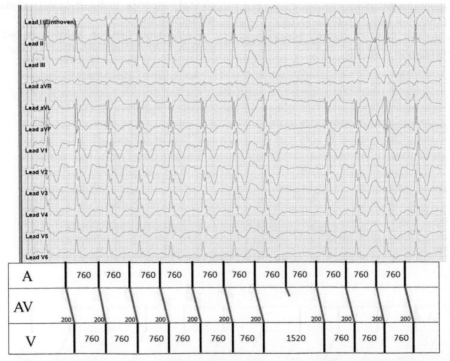

A	760	760	760	760	760	760	760	760	760	760	760
AV	200	200	200	200	200	200	200	200	200	200	200
V	760	760	760	760	760	760	1520		760	760	760

Fig. 11. Second-degree AVB type II. Sinus rhythm with stable PP interval of 760 msec, PR of 200 msec, and a wide QRS with RBBB morphology. A nonpremature P is blocked; the PR interval of the conducted beat immediately preceding and immediately following the nonconducted P is the same. The presence of an HPS conduction delay, RBBB, with a fixed PR localizes the level of block at the HPS level. This initially asymptomatic block will most likely progress to CHB, and a prophylactic PPM implant is required at this stage.

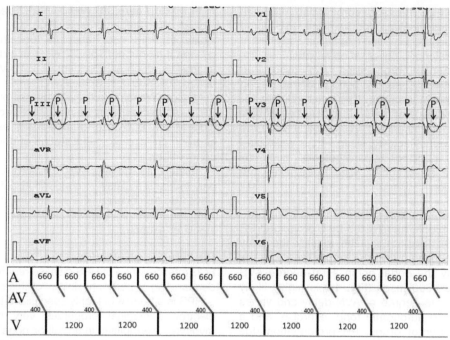

A	660	660	660	660	660	660	660	660	660	660	660	660	660	660	660
AV	400		400		400		400		400		400		400		400
V		1200		1200		1200		1200		1200		1200		1200	

Fig. 12. AVB 2:1. Sinus rhythm with PP interval of 660 msec. A pattern of 2:1 AV conduction is present with one in every 2 P waves conducting to the ventricles with an RBBB. In this case, the level of block cannot be clearly identified, because both AVN and HPS disease can lead to 2:1 AVB. The presence of a BBB does not help to localize the level of block. Observing, in the same patient, evidence of AVN (ie, periods of Wenckebach phenomenon) or HPS (ie, type II second-degree AVB) localize the 2:1 block at the same anatomic level (see also **Figs. 15** and **16**).

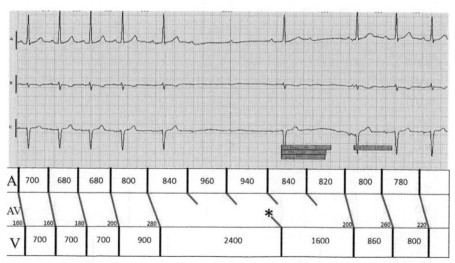

A	700	680	680	800	840	960	940	840	820	800	780
AV	160	160	180	200	280		*		200	260	220
V	700	700	700	900		2400		1600		860	800

Fig. 13. Paroxysmal AVB. Sinus rhythm with narrow QRS and increasing prolongation of PP interval in the first 5 beats with the last conducted beat having a longer PR. This is followed by 2 nonconducted P waves and a third followed by a QRS. The subsequent P wave is again nonconducted, and conduction resumes with a variable PR in the following 3 beats. With resumption of stable conduction PR is shorter as it would be expected with recovery of AVN conduction. This observation, together with slowing of sinus rate and the prolongation of AV conduction just preceding the PAV, strongly suggest AVN as the site of block. It is unclear whether the sixth QRS represents a junctional escape with an intrinsic rate of 2.4 seconds or it is a conducted beat form the preceding P wave. The long PR of this beat, the persisting nonconduction of the following P, and a short PR of the beat associated with resumption of conduction suggest that the sixth beat is a junctional escape (*asterisk*).

AVB (see **Fig. 12**), and paroxysmal AVB (see **Fig. 13**). These findings tend, with time, to become more frequent to the point that all may be present during a prolonged period of observation.

To document progression and associated symptomatology, lengthy periods of monitoring are therefore necessary. Their interpretation requires knowledge of medical therapy as well as a conjecture on the patient's vagal influence at the time; rest versus activity, sleep versus wake, and situations inducing hypervagotonia, such as straining or sleep apnea, need to be taken into consideration.

First-degree atrioventricular nodal block First-degree AVN block, manifested by a prolonged PR (see **Fig. 9**), does not, in itself, localize the delay at the AVN except that the longer the delay the more likely the nodal origin. First-degree AVB longer than 300 msec (**Fig. 14**) is highly likely to have some degree of AVN delay and varies according to autonomic tone, exercise, and a large number of drugs. PR prolongation due to HPS delay is usually, but not always, accompanied by BBB frequently of advanced degree and it is not usually affected by autonomic tone.

Typical and atypical Wenckebach Presence of typical Wenckebach (see **Fig. 10**; **Fig. 15**) localizes, with near absolute certainty, other concomitant but nonspecific electrocardiographic anomalies, such as first-degree, 2:1 AV block or periods of AV block, to the AVN.

Atypical Wenckebach,[3] with its less predictable PR prolongation, may require construction of a laddergram, but once identified it is as specific as the more classic manifestation of decremental conduction.

Isolated first-degree AVB, 2:1 AVB, and PAVB only indicate a delay of conduction but in themselves do not localize where it occurs, and identifying the anatomic level will be discussed in detail in a later section.

His-Purkinje system disease
ECG interpretation of HPS disease requires an understanding of pathophysiology of this structure.

HPS is a bundle of highly specialized fibers with electrophysiological properties very similar to myocytes exemplified in an "all-or-none" conduction. The presence of a higher number of Na channels increases its velocity of conduction, whereas the difference in refractory period of R and L branch of the HPS is due to their dissimilar

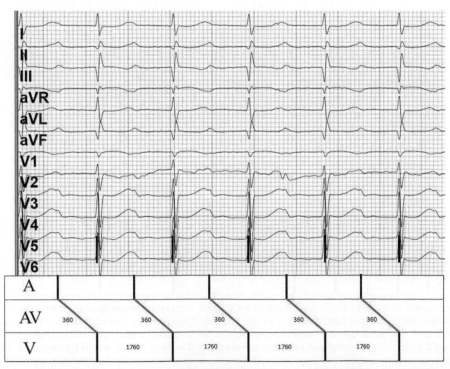

Fig. 14. P waves playing hooky. First-degree AVB. This figure shows a regular QRS at CL 1760 msec with what seems to be a long QT. No P wave is immediately visible, suggesting a diagnosis of junctional rhythm with long QT. The slight morphologic changes (see third T wave) of the second component of the T wave exclude a U wave and makes a hidden P wave far more likely in this case of marked first-degree AVB.

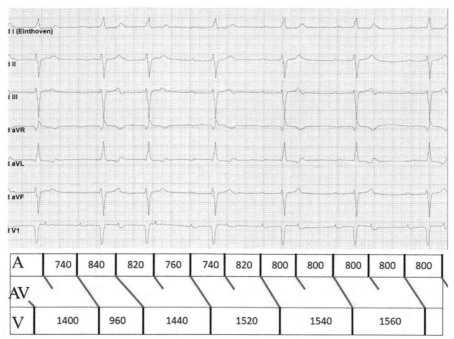

Fig. 15. To find the truth keep on looking. 2:1 AVN and Wenckebach. Regular sinus rhythm with mostly 2:1 conduction with, in the conducted beat, long PR and wide QRS with left bundle branch block (LBBB) and left anterior descending pattern. Just observing the 2:1 periods of conduction is impossible to define the level of block prognosis and management depend on this information; the presence of advanced HPS disease may suggest a block at this level but it is not sufficiently specific. The second, third and fourth P demonstrate a different type of conduction characterized by a prolongation of the PR with block on the third beat and resumption of 2:1. The presence of decremental conduction (Wenckebach phenomenon) localizes the 2:1 block at the AVN level.

distribution of K channels. A premature depolarization can therefore block completely in common bundle or in 1 of the 3 branches of the HPS with ECG manifestations of BBB and its variations.

CHB due to HPS is due to progressive deterioration of conduction in its 3 branches and when fully manifested has very serious clinical implications and long-term prognosis. Therefore, assessment of conduction dysfunction within the HPS is far more important than in the case of AVN disease.

AVN has a great deal of functional reserve that make assessment of severity of its dysfunction difficult, whereas evidence of progressive disease of the trifascicular structure of the HPS can be ascertained with a higher precision.

A normal ECG does not exclude advanced HPS disease, because an intra-His block before the bundles division will show a normal QRS duration. Persistent BBB present during SR have prognostic implications as discussed elsewhere.[4]

Progressive His-Purkinje system disease HPS disease evolution can be easily recognized in the case of abnormalities present during normal SR as is in the case of right bundle branch block (RBBB) progressing to, RBBB and hemiblock

(bifascicular block) later showing PR prolongation (by some called trifascicular block).[4]

Manifestations of progressive HPS conduction failure will occur sporadically often without any apparent triggers and may progress in well-recognizable patterns:

Mobitz type II atrioventricular block Sudden failure of sinus P conduction without any PR changes of the beats immediately preceding or following the block (Mobitz type II) (see **Fig. 11**) is a behavior characteristic of advanced HPS disease. Blocked APC, likely to be a physiologic response, needs to be excluded by measurement of preceding PP intervals.

2:1 Atrioventricular block This conduction abnormality is not specific for either AVN or HPS block, because it is observed in advanced HPS and AVN dysfunction. Observing PR variations (shortening of post block PR following resolution of 2:1 block) and ruling out vagal influences, as previously described, is the diagnostic key distinguishing AVN and HPS behavior.

Furthermore, during 2:1 conduction, a PR less than 160 msec in the conducted beat, particularly if occurs with a normal QRS, is virtually diagnostic

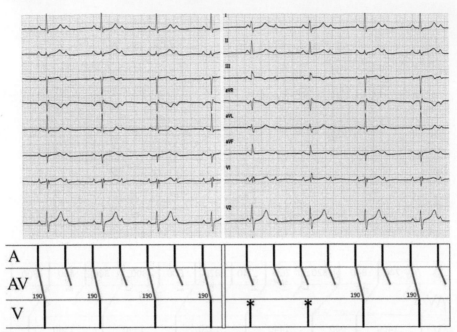

Fig. 16. To find the truth keep on looking. 2:1 AVN block at common His bundle. These are 2 tracings recorded at different times in the same patient. Fig A shows SR CL 720 msec with 2:1 AV block and narrow QRS. As previously noted, there are no specific features helping in localizing the level of block. Tracing B shows a period of PAVB during SR at 680 msec. The first 2 narrow QRS have a slower CL than the following 2 QRS, which together with a variable PR suggests that they are junctional escape beats. The last 4 P are conducted with 2:1 block similar to Fig A. Observations localizing the level of block to common His are presence of high-degree AV block, no PR prolongation, and fixed PR interval less than 160 msec with narrow QRS.

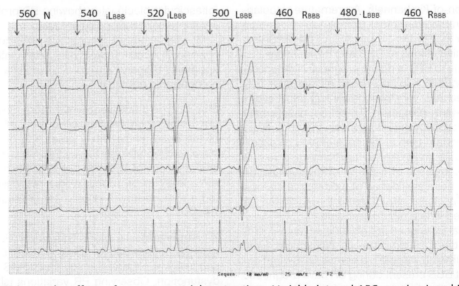

Fig. 17. HPS input: the effects of premature atrial contractions. Variable interval APCs causing L and RBBB: ECG manifestations. This figure shows sinus rhythm with APCs in a pattern of bigeminy occurring at variable intervals. Depending on the degree of premature depolarization of the HPS, different degrees of bundle branch block are observed: from normal conduction (first beat P-APC 560 msec), to incomplete LBBB (second APC with an interval P-APC of 540 msec), to complete LBBB morphology (P-APC of 520 and 540 msec). The fifth and seventh APC come with increased prematurity (P-APC 460 msec) and conduct with RBBB morphology. Most likely explanation of this finding is an unchanged conduction delay in LB and more marked delay in the R bundle (see following figure and laddergram).

of common His block, because this type of block presents with normal QRS and minimal conduction delay hence the normal PR (**Fig. 16**). On the contrary, if AVN disease is responsible for 2:1 block, some degree of delay will be present in the conducted beat. A PR of greater than 300 msec in the conducted beat localizes the block at AVN level (see **Fig. 14**).

Wide QRS with 2:1 block it is not helpful, as it can occur in both AVN block with preexisting BBB or intra-His block.

HPS and AVN conduction respond in opposite ways to vagal maneuvers and exercise and use of maneuvers increasing sympathetic or vagal tone can also be useful in distinguishing the level of block. The reason for this opposite response is the increased AVN conduction delay induced by hypervagotonia. This effect will further increase nodal block delaying AVN conduction. The same

delay will allow more time for HPS recovery, improving or leaving unchanged the 2:1 block. Sympathetic stimulation, by increasing AVN conduction, will have the opposite final effect with improvement of AVN block and deterioration of HPS conduction.

Paroxysmal atrioventricular block PAVB is the stage immediately preceding CHB. Its distinctive feature is a sudden change from apparently normal 1:1 AV conduction to a repetitive block of atrial impulse progression to the ventricles. This is frequently observed during periods of increased heart rate (tachycardia-dependent PAVB) or following a postextra systolic pause mediated by atrial or ventricular ectopic beats (bradycardia-mediated PAVB).[5]

Absence of an escape rhythm with asystole is frequently observed. Both cases are often due to

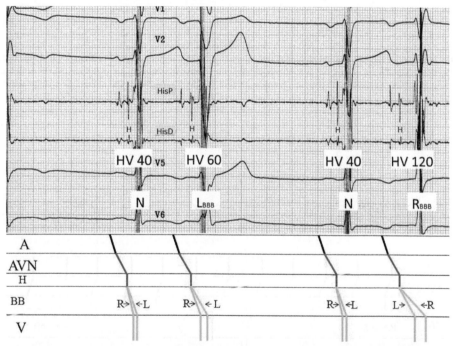

Fig. 18. Confirmation of astute ECG interpretation. Variable interval APCs causing L and RBBB: intracardiac recordings. This figure shows intracardiac recording in the same patient during APCs. The response of the HPS will depend on the refractory period of each of its branches. To end the refractory interval and recover excitability each branch will require a minimum period of time between two subsequent stimulations. This time lag is different for R and LB and can be only approximated from surface ECG measuring the RR interval. Intracardiac recording can, by recording His potential, demonstrate exactly when the HPS was depolarized. If this time is shorter than a specific bundle branch refractory period, that branch will either fail to be depolarized or it will conduct with slower propagation velocity. On the ECG both cases will demonstrate a variable degree of BBB. The intracardiac recordings in this figure show clearly the variable responses for a changing HH interval. The HV interval represents total HPS conduction time; this interval is 70 msec during LBBB and increases to 110 msec during RBBB. As suspected during ECG analysis and clearly shown in the laddergram later, this increased HV interval is the manifestation of a progressive RB conduction delay becoming longer than the LB conduction time. Maintenance of conduction, albeit very slow, is still maintained demonstrating again that conduction in the branches is only delayed and not completely blocked.

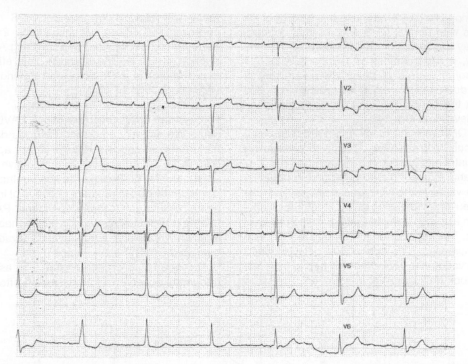

Fig. 19. Varying PR and QRS morphology. Regular sinus rhythm CL 600 msec with QRS of variable morphologies, 2:1 AVB, and different PR intervals on the conducted beats. Close inspection of the tracing reveals a progressive PR lengthening while QRS morphology changes from RBBB to normal to LBBB. See **Fig. 20** for further explanation.

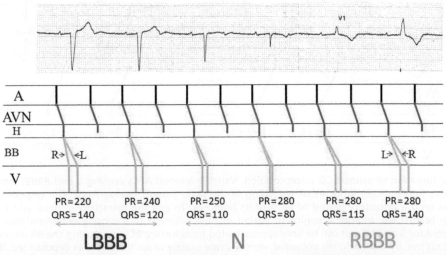

Fig. 20. Varying PR and QRS morphology: when rules are bent. Bilateral BB delay with RB Wenckebach (same ECG of **Fig. 19**). The laddergram illustrates this unusual ECG is due to a fixed LBB delay accompanied by a progressive RBB delay. The effect of delay variation in the 2 branches explains an initial LBBB morphology, with progressive QRS narrowing as the delay between the 2 branches equalizes rendering the activation of both ventricles synchronous again (N). When RB conduction becomes slower than LB, an RBBB morphology becomes evident. These findings strongly suggest the RB progressive delays conduction, showing a behavior similar to Wenckebach phenomenon. PR lengthening reflects the increased time necessary to reach the ventricles as impulse conduction is progressively slowed in both L and R His-Purkinje branches.

advanced HPS disease, and BBB is often present at baseline ECG. The electrophysiologic alterations in HPS cells are secondary to abnormal Na current kinetics leading to prolonged postrepolarization refractoriness, rate-dependent concealed conduction, and spontaneous phase 4 depolarization.[6]

Although due to HPS disease, in most cases, this advanced block is nonspecific as can also be due to AVN block during heightened vagal tone and carries, in this case, a more benign outlook (see **Fig. 13**)

A clear distinction between the 2 is not always possible, but diagnosing level of block is important because HPS block requires a pacemaker implant, although no studies have shown benefit of prophylactic pacemaker implantation in vagal PAVB.

- Observations supporting PAVB due to HPS disease include
  1. PAVB initiated by an extrasystole
  2. PAVB occurring at the beginning of SVT or sinus tachycardia
  3. Observing in the same patient episodes of Mobitz type II
  4. Retrograde conduction following VPC during PAVB often with atrial resetting and termination of the asystolic episode
- Observations suggesting vagally mediated AVN block are
  1. Normal QRS, particularly if accompanied by a long PR
  2. Significant PR prolongation on resumption of AV conduction
  3. Marked PR prolongation or Wenckebach before initiation of AVB
  4. PP interval prolonging during asystole
  5. Recovery of conduction on sinus acceleration
  6. Shortening of the PR of first conducted beat, compared with the one preceding PAVB

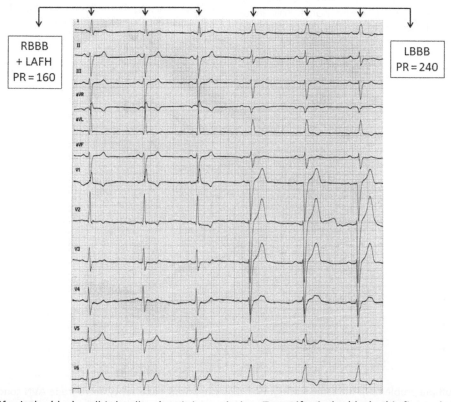

RBBB
+ LAFH
PR = 160

LBBB
PR = 240

Fig. 21. Trifascicular block: call it loudly when it is convincing. True trifascicular block: this figure demonstrates the essence of a diagnosis of trifascicular block. Rhythm is sinus with a steady rate of 1280 msec; the first 3 beats show conduction with an RBBB and left anterior fascicular block (LAFB) followed by a sudden change to LBBB. PR prolongs from 160 to 240 msec. In the last 3 beats more than just the LAF conduction is delayed as the ECG assumes the morphology of LBBB. Conduction is therefore longer than when only RBBB and LAFB were affected. The increasing PR demonstrates, akin to a prolongation of the HV interval, a lengthening of total HPS conduction time. Because this occurs during stable sinus rate, conduction fatigue in the LB is the most likely explanation for this observation.

7. PAVB occurring during situations that suggest heightened vagal tone (ie, cough, micturition, phlebotomy, etc.)
8. No retrograde activation of the His bundle with a ventricular or His extrasystole to reset and abolish AVB

Subtle evidence of advanced His-Purkinje system disease. Delay or block? The ECG patterns described earlier constitute a well-standardized pattern of conduction dysfunctions. They occur during stable circumstances without obvious precipitating factors and often observed serendipitously. The major difficulty in their interpretation is often the localization to AVN or HPS necessary, as previously discussed, to formulate a correct prognosis and therapy.

Several other ECG findings in response to obvious triggers, such as premature stimulation or a change in stimulation rate, represent subtle evidence of abnormal HPS behavior. HPS has a trifascicular structure, variable electrophysiologic proper among the branches, and a conduction that is an all-or-none phenomenon hardly influenced by autonomic tone. The ECG changes

discussed in the next section (**Figs. 17–24**) represent uncommon findings of advanced HPS disease during common physiologic challenges to the conduction properties of the HPS. These abnormalities need to be carefully evaluated, because, in view of the HPS little functional reserve, they carry an ominous prognostic significance.

Premature excitation and aberrancy Subtler, yet probably equally relevant, are conduction changes induced by premature stimulation (see **Fig. 17**) or by abrupt rate increase occurring during maintained AV conduction. In these cases, latent dysfunction of HPS ramifications will become manifest revealing disease more severe than previously suspected.

Premature beats, most often APCs, can increase conduction delay or induce block in a His-Purkinje branch able to conduct normally during steady sinus rhythm (see **Fig. 18**). Abnormal responses to premature atrial contractions include appearance of a hemiblock during a stable RBBB, varying hemiblocks or shift from RB to LB, and normalization of QRS.

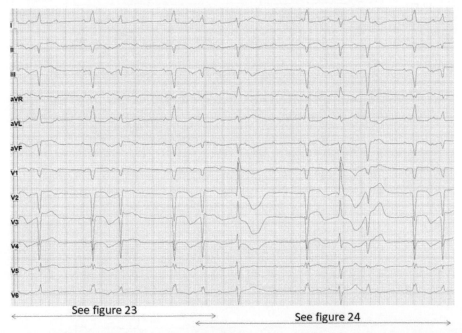

See figure 23

See figure 24

Fig. 22. Multiple problems in the same tracing. Wenckebach, phase 4 aberrancy, retrograde AVN concealed conduction. Figure shows sinus rhythm CL 640 msec, with variable AV conduction and varying QRS morphologies. There is periodic group beating involving QRS 2 and 3, 4 and 5, and 10 and 11. The group beating is characterized by similar RR intervals, progressive PR prolongation followed by a nonconducted P that suggests Wenckebach periodicity. The first QRS of the 2 beats has an LBBB morphology, whereas the second QRS is narrower. There are 2 QRS with RBBB morphology, beat 6 and 8, with no clear relationship with the preceding P and most likely represent VPCs. After the first VPC there are 2 nonconducted Ps. The following ECG is presented in complete form in **Fig. 21**; because of the number of findings it is further divided in 2 sections (**Figs. 23** and **24**) both analyzed with a laddergram.

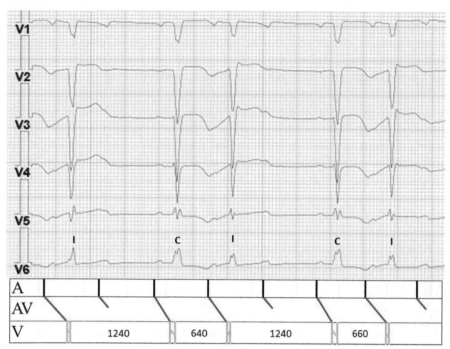

Fig. 23. Multiple problems in the same tracing (left side of **Fig. 22**). This section demonstrates the Wenckebach periodicity; QRS morphology is variable with the first beat having a near normal appearance followed by a wide QRS with LBBB and a third beat with an incomplete LBBB morphology. These changes are best explained with a phase 4 aberrancy due to spontaneous diastolic depolarization of the LB during periods of prolonged RR intervals. The longer the interval the more marked the degree of aberrancy. In the laddergram the delay of the LB is expressed by an increased interval between green, representing RB conduction, and orange bar, representing LB conduction.

APC encroachment in the branch effective refractory period explains these findings, which may occur at different intraectopic intervals as action potential duration can vary depending on stimulating rate (Ashman phenomenon).

Delay or block? Decremental conduction in His-Purkinje system Although it is customary to define block in the ECG manifestations of nonconduction along one or more of its branches, very often the block is not a full electrical interruption of these HPS ramifications (see **Figs. 19** and **20**).[7]

The electrocardiographic features of BBB will be similar and reproducible whether due to complete interruption or relative delay of conduction of an HPS branch.

Yet considering the "block" a dynamic phenomenon with different degrees of conduction slowing will allow us to explain findings that would otherwise be uninterpretable.

A narrow QRS is due to simultaneous activation of both ventricles; this occurs during normal activation or in any other situation where R and LB delay is equal.

A wide QRS is due to a delay of activation of regions of one or both ventricles and the ECG will mostly represent depolarization of the ventricle supplied by the most delayed branch/branches. If a conduction slowing in a branch is added to a preexisting block in the other, the resultant ECG shows an initial dominant BBB, followed by normalization of QRS duration when delay in both branches is similar, and finally emergence of a different BBB (see **Fig. 19**). Keeping this approach in mind can explain very uncommon behavior of the HPS cells, which, when severely diseased, change their "all-or-none" conduction to a decremental one very similar to AVN behavior (see **Fig. 20**). This abnormality is probably due to alterations in gap junction function and Na channels kinetics and not due to predominance of Ca channels behavior as in AVN cells.[8,9] PR prolongation can also be observed as manifestation of the overall increases in conduction time along the HPS.

Acceleration-dependent block Aberrant conduction induced by minimal acceleration of heart rate is due to failure of the AP to shorten or at times even prolong.[10] This aberration, which most frequently affects the LB, appears at rates below 100 bpm, and it is due to inability of HPS cells to

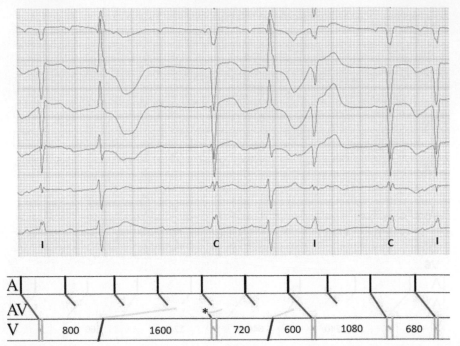

Fig. 24. Multiple problems in the same tracing (right side of **Fig. 22**). This second figure represents the following portion of **Fig. 21** ECG. In this tracing, the normal sinus rhythm is interrupted by a VPC, red bar, which most likely conducts retrogradely penetrating into the AVN/HPS. The following 2 P waves are blocked as a result of AVN/HPS conduction delay. The following QRS with LBBB represents a junctional beat with phase 4 aberrancy as previously discussed. Next P blocks in the AVN depolarized by the preceding junctional beat. A VPC follows but it is too close to the previous P wave and therefore unable to penetrate retrogradely into the AVN recovering from prior depolarization induced by the previous junctional/P wave combination. Next P wave conduces with a long PR and the following blocks as part of Wenckebach periodicity. The last 2 beats begin anew the 3:1 Mobitz type I block. *Laddergram Legend*: A, atrium; AV, atrioventricular; *V,* ventricular. *Black bar*: antegrade interatrial conduction. *Blue Bar*: antegrade AVN conduction. *Green Bar*: antegrade RB conduction. *Orange Bar*: antegrade LB conduction. The distance between green and orange bars expresses the relative delay of each bundle. *Red Bar*: retrograde HPS conduction. *Pale Blue Bar*: retrograde AVN conduction. *Asterisk*: junctional beat. *C:* complete LBBB. *I:* incomplete LBBB.

adequately shorten APD in response to heart rate acceleration (same electrophysiologic abnormalities causing PAVB). In more advanced HPS disease, alternating BBB can be observed for minimal increase in rate (see **Fig. 21**) typifying the true meaning of trifascicular block.

Deceleration-dependent block Deceleration-dependent BBB is much less common than aberrancy due to acceleration of the heart rate, can affect both bundles, and is associated with severe HPS disease. The mechanism for this aberrancy[11,12] is abnormal spontaneous diastolic (phase 4) depolarization of a diseased conduction system. Because of spontaneous depolarization, more prominent after longer cycles, the cells are activated from a less negative resting membrane potential and conduction delay or block may result (see **Figs. 22–24**). The block is not an all-or-none phenomenon but can result in incomplete BBB progressing to complete

BBB as the duration of the preceding pause increases.

Therapy Bradycardia's therapy, once possible reversible causes are eliminated, is based on implant of permanent pacemakers. Pharmacologic therapy, often used in emergent situations, that is, atropine or catecholamines, does not represent definitive treatment. Device therapy is indicated in every symptomatic bradycardia or in the presence of findings with malignant prognostic significance such as Mobitz type II, trifascicular blocks, and paroxysmal AVB due to His-Purkinje disease. These conditions often evolve to symptomatic or lethal CHB and placement of ppm drastically changes patient's clinical outcome. On the other hand, physiologic asymptomatic bradycardias occurring in young subjects, in athletes, during the night or secondary to sinus depressive therapies should not be treated with device implant regardless of the apparent severity of the findings.

12 lead ECG or longer periods of monitoring should, in most cases, guide toward a therapeutic decision leaving a handful of cases to be further evaluated by intracardiac recordings.

Guidelines of pacemaker therapy are well standardized and for full review of this topic the reader is referred to published guidelines.[13,14]

The authors would like to thank Dr Ezio Mesolella, Dr Dario Turturiello, and Claudia Bartolini for their help in collecting the ECG shown in **Fig. 19** (E.M. and D.T.) and in **Fig. 22** (C.B.).

REFERENCES

1. Locati ET, Bagliani G, Padeletti L. Normal ventricular repolarization and QT interval: ionic background, modifiers and measurements. Card Electrophysiol Clin 2017;9:487–513. Normal Electrophysiology, Substrates and the Electrocardiographic Diagnosis of Cardiac Arrhythmias: Part I.

2. De Ponti R, Marazzato J, Bagliani G, et al. Sick sinus syndrome. Card Electrophysiol Clin 2017;9:183. Bradycardias, Tachycardias and Clinical Arrhythmias: the Role of eELectrocardiogra0phy Part II.

3. Bagliani G, Leonelli FM, De Ponti R, et al. Atrio ventricular nodal conduction disease. Card Electrophysiol Clin 2017;9:197. Bradycardias, Tachycardias and Clinical Arrhythmias: the Role of eELectrocardiogra0phy Part II.

4. Leonelli FM, Bagliani G, De Ponti R, et al. Intraventricular delays ansd blocks. Card Electrophysiol Clin 2017;9(3):211. Bradycardias, Tachycardias and Clinical Arrhythmias: the Role of eELectrocardiogra0phy Part II.

5. Lee S, Wellens HJJ, Josephson ME. Paroxysmal atrioventricular block. Heart Rhythm 2009;6:1229–34.

6. El-Sherif N, Jalife J. Paroxysmal atrioventricular block: are phase 3 and phase 4 block mechanisms or misnomers? Heart Rhythm 2009;6(10):1514.

7. Cranfield PF, Klein HO, Hoffman BF. Conduction of the cardiac impulse. I. Delay, block and one way block in depressed Purkinje fibers. Circ Res 1971; 28:199–209.

8. Singer DH, Lazzara R, Hoffman BF. Conduction disturbances due to enhanced phase 4 depolarization of automatic cells [abstract]. Am J Cardiol 1966; 17:138.

9. Singer DH, Lazzara R, Hoffman BF. Interrelationships between automaticity and conduction in Purkinje fibers. Circ Res 1967;21:537.

10. Jalife J, Antzelevitch C, Lamanna V, et al. Rate-dependent changes in excitability of depressed cardiac Purkinje fibers as a mechanism of intermittent bundle branch block. Circulation 1983;67: 912–22.

11. Fish C, Miles WM. Deceleration dependent left bundle branch block: a spectrum of bundle branch delay. Circulation 1982;65:1029.

12. Massumi RA. Bradycardia-dependent bundle branch block. A critique and proposed criteria. Circulation 1968;38:1066.

13. The Task Force on cardiac pacing and resynchronization therapy of the European Society of Cardiology (ESC). Developed in collaboration with the European Heart Rhythm Association (EHRA). 2013 ESC Guidelines on cardiac pacing and cardiac resynchronization therapy. Eur Heart J 2013; 34:2281.

14. A Report of the American College of Cardiology/ American Heart Association Task Force on Practice Guidelines (Committee on Pacemaker Implantation) ACC/AHA guidelines for implantation of cardiac pacemakers and antiarrhythmia devices. J Am Coll Cardiol 1998;31(5):1175–209.

Challenges in Narrow QRS Complex Tachycardia Interpretation

Roberto De Ponti, MD, FHRS[a],*, Jacopo Marazzato, MD[a],
Raffaella Marazzi, MD[a], Matteo Crippa, MD[a],
Giuseppe Bagliani, MD[b,c], Fabio M. Leonelli, MD[d]

KEYWORDS

- Narrow QRS complex tachycardia • Atrioventricular nodal reentrant tachycardia
- Junctional tachycardia • Dual atrioventricular node pathway • Inappropriate sinus tachycardia
- Ventricular tachycardia

KEY POINTS

- Peculiar arrhythmogenic substrates may generate a narrow QRS complex tachycardia different from the those commonly encountered in clinical practice.
- These arrhythmias could be misdiagnosed if the surface ECG is not accurately interpreted to orient the diagnosis, eventually confirmed by invasive electrophysiologic study.
- Misdiagnosis may have a major impact on correct patient management, with potentially severe consequences.
- Dual atrioventricular node physiology may be responsible for different forms of these uncommon narrow QRS complex tachycardia, also without a re-entrant arrhythmogenic mechanism.
- A narrow QRS complex during tachycardia does not exclude a ventricular origin; ventricular tachycardia from the upper ventricular septum may have a direct involvement of the specific conduction system and narrow QRS complex.

INTRODUCTION

Narrow QRS complex tachycardia (NCT) is the most common form of cardiac arrhythmia encountered in clinical practice, generally with a supraventricular origin. Although different algorithms recently have been proposed to guide clinicians in the differential diagnosis of such cardiac arrhythmias,[1,2] some peculiar and uncommon forms of NCT may be misdiagnosed if unknown. **Box 1** shows a list of these uncommon forms of NCT, subdivided according to anatomic origin and type of arrhythmogenic substrate.[3–6] Despite the rarity of these cardiac arrhythmias in common clinical practice, their recognition should not be regarded as a mere academic speculation. The management of patients presenting in an emergency department or in any other clinical setting with these arrhythmias may change dramatically, if these peculiar forms are not properly diagnosed

Conflicts of Interest Disclosure: Dr R. De Ponti received lecture fees from Biosense Webster and Biotronik and educational grants from Biosense Webster, Biotronik, Medtronic, Abbott, and Boston Scientific; none for the other authors.
No funding sources to be acknowledged.
[a] Department of Heart and Vessels, Ospedale di Circolo and Macchi Foundation, University of Insubria, Viale Borri, 57, Varese 21100, Italy; [b] Arrhythmology Unit, Cardiology Department, Foligno General Hospital, Via Massimo Arcamone, Foligno, Perugia 06034, Italy; [c] Cardiovascular Disease Department, University of Perugia, Piazza Menghini 1, Perugia 06129, Italy; [d] Cardiology Department, James A. Haley Veterans' Hospital, University of South Florida, 13000 Bruce B Down Boulevard, Tampa, FL 33612, USA
* Corresponding author.
E-mail address: roberto.deponti@uninsubria.it

Card Electrophysiol Clin 11 (2019) 283–299
https://doi.org/10.1016/j.ccep.2019.02.003
1877-9182/19/

and treated. Nevertheless, the correct ECG interpretation of these uncommon forms of arrhythmia could be particularly challenging.

Four cases of these uncommon NCT are presented, focusing on surface ECG interpretation and on the findings at the subsequent invasive electrophysiologic study (EPS).

CASE 1. DUAL ATRIOVENTRICULAR NODAL NONREENTRANT TACHYCARDIA
Clinical Presentation

A 45-year old man with history of paroxysmal palpitations in the past 5 years was referred for the worsening of symptoms. A single-lead ECG showed an NCT with spontaneous termination (**Fig. 1**). Transthoracic echocardiogram showed severely reduced left ventricular function with ejection fraction of 30%; coronary angiography excluded coronary artery disease. The patient received angiotensin-converting enzyme inhibitors and carvedilol, with no improvement of symptoms. On admittance, 12-lead ECG showed a regular NCT at 125 beats per minute (**Fig. 2**).

Electrocardiogram Interpretation

Analyzing the single-lead tracing (see **Fig. 1**), at first sight, no clearly distinguishable P wave during tachycardia is observed before transient sinus rhythm restoration; afterward, a P wave seems present every 2 beats. Moreover, there is a clear alternans of the QRS complex, because its morphology is slightly different in every second beat. The R-R interval between the 2 QRS morphologies progressively increases up to 40 ms before disappearance of the second morphology and transient sinus rhythm restoration; thereafter, the R-R interval becomes alternant, with a sequence of shorter and longer cycles. The 12-lead ECG (see **Fig. 2**) helps find the P wave, which is clearly seen in the right precordial leads every 2 QRS complexes, has a morphology consistent with sinus origin, and is conducted with a normal P-R interval to the QRS complex with the first morphology. This leads to the working hypothesis of sinus rhythm with bigeminal junctional ectopy or dual atrioventricular (AV) nodal nonreentrant tachycardia (DAVNNRT), in which a single sinus impulse is simultaneously conducted over both the fast and slow pathways, generating 2 QRS complexes. The observation that the R-R interval progressively prolongs before transient disappearance of the second beat, with subsequent shortening of the coupling interval between the first and second beats (see **Fig. 1**), favors the hypothesis of DAVNNRT, because this may be indicative of a Wenckebach phenomenon over a very slow AV node pathway.

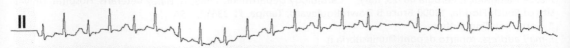

Fig. 1. Case 1: single-lead ECG during tachycardia.

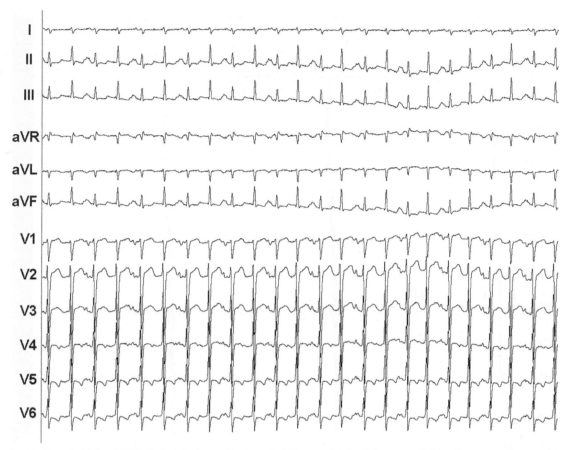

Fig. 2. Case 1: 12-lead ECG during tachycardia. Inverted T waves in the left precordial leads are consistent with tachycardiocardiomyopathy.

At EPS, the diagnosis of DAVNNRT was confirmed. At baseline (**Fig. 3**), a single sinus impulse reproducibly generated 2 QRS complexes with the same H-V interval. Moreover, during programmed atrial stimulation at 500-ms cycle length, the conduction over the slow pathway progressively prolonged, with a prolongation of the A-H″ interval, up until it was blocked at a critical S1S2 coupling interval (**Fig. 4**). Retrograde conduction was absent during right ventricular pacing. Finally, ablation of the slow pathway immediately after initiation of energy delivery suppressed the tachycardia (**Fig. 5**). During follow-up, the patient was on normal sinus rhythm and after 3 months left ventricular ejection fraction improved to 55%.

Clinical Considerations

DAVNNRT is rare but not impossible to encounter in clinical practice, and this represents a diagnostic challenge, which begins at the time of surface ECG interpretation. Several cases have been described over the past decades,[7,8] and 68 cases have been collected in the last published review.[8] Simultaneous conduction over the fast and slow AV node pathways on induction of typical atrio-ventricular nodal re-entrant tachycardia (AVNRT)[9] shares some pathophysiologic aspects with the arrhythmia described and is observed more commonly. DAVNNRT can be easily misdiagnosed as atrial fibrillation, atrial tachycardia, or junctional ectopies, with potentially harmful consequences. Bigeminal junctional ectopies usually show more irregular variations of the coupling interval with the previous sinus beat. Differential diagnosis is critical, because ablation of Hisian ectopies requires different techniques with higher risk for the normal AV conduction system. When aberrant conduction in the DAVNNRT is present, this arrhythmia can be misdiagnosed as ventricular in origin, and this may lead to implantable cardioverter/defibrillator implantation when depressed ventricular function is associated with possibly inappropriate shocks during follow-up. Delay in diagnosis and appropriate treatment can lead to tachycardiomyopathy,[8] as in this case, which recovers after regular sinus rhythm restoration. Alternans of 2 slightly different QRS complex

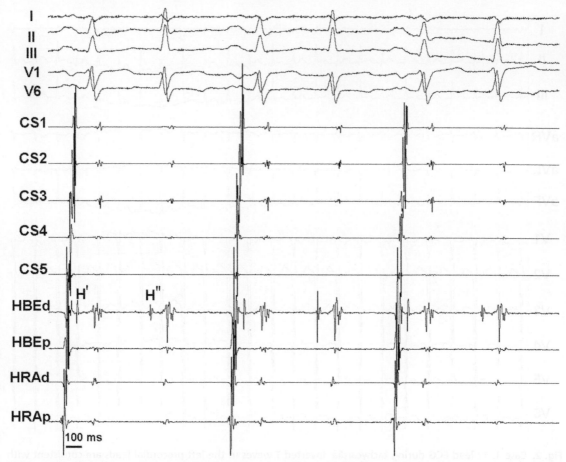

Fig. 3. Case 1: baseline tracings during EPS. In this, as in **Figs. 4**, **8A,12,15,16**, and **17**, tracings are displayed from top to bottom as follows: surface ECG, bipolar recordings of the coronary sinus catheter, from distal (CS1) to proximal (CS5), of the distal (HBEd) and proximal (HBEp) His bundle catheter, and of the distal (HRAd) and proximal (HRAp) high right atrium catheter. A sinus impulse is present every 2 ventricular beats, generated by simultaneous conduction over a fast and slow AV node pathways giving origin to H′ and H″, respectively. A-H′ interval measures 67 ms, A-H″ interval 525 ms and both H′-V and H″-V intervals measure 50 ms. CS1, distal coronary sinus catheter; CS5, proximal coronary sinus catheter; HBEd, distal His bundle catheter; HBEp, proximal His bundle catheter; HRAd, distal high right atrium catheter; HRAp, proximal high right atrium catheter.

morphologies in dual AV nodal nonreentrant tachycardia has been already reported,[8] also including patients with bundle branch block.[10] This could be due to a different input of the fast and slow pathway into the His bundle, corroborating the hypothesis that in the presence of dual AV node physiology there might be a longitudinal dissociation, which extends to the distal part of the AV conduction pathway.[11]

Finally, as previously reported for this arrhythmia,[7,8] catheter ablation of the slow pathway is safe and curative.

CASE 2. JUNCTIONAL TACHYCARDIA
Clinical Presentation

A 56-year-old male hypertensive patient with prior history of paroxysmal palpitations for 6 months

presented at the emergency department for a prolonged episode. On admittance, the 12-lead ECG showed an NCT, with a heart rate of 165 beats per minute (**Fig. 6**). The arrhythmia was then terminated by intravenous administration of 5 mg of metoprolol with sinus rhythm restoration (**Fig. 7**). Because the arrhythmia was recurrent, the patient was admitted to the ward for further noninvasive and invasive evaluation. Transthoracic echocardiogram showed mild left ventricular hypertrophy with normal ejection fraction and mild mitral valve prolapse with no regurgitation. Exercise stress test was unremarkable. Then, the patient underwent EPS.

Electrocardiogram Interpretation

Generally, when a patient with an NCT is approached, AVNRT or AV reentrant tachycardia

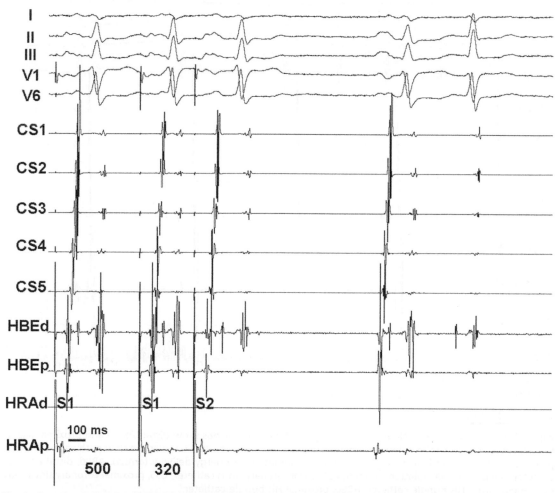

Fig. 4. Case 1: programmed high right atrial stimulation at a drive of 500 ms (S1) and a premature (S2) beat with a coupling interval of 320 ms. Although with longer coupling intervals the A-H″ interval progressively prolonged to a maximum of 585 ms, now conduction over the slow pathway is blocked at this critical S1-S2 interval. CS1, distal coronary sinus catheter; CS5, proximal coronary sinus catheter; HBEd, distal His bundle catheter; HBEp, proximal His bundle catheter; HRAd, distal high right atrium catheter; HRAp, proximal high right atrium catheter.

(AVRT) is first hypothesized. In these arrhythmias, a retrograde P wave can be clearly identified after each QRS complex. This is not the case in the ECG of this patient. Not only is there no clearly distinguishable P wave after the QRS complex, but also a dissociated P wave can be detected especially in lead V1, which excludes AVRT. Moreover, comparing the ECGs during arrhythmia and sinus rhythm, the QRS complex has approximately the same duration, but the QRS axis is definitely more vertical during tachycardia. Although in rare cases a dissociated atrial activity during AVNRT is possible, it is usually intermittent and reversed by isoproterenol infusion.[12] On the other hand, in this case, the combined findings of dissociated P waves and slightly different morphology of the QRS complex during tachycardia are against AVNRT and highly

in favor of junctional tachycardia. This diagnosis was confirmed at the EPS: ventriculoatrial dissociation during ventricular pacing was present even during isoproterenol infusion, with no evidence of dual AV node physiology. During β-adrenergic stimulation, the clinical arrhythmia could be induced only by burst ventricular pacing. Tachycardia also initiated spontaneously during isoproterenol infusion with iterative presentation. During tachycardia, the H-V interval was shorter than in sinus rhythm, and a distal to proximal activation of the His bundle was observed (**Fig. 8**). Moreover, accurate mapping of the right and left side of the upper septum identified the earliest activated ventricular area on the left side, in strict anatomic relationship with the left bundle branch (**Fig. 9**). For the high risk of AV conduction damage, ablation was not performed and therapy

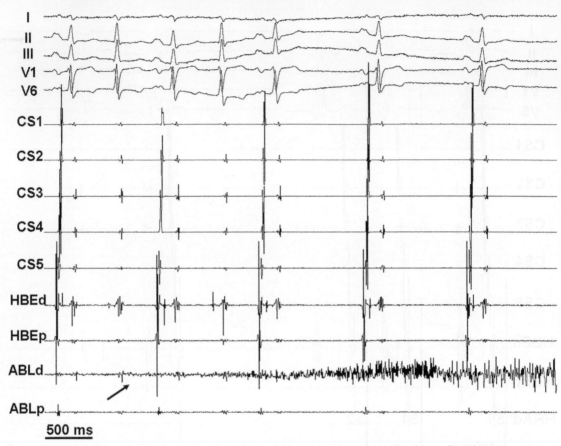

Fig. 5. Case 1: slow pathway ablation. In this figure, the last 2 tracings show distal (ABLd) and proximal (ABLp) bipolar recordings from the ablation catheter. Suppression of the conduction over the slow pathway with disappearance of the second beat is observed soon after initiation of energy delivery (*arrow*). ABLd, distal ablation catheter; ABLp, proximal ablation catheter; CS1, distal coronary sinus catheter; CS5, proximal coronary sinus catheter; HBEd, distal His bundle catheter; HBEp, proximal His bundle catheter.

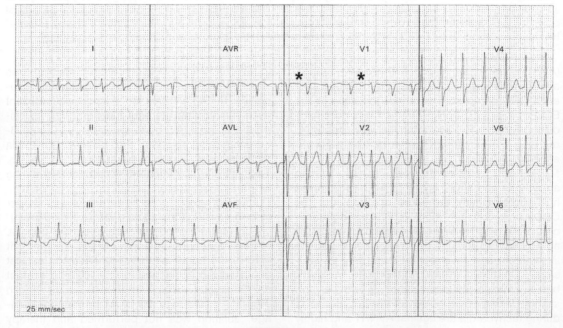

Fig. 6. Case 2: 12-lead ECG during tachycardia. Asterisks identify dissociated P waves.

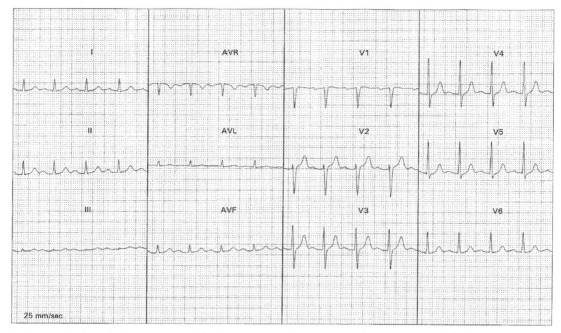

Fig. 7. Case 2: sinus rhythm is restored by intravenous administration of 5 mg of metoprolol; the longer P-R interval is related to β-blocker administration. CS1, distal coronary sinus catheter; CS5, proximal coronary sinus catheter; HBEd, distal His bundle catheter; HBEp, proximal His bundle catheter; HRAd, distal high right atrium catheter; HRAp, proximal high right atrium catheter.

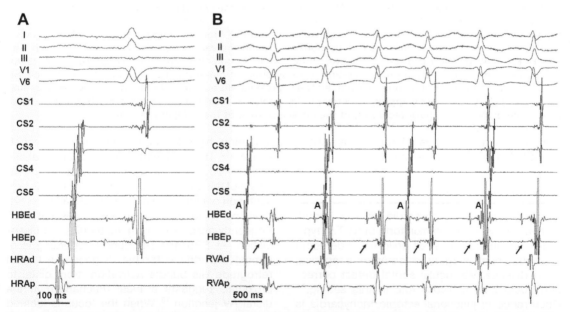

Fig. 8. Case 2: intracavitary recordings during EPS; tracings are displayed (as in **Fig. 3**) with the only difference the last 2 tracings show distal (RVAd) and proximal (RVAp) bipolar recordings from the catheter positioned in the right ventricular apex (*B*). A-H and H-V intervals are 110 and 45 ms, respectively (*A*). During tachycardia (*B*), the atrial activity (*A*) is dissociated from the ventricular; the H-V interval is 28 ms, shorter than during sinus rhythm; and a distal to proximal activation of the His bundle is observed. The first beat is the result of minor fusion between the junctional tachycardia and sinus beat; the activation sequence of the His bundle is inverted compared with the other beats, and the morphology of the QRS complex slightly changes with a less vertical axis compared with the other beats. Conversely, the third sinus beat (third *A*) occurs too late and is unable to modify the His bundle sequence and the surface ECG as the first beat did. Arrows indicate proximal His bundle deflection. CS1, distal coronary sinus catheter (CS1); CS5, proximal coronary sinus catheter; HBEd, distal His bundle catheter; HBEp, proximal His bundle catheter; HRAd, distal high right atrium catheter; HRAp, proximal high right atrium catheter; RVAd, distal right ventricular apex catheter; RVAP, proximal right ventricular apex catheter.

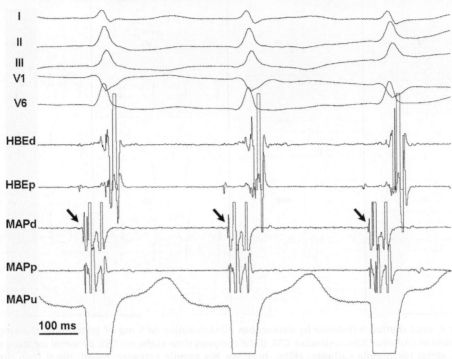

Fig. 9. Case 2: mapping of the left upper ventricular septum, reached transeptally. From top to bottom, the following tracings are displayed: surface ECG, distal and proximal bipolar recordings of the His bundle (HBEd and HBEp) and mapping (MAPd and MAPp) catheters, and the unipolar recording of the distal electrode of the mapping catheter (MAPu). The site of earliest ventricular activation is shown in MAPd, where a high-frequency prepotential likely related to the proximal left bundle branch is present (*arrows*). MAPu shows a concomitant steep negative intrinsicoid deflection, confirming the earliest ventricular activation in this site. The HBEp, now positioned distally, however, shows a His bundle deflection, which precedes by 15 ms the earliest ventricular activation, suggesting a tachycardia origin from the very distal part of the His bundle/fascicle. HBEd, distal His bundle catheter; HBEp, proximal His bundle catheter; MAPd, bipolar recording of the distal electrode of the mapping catheter; MAPp, bipolar recording of the proximal electrode of the mapping catheter; MAPu, unipolar recording of the distal electrode of the mapping catheter.

with oral metoprolol was initiated. The subsequent follow-up was uneventful.

Clinical Considerations

Junctional ectopic tachycardia or His bundle tachycardia is an uncommon form of NCT,[13] typically encountered in small children undergoing corrective heart surgery for complex congenital heart disease. Ventricular septal defect correction could play a pivotal role in this setting.[14] Occurrence of junctional ectopic tachycardia is particularly worrisome in this pediatric population because it is associated with a rapid ventricular rate, potentially causing acute heart failure. If this tachycardia is considered uncommon in a pediatric population with structural heart disease, it is particularly rare in patients without heart disease and even less common in adults.[12] In the latter setting, silent automatic foci close to the His bundle region could be unmasked by specific situations, such as fever, or other conditions,

triggering high levels of circulating catecholamines.[12] This suggests enhanced automaticity or triggered activity as a pathophysiologic mechanism of this tachycardia.[12] The typical ECG presentation of junctional arrhythmias is a fast (>170 beats per minute), in some cases incessant, NCT frequently associated with ventriculoatrial dissociation. At EPS, the His bundle recording is of utmost importance for the diagnosis: a typical retrograde His bundle activation, from distal to proximal, suggests a focal mechanism in the distal AV junction.[15] When the focus is located distally in the His bundle/fascicle, the H-V interval during tachycardia is shorter than that recorded during sinus rhythm, because there is an overlap in the timing of the His bundle and ventricular activation.[16] In cases affected by very frequent Hisian ectopies, it has been suggested that the accurate standard and 3-D mapping of the right and left upper septal regions could be useful to accurately definite the site of arrhythmia origin.[17,18] Catheter ablation of junctional

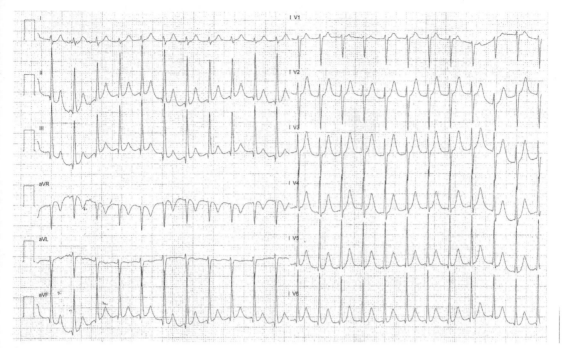

Fig. 10. Case 3: 12-lead ECG during tachycardia.

tachycardia could be particularly harmful due to the close proximity of these ectopic foci to the His bundle and compact AV node. For this reason, cryoablation should be considered for the well-known safe and effective profile.[16,19]

CASE 3. SINUS TACHYCARDIA RELATED TO LONG P-R INTERVAL
Clinical Presentation

A 21-year-old female patient came to medical attention for recurrent effort related episodes of palpitations. Symptoms started several years before but worsened over the past months. The rest 12-lead ECG was unremarkable, as was the transthoracic echocardiogram. Effort stress test reproduced symptoms during the postexercise phase and the NCT (shown in **Fig. 10**) was recorded. The arrhythmia spontaneously terminated after a few minutes. The patient was then referred for EPS and catheter ablation of these supraventricular tachycardia.

Electrocardiogram Interpretation

During tachycardia (see **Fig. 10**), the heart rate is 136 beats per minutes and no clearly visible P

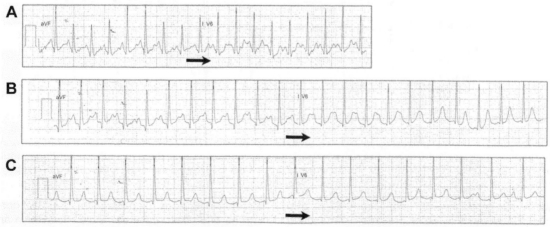

Fig. 11. Case 3: sequential (*arrow*) ECG recording in lead aVF and V6 of the maximal heart rate during effort test (*A*), after 2 minutes (*B*), and 10 (*C*) minutes from effort test termination. See text for further explanations.

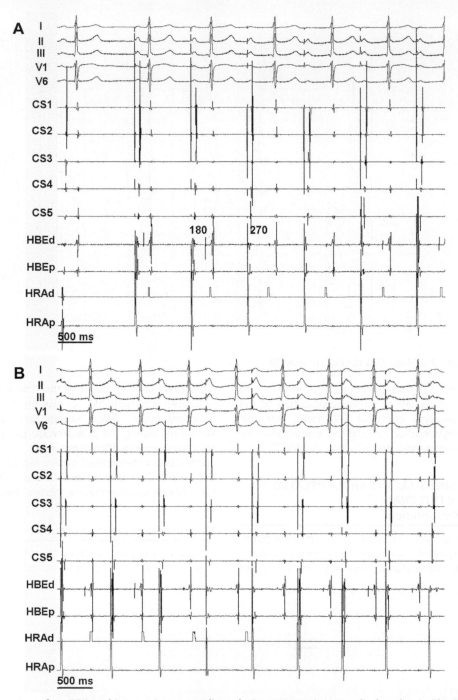

Fig. 12. Case 3: surface ECG and intracavitary recordings during EPS; tracings are displayed as in **Fig. 3**. At baseline, the A-H interval is normal and when incremental atrial pacing is started at a cycle length of 800 ms (*A*), a sudden jump of the A-H interval up to 270 ms is observed for the transition of conduction from the fast pathway to the slow pathway. Subsequently, at a shorter pacing cycle, conduction over the slow pathway continues until, at a pacing cycle length of 680 ms (*B*), the stimulated P wave hides into the T wave of the preceding QRS complex, reproducing what was spontaneously observed. Wenckebach point was at a pacing cycle length of 520 ms.

wave can be observed. A deflection that can be interpreted as a P wave precedes the second QRS complex, but this is not reproducibly and regularly observed in the following beats and, therefore, this leads to conclude for an artifact during the effort test. Lack of visible P waves in an NCT is highly suggestive of an AVNRT.[20] More information can be gathered, however, analyzing the

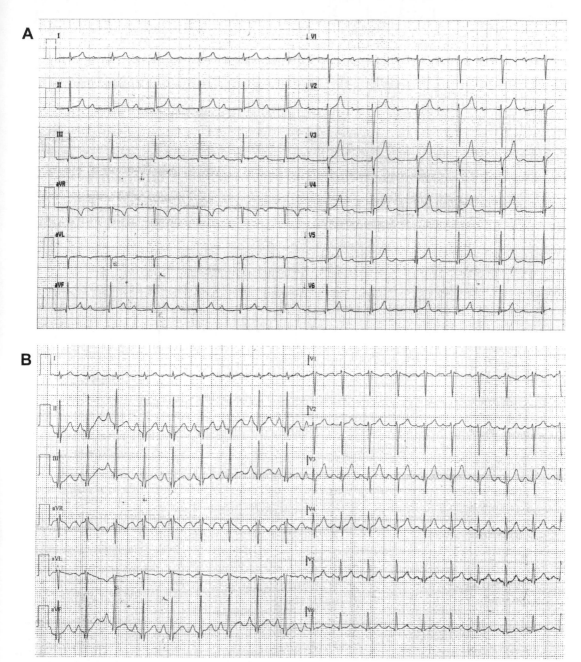

Fig. 13. Example in another patient of dual AV node pathway manifest during sinus rhythm without relevant symptoms. At rest (*A*), at a heart rate of 68 beats per minute, a first-degree AV block with a P-R interval of 400 ms is present, which represents the expression of AV conduction over a slow pathway. During mild effort (*B*), the sinus rate increases to 109 beats per minutes and the P-R interval normalizes (150 ms), as now AV conduction occurs over a fast pathway, which, under sympathetic stimulation, decreases its effective refractory period.

modality of onset and termination of the tachycardia during the effort stress test. During the test, the sinus rate increases up to a maximum of 176 beats per minute with a normal P-R interval (**Fig. 11**A). After 2 minutes from exercise termination, the sinus rate decreases to 136 beats per minutes and, concomitantly, the P-R interval progressively prolongs, so that the sinus P wave remains hidden in the T wave of the previous beat, mimicking a supraventricular tachycardia (**Fig. 11**B). The tachycardia continues for approximately 10 minutes with a progressive slowing of

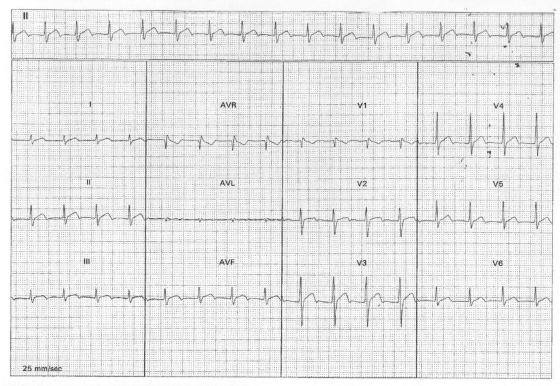

Fig. 14. Case 4: 12-lead ECG during palpitations.

the heart rate, until, at a rate of 100 beats per minute, the P-R interval suddenly shortens and the sinus P wave becomes manifest before the QRS complex (**Fig. 11**C). Then, the following P-P cycle is suddenly longer, probably for a respiratory sinus arrhythmia, and the last beat in **Fig. 11**C shows a normal P-R interval. Symptoms, possibly related to the AV contraction dyssynchrony, disappear at the time of P-R interval normalization. The diagnosis of sinus tachycardia is corroborated by the observation that the P-wave morphology does not change on the 12-lead ECG at the time of tachycardia initiation and termination and by the lack of a pause, which is typically observed on termination of a supraventricular tachycardia. EPS was performed to further exclude supraventricular arrhythmias. Dual AV node physiology was evident even at longer atrial pacing cycles, with a jump from the fast pathway to the slow pathway at cycle length of 800 ms (**Fig. 12**). Even during isoproterenol infusion, retrograde conduction over the AV node was absent and no arrhythmia was induced by aggressive stimulation protocols. During follow-up, symptoms were markedly improved by administration of low dose ivabradine.

Clinical Considerations

Inappropriate sinus tachycardia is a clinical entity defined by fast sinus rates without any clear explanation or out of proportion to any known stressor.[21] Inappropriate sinus tachycardia has been described after both radiofrequency[22] and cryothermal energy[23] ablation of AVNRT. This complication occurs more frequently when the fast pathway is damaged; in these cases, a good response to pharmacologic treatment with ivabradine[24] suggests a pivotal role of the sinus node in the pathophysiology of this phenomenon. Previous studies indicate parasympathetic denervation as a possible mechanism.[22,23]

In the clinical case presented, the possible mechanism leading to sinus tachycardia perceived by the patient as palpitations seems different. The patient had not previously undergone any ablation; therefore, the mechanism of this tachycardia associated with a long P-R interval must be different from that proposed previously. To the authors' knowledge, similar cases have not been previously described and, therefore, the pathophysiology of this condition has not been thoroughly investigated. These cases, however, deserve some considerations, because, in the authors' experience, some of these young patients are referred for invasive arrhythmia evaluation.

It is well known that dual AV node physiology can be evident spontaneously during sinus rhythm, giving origin to P-R intervals markedly different during sinus rhythm, mimicking an intermittent first-degree AV block (**Fig. 13**). In some juveniles, the Wenckebach cycle length can be longer than 600 ms and the effective refractory

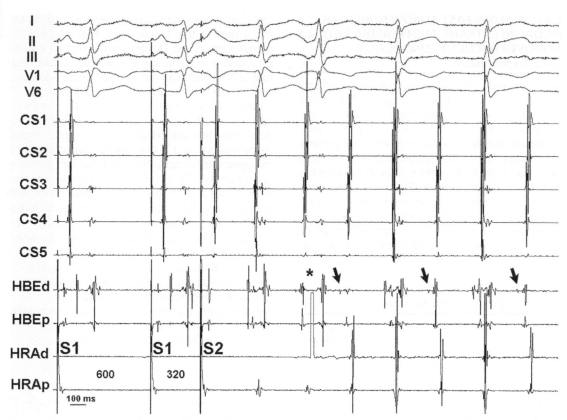

Fig. 15. Case 4: in this and in **Fig. 16** and **17**, the display of surface and intracavitary recordings is as in **Fig. 3**. During programmed atrial stimulation at 600-ms cycle length, a premature beat with a coupling interval of 320 ms critically prolongs the A-H interval and induces the AVNRT. In the first tachycardia beat, the His bundle potential followed by an atrial deflection is well evident with an H-V interval of 40 ms, whereas in the second beat (*asterisk*), it shows a minimal amplitude and the H-V interval is prolonged. Afterward, 2:1 AV conduction occurs with a His bundle potential (*arrows*) preceding an atrial deflection in the distally blocked beat. In the blocked beats, the amplitude of the His bundle is smaller compared with the one of the conducted beats. CS1, distal coronary sinus catheter; CS5, proximal coronary sinus catheter; HBEd, distal His bundle catheter; HBEp, proximal His bundle catheter; HRAd, distal high right atrium catheter; HRAp, proximal high right atrium catheter.

period of the fast pathway longer than 500 ms, although fast pathway conduction markedly improves during β-adrenergic stimulation and after successful ablation of the slow pathway in patients with AVNRT.[25] During sinus rhythm, when AV conduction occurs persistently over the slow pathway with a longer P-R interval, the sinus P wave is very close or even superimposed to the T wave of the preceding beat. This has 2 consequences that may explain both the symptoms and perpetuation of a higher sinus rate. The first is that the atrial contraction occurs when the AV valves are closed and this increases atrial pressure in the thoracic veins, possibly leading to the perception of palpitations. The second is that, in this circumstance, atrial contraction causes also atrial distension and this could lead to perpetuation of a higher sinus rate due to

Bainbridge reflex, although in humans its role is not completely clear.[26] Symptoms disappear when P-R interval normalizes. The good response to ivabradine further suggests the involvement of the sinus node in the maintenance of the arrhythmogenic mechanism.

Although there is some evidence that slow pathway ablation in children with AVNRT improves fast pathway conduction capability, potentially suppressing manifest dual AV node physiology during sinus rhythm, slow pathway ablation in the absence of AVNRT, as in the authors' case, is questionable and should be avoided. Further studies are needed to better investigate this phenomenon. Meanwhile, electrophysiologists should take into consideration the possibility of such a tachycardia, to avoid potentially harmful ablation of the sinus node.

CASE 4. SLOW-FAST ATRIOVENTRICULAR NODAL REENTRANT TACHYCARDIA WITH 2:1 ATRIOVENTRICULAR CONDUCTION
Case Presentation

A 17-year-old male patient without prior significant clinical history came to the emergency department for sudden onset of palpitations. On admittance, symptoms slightly improved, but palpitations, especially localized in the neck, were still present. A 12-lead ECG showed a slow NCT with a ventricular rate of 100 beats per minutes and incomplete right bundle branch block (**Fig. 14**). Carotid sinus massage promptly restored sinus rhythm, still conducted with incomplete right bundle branch block. Echocardiogram showed no evidence of structural heart disease; routine blood sample analysis was unremarkable. Thereafter, the patient was referred for EPS.

Electrocardiogram Interpretation

A narrow P wave, negative in the inferior and lateral leads, can be detected in the middle of 2 QRS complexes, partially superimposed to the terminal part of the T wave (see **Fig. 14**). For the morphology of the P wave, sinus rhythm can be excluded. For the longer P-R interval at this heart rate, a 1:1 atrial tachycardia also can be excluded. The 2 most likely hypothesis are a 2:1 atrial tachycardia or AVNRT, with 2:1 distal conduction block. The narrow P wave suggests a concentric atrial activation possibly related to a septal focus/reentry circuit, but it also fits the hypothesis of a retrograde atrial activation over the fast pathway during an AVNRT. Finally, although rarer, atypical (slow-slow) AVNRT and orthodromic AVRT with retrograde conduction over a very slow/decremental AV accessory pathway cannot be excluded. The slow tachycardia rate, however, almost rules out these hypotheses and, once terminated, the tachycardia did not show an iterative presentation, as frequently observed in the previously discussed form of arrhythmia.

During EPS, dual AV node pathway was evident with a normal Wenckebach cycle length. Programmed atrial stimulation (**Fig. 15**) induced the

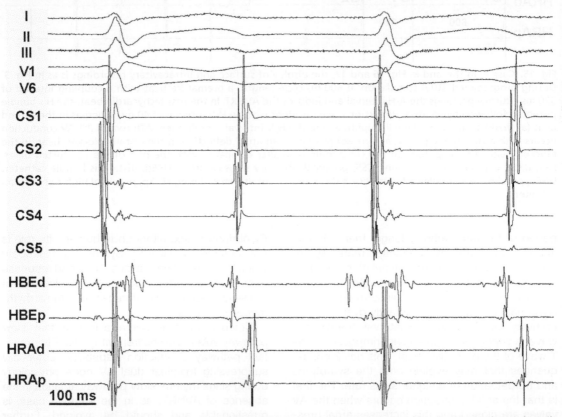

Fig. 16. Case 4: 2:1 AVNRT at a higher sweep speed. Both in the conducted beat and blocked beat, the His bundle precedes the atrial deflection with a short H-A interval, whereas the atrial activation sequence is consistent with a slow-fast AVNRT. The amplitude of the His bundle potential is invariably lower in the blocked beat, with a regular alternans of higher and lower amplitude of the His bundle potential. CS1, distal coronary sinus catheter; CS5, proximal coronary sinus catheter; HBEd, distal His bundle catheter; HBEp, proximal His bundle catheter; HRAd, distal high right atrium catheter; HRAp, proximal high right atrium catheter.

clinical arrhythmia when a sudden jump in the A-H interval was observed in the premature beat. The modality of induction, the H-A interval, and the sequence of atrial activation during tachycardia associated with the presence of a 2:1 AV block distal to the His bundle deflection confirm the diagnosis of typical AVNRT (see **Fig. 15**; **Fig. 16**). Atrial burst pacing during tachycardia with 2:1 AV conduction transiently prolonged the A-H interval and favored the recovery of refractoriness of the distal AV conduction pathway, so that 1:1 conduction was possible with the typical aspect of AVNRT (**Fig. 17**). Slow pathway ablation suppressed the arrhythmia induction and permanently cured the patient.

Clinical Considerations

Clinically, it is important to keep in mind that 2:1 AV conduction during tachycardia does not exclude the hypothesis of an AVNRT. A lower prevalence of AVNRT, with 2:1 conduction block, has been reported in adults[27] compared with children[28] (9% vs 17%, respectively). Development changes in autonomic tone and conduction physiology might contribute to this phenomenon.[28] Different studies have investigated the possible location of the site of block in these patients. Although in several cases the site of conduction block can be relatively proximal, between the AV node and the proper His bundle,[29] other reports suggest an intra-Hisian or infra- Hisian location of the site block due to the high prevalence of cases with a His bundle potential in the blocked beats at EPS during tachycardia, varying from 62% to 75%.[27,30,31] Moreover, the lack of response to atropine corroborates the hypothesis that this phenomenon during tachycardia is due to a distal block.[27] Regardless of the site of conduction block, there is strong evidence that mechanism of block is based on a functional phenomenon. The difference in refractoriness between the input in the proximal His bundle of the slow pathway, with longer effective refractory period, and the the input in the proximal His bundle of the fast pathway, with shorter effective refractory period, can play a major role in the genesis of this functional phenomenon.[29,32] Moreover, the shorter tachycardia cycle length frequently observed in these cases favors a functional 2:1 AV conduction block.[27,28] In addition, the observation of spontaneous conversion from 2:1 AV conduction to 1:1 AV conduction through a phase of aberrant conduction, with transient prolongation of the H-V interval,

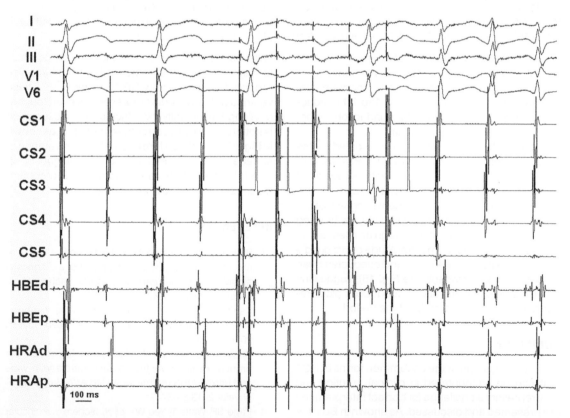

Fig. 17. Case 4: coronary sinus burst pacing at 240 ms during 2:1 AVNRT minimally but critically prolongs the A-H interval in the last paced beat and allows recovery from refractoriness of the distal His bundle and, therefore, 1:1 AV conduction during tachycardia.

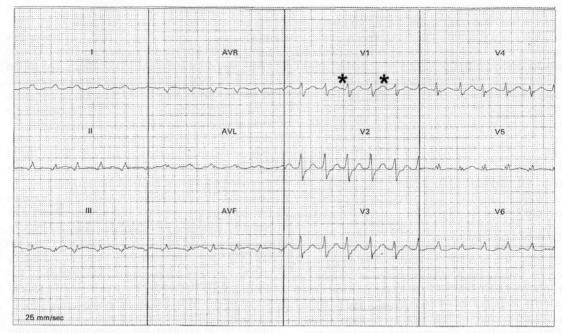

Fig. 18. Twelve-lead ECG of a ventricular tachycardia with a relatively narrow QRS complex (108 ms) in a patient with prior inferior myocardial infarction. Dissociated P waves are evident, especially in lead V1 (*asterisks*). At EPS, ventriculoatrial dissociation was confirmed; reentry circuit involving a low-voltage area in the upper left septum was identified and successfully ablated with no damage to the distal conduction system. For the ventricular rate of 140 beats per minute, the arrhythmia was misdiagnosed as atrial flutter by the attending physician. Notches in the terminal part of the QRS complex in lead V2-V4 also can be misinterpreted as retrograde P waves, leading to the possible misdiagnosis of a reentrant supraventricular arrhythmia.

suggests a proximal migration of the site of block, to be interpreted as a functional phenomenon.[30] Finally, the observation that a ventricular premature depolarization may convert from 2:1 to 1:1 conduction by resetting the distal AV conduction further supports a functional mechanism.

Another interesting feature is represented by the variable amplitudes of the His bundle potential during 2:1 conduction of AVNRT, with evidence of lower amplitude in nonconducted beats.[27,30] This finding may be explained by variable degrees of impulse penetration in the His bundle in the blocked beats. In the authors' case, a regular alternans of small amplitude and normal amplitude of His bundle potential in each blocked beat and conducted beat, respectively, was evident (see **Fig. 16**), suggesting that in some cases the site of conduction block remains constant over a certain time period.

SUMMARY

In this article, some of the uncommon forms of NCT that can be encountered in clinical practice and may represent a challenge for correct interpretation are presented and discussed. As shown in **Box 1**, a ventricular substrate also may generate a narrow QRS complex, if this substrate is close to or directly

involves the proximal part of the specific conduction system, which is responsible for fast impulse propagation and narrow QRS complex.[3,4,6] These ventricular tachycardias represent an even tougher challenge, especially if ventriculoatrial dissociation is not present or not correctly recognized, as shown in **Fig. 18**. In all these forms, careful interpretation of surface ECG is useful for correct diagnosis. In several cases, invasive EPS is needed to confirm diagnosis and cure the arrhythmia.

REFERENCES

1. Buttà C, Tuttolomondo A, Di Raimondo D, et al. Supraventricular tachycardias: proposal of a diagnostic algorithm for the narrow complex tachycardias. J Cardiol 2013;61:247–55.
2. Katritsis DG, Josephson ME. Differential diagnosis of regular, narrow-QRS tachycardias. Heart Rhythm 2015;12:1667–76.
3. Kusa S, Tamiguchi H, Hachiya H, et al. Bundle branch reentrant ventricular tachycardia with wide and narrow QRS morphology. Circ Arrhythm Electrophysiol 2013;6:e87–91.
4. Page SP, Watts T, Yeo WT, et al. Ischemic ventricular tachycardia presenting as a narrow complex tachycardia. Indian Pacing Electrophysiol J 2014;14:203–10.

5. Katritsis DG, Boriani G, Cosio FG, et al. European Heart Rhythm Association (EHRA) consensus document on the management of supraventricular arrhythmias, endorsed by Heart Rhythm Society (HRS), Asia-Pacific Heart Rhythm Society (APHRS), and Sociedad Latinoamericana de Estimulacion Cardiaca y Electro-fisiologia (SOLAECE). Europace 2017;19:465–511.

6. Guo XG, Liu X, Zhou GB, et al. Clinical, electrocardiographic, and electrophysiological characteristic of the left upper septal fascicular ventricular tachycardia. Europace 2018;20:673–81.

7. Wang NC. Dual atrioventricular nodal nonreentrant tachycardia: a systematic review. Pacing Clin Electrophysiol 2011;34:1671–81.

8. Peiker C, Pott C, Eckardt L, et al. Dual atrioventricular nodal non-re-entrant tachicardia. Europace 2016;18:332–9.

9. Tomasi C, De Ponti R, Tritto M, et al. Simulataneous dual fast and slow pathway conduction upon induction of typical atrioventricular nodal reentrant tachycardia: electrophysiologic characteristics in a series of patients. J Cardiovasc Electrophysiol 2005;16:594–600.

10. Li VH, Mallick A, Concannon C, et al. Wide complex tachycardia causing congestive heart failure. Pacing Clin Electrophysiol 2011;34:1154–7.

11. Zhang Y. His electrogram alternans (Zhang's phenomenon) and a new model of dual pathway atrioventricular node conduction. J Interv Card Electrophysiol 2016;45:19–28.

12. Brochu BD, Abdi-Ali A, Shaw J, et al. Successful radiofrequency ablation of junctional ectopic tachycardia in an adult patient. HeartRhythm Case Rep 2018;4:251–5.

13. Di Biase L, Gianni C, Bagliani G, et al. Arrhythmias involving the atrioventricular junction. Card Electrophysiol Clin 2017;9:435–52.

14. Haas NA, Plumpton K, Justo R, et al. Postoperative junctional ectopic tachycardia (JET). Z Kardiol 2004;93:371–80.

15. Choi KJ, Shah DC, Jais P, et al. Successful ablation of Hisian ectopy identified by a reversed His bundle activation sequence. J Interv Card Electrophysiol 2002;6:183–6.

16. Eizmendi I, Almendral J, Hadid C, et al. Successful catheter cryoablation of Hisian ectopy using 2 new diagnostic criteria based on unipolar and bipolar recordings of the His electrogram. J Cardiovasc Electrophysiol 2012;23:325–9.

17. Yamashita S, Hooks DA, Hocini M, et al. Ablation of parahisian ventricular focus. HeartRhythm Case Rep 2015;1:64–7.

18. Pathak RK, Betensky BP, Santangeli P, et al. Distinct electrocardiographic form of idiopathic ventricular arrhythmia originating from the left bundle branch. J Cardiovasc Electrophysiol 2017;28:115–9.

19. Law IH, Von Bergen NH, Gingerich JC, et al. Transcatheter cryothermal ablation of junctional ectopic tachycardia in the normal heart. Heart Rhythm 2006;3:903–7.

20. Rivera S, De La Paz Ricapito M, Conde D, et al. The retrograde P-wave theory explaining ST segment depression in supraventricular tachycardia by retrograde AV node conduction. Pacing Clin Electrophysiol 2014;37:1100–5.

21. Olshansky B, Sullivan RM. Inappropriate sinus tachycardia. Europace 2019;21:194–207.

22. Skeberis V, Simonis F, Tsakonas K, et al. Inappropriate sinus tachycardia following radiofrequency ablation of AV nodal tachycardia: incidence and clinical significance. Pacing Clin Electrophysiol 1994;17:924–7.

23. De Sisti A, Tonet J, Benkaci A, et al. A case of inappropriate sinus tachycardia after atrio-ventricular nodal reentrant tachycardia cryoablation successfully treated by ivabradine. Europace 2010;12:1029–31.

24. Capulzini L, Sarkozy A, Semeraro O, et al. Ivabradine to treat inappropriate sinus tachycardia after the fast pathway ablation in a patient with severe pectus excavatum. Pacing Clin Electrophysiol 2010;33:e32–5.

25. Van Hare GF, Chiesa NA, Campbell RM, et al. Atrioventricular nodale re-entrant tachycardia in children: effect of slow pathway ablation on fast pathway function. J Cardiovasc Electrophysiol 2002;13:203–9.

26. Kuhtz-Buschbeck JP, Schaefer J, Wilder N. Mechanosensitivity: from Aristotle's sense of touch to cardiac mechano-electric coupling. Prog Biophys Mol Biol 2017;130:126–31.

27. Man KC, Brinkman K, Bogun F, et al. 2:1 atrioventricular block during atrioventricular node reentrant tachycardia. J Am Coll Cardiol 1996;28:1770–4.

28. Mahajan T, Berul CI, Cecchin F, et al. Atrioventricular nodal reentrant tachycardia with 2:1 block in pediatric patients. Heart Rhythm 2008;5:1391–5.

29. Bagliani G, Leonelli FM, De Ponti R, et al. Advanced concepts of atrioventricular nodal electrophysiology: observations on the mechanism of atrioventricular nodal reciprocating tachycardias. Card Electrophysiol Clin 2018;10:277–97.

30. Lee SH, Tai CT, Chiang CE, et al. Spontaneous transition of 2:1 atrioventricular block to 1:1 atrioventricular conduction during atrioventricular nodal reentrant tachycardia: evidence supporting the intra-Hisian or infra-Hisian area as the site of block. J Cardiovasc Electrophysiol 2003;14:1337–41.

31. Wellens HJJ, Wesdorp JC, Duren DR, et al. Second degree block during reciprocal atrioventricular nodal tachycardia. Circulation 1976;53:595–9.

32. Zhang Y, Bharati S, Mowrey KA, et al. His electrogram alternans reveal dual-wavefront inputs into and longitudinal dissociation within the bundle of His. Circulation 2001;104:832–8.

Challenging Cases of Wide Complex Tachycardias
Use and Limits of Algorithms

Alessandra Tordini, MD[a],*, Fabio M. Leonelli, MD[b],
Roberto De Ponti, MD, FHRS[c], Giuseppe Bagliani, MD[d],
Stefano Donzelli, MD[a], Ludovico Lazzari, MD[a],
Chiara Marini, MD[a], Marco M. Pirrami, MD[a],
Giovanni Carreras, MD[a]

KEYWORDS

- Wide QRS complex tachycardia • Ventricular tachycardia • Aberrant ventricular conduction
- Arrhythmogenic right ventricular cardiomyopathy • Epsilon wave
- Right branch ventricular tachycardia • Outflow tract ventricular tachycardia

KEY POINTS

- Electrocardiographic algorithms allow in most cases a differential diagnosis between supraventricular and ventricular arrhythmia.
- Particular situations such as the presence of accessory pathways, use of antiarrhythmic drugs, congenital heart diseases, and artificial pacing make the interpretation of the electrocardiogram complex.
- Ventricular tachycardias arising within the conduction system generate a relatively narrow QRS, which may be confused with supraventricular arrhythmia.
- In conditions of hemodynamic stability, the use of drugs such as adenosine can be helpful in interpreting the ECG.

INTRODUCTION

Wide QRS complex tachycardias (WCT) are cardiac rhythm disorders of 3 or more consecutive beats, with rates exceeding 100 beats per minute and a QRS duration of 120 milliseconds or greater. The width of the QRS complex should be verified in all leads, because the QRS complex can often be narrower in 1 or 2 of the 12 leads. WCT could be due to aberrant atrioventricular (AV) conduction, ventricular origin, ventricular pre-excitation, or ventricular pacing.[1]

Palpitation, syncope, angina, and the patient's hemodynamic state during tachycardia are important, but they are not helpful in determining the mechanism of the arrhythmia.

Careful step by step analysis of the electrocardiogram (ECG) can lead us to the correct diagnosis in most cases (**Box 1**).[1–7]

Some conditions, such as electrolyte imbalance, administration of antiarrhythmic drugs (AADs), or accessory AV pathways, can make the differential diagnosis difficult, and knowledge of

No relevant conflict to disclose for any of the authors.
No funding sources received for any of the authors.
[a] Arrhythmology Unit, Cardiology Department, Terni Hospital, Piazzale Tristano da Joannuccio, 1, Terni 05100, Italy; [b] Cardiology Department, James A. Haley Veterans' Hospital, University South Florida, Tampa, FL, USA; [c] Department of Cardiology, School of Medicine, University of Insubria, Viale Borri, 57, Varese 21100, Italy; [d] Arrhythmology Unit, Cardiology Department, Foligno General Hospital, Via Massimo Arcamone, Foligno, Perugia 06034, Italy
* Corresponding author.
E-mail address: alessandratordini@gmail.com

Card Electrophysiol Clin 11 (2019) 301–314
https://doi.org/10.1016/j.ccep.2019.02.008

Box 1
Electrocardiographic criteria to discriminate between ventricular and supraventricular origin in wide QRS complex tachycardia

- Identification of atrial activity
- Relationship between atrial and ventricular activity
  - AV dissociation = VT
- Morphologic changes of the wide QRS complex during tachycardia
  - Capture and fusion beats = VT
  - Ashman phenomenon (aberrant conduction related to variations of the preceding cardiac cycle length) = SVT
- Detailed morphologic analysis of the wide QRS complex
  - Brugada algorithm
    - Absence of RS complex in all the precordial leads or negative/positive concordance → VT
    - Longest interval from R onset to S > 100 milliseconds in any precordial lead → VT
    - Further analysis of QRS complex morphology in V1, V2, and V6
      - RBBB or LBBB pattern (Sandler and Marriott criteria)[2]
        - Initial vector of the QRS complex identical to sinus rhythm → SVT
        - rSR′ complex with S crossing isoelectric line → SVT
        - Triphasic QRS complex in V1 → SVT
      - RBBB pattern (Wellens criteria)[3]
        - QRS width >140 milliseconds and left axis deviation → VT
        - QR, R, RSr′ (with S not crossing the isoelectric line) in V1 → VT
        - R/S < 1 or QS in V6 → VT
      - LBBB pattern (Kindwall criteria)[4]
        - R wave in V1 or V2 > 30 milliseconds → VT
        - Interval between QRS onset and nadir of the S wave in V1 or V2 >60 milliseconds → VT
        - Notch on the downstroke of the S wave in V1 or V2→ VT
        - Any Q wave in V6 → VT
      - Vereckei algorithm[6]
        - Initial, dominant R wave in aVR → VT
        - Initial, nondominant q or r in aVR >40 milliseconds → VT
        - Notch on the initial downstroke in aVR → VT
        - in aVR: Amplitude of the first 40 milliseconds of the QRS complex lover then amplitude of the last 40 milliseconds (V1/Vt < 1) → VT

Abbreviations: →, suggests diagnosis of; AV, atrioventricular; LBBB, left bundle branch block; RBBB, right bundle branch block; SVT, supraventricular tachycardia; VT, ventricular tachycardia.

Data from Refs.[1–6]

---

the patient's medical history plays a fundamental role in the diagnostic process.

Class IC AADs may cause unusual forms of aberrant conduction during supraventricular tachycardia (SVT) mimicking ventricular tachycardia (VT). The occurrence of bizarre bundle branch blocks (BBBs) during treatment with class IC AADs is likely due to use-dependent conduction delay, especially in the ventricular myocardium.[8] Class III AADs, especially dofetilide (pure IKr blockers), may cause alternating BBBs, which may be easily misdiagnosed as multiple monomorphic VTs. This may be related to cycle length-dependent bundle branch delay and retrograde penetration in the ipsilateral bundle.[9]

In the case of hemodynamic stability and uncertain diagnosis it may be useful to administer drugs such as adenosine triphosphate for diagnostic maneuver.[10]

This article presents challenging cases of wide QRS complex tachycardia with an analysis of the mechanism based on ECG findings.

CASE 1. ARRHYTHMOGENIC RIGHT VENTRICULAR CARDIOMYOPATHY
Case Presentation

A 60-year-old man arrived at the emergency room following an aborted cardiac arrest. Initial ECG showed a sustained monomorphic tachycardia suggestive of VT (**Fig. 1**). The patient was cardioverted to sinus rhythm (SR).

Morphologic analysis of the tracing shows a WCT with cycle length of 280 milliseconds, a QRS duration of 160 milliseconds, left bundle branch block (LBBB) morphology in lead V1 with the interval between QRS beginning and nadir greater than 60 milliseconds (110 ms) and downstroke notch (red arrow) in the same lead (Kindwall criteria, see **Box 1**). The precordial transition in lead V5 and the axis suggest a VT exit site from the right ventricular outflow tract.

Echocardiography and coronary angiography were normal. Cardiac magnetic resonance showed increased right ventricular (RV) dimension, reduced (43%) RV ejection fraction (EF), dyssynergic areas in the free wall of the RV, adipose

infiltration, and fibrosis areas in the lower and free walls of the RV. The resting ECG showed, for the first time, an epsilon wave (**Fig. 2**B). Combining the 3 major criteria (cardiac magnetic resonance evidence of dyssynergic areas, epsilon wave, and sustained VT) and the minor criteria (reduction of EF and the increased dimension of the RV), a reliable diagnosis of arrhythmogenic RV cardiomyopathy was made.

The patient underwent placement of an implantable cardioverter-defibrillator (ICD).

Clinical Considerations

Arrhythmogenic RV cardiomyopathy is a progressive hereditary heart muscle disorder mostly inherited as an autosomal dominant disease caused by mutations of genes encoding for the desmosomal protein plkophilin-2 (PKP2),[11] resulting in progressive loss of myocardial cells replaced by fatty tissue predominantly affecting the RV. This abnormality induces areas of slow conduction and altered refractoriness leading to re-entrant ventricular arrhythmias (VAs).

The epsilon wave is an electrical potential of small amplitude that occurs at the end of the QRS complex and at the beginning of the ST segment in the right precordial leads (V1-V3). A high pass filter of 40 Hz, an increase of gain to 20 mV/mm, and a recording speed to 50 mm/s help identification of the epsilon wave. It represents areas of delayed activation (usually localized

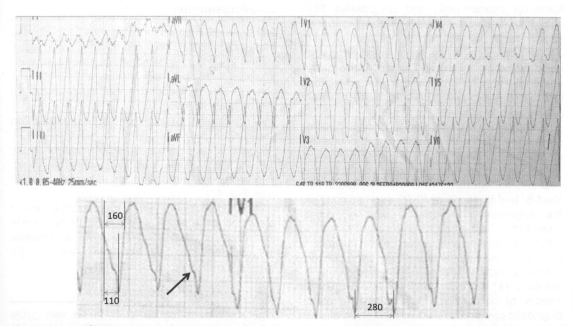

Fig. 1. Case 1. The ECG recorded at the time of admission. It shows a WCT with left bundle branch block (LBBB) morphology. See text for figure explanation.

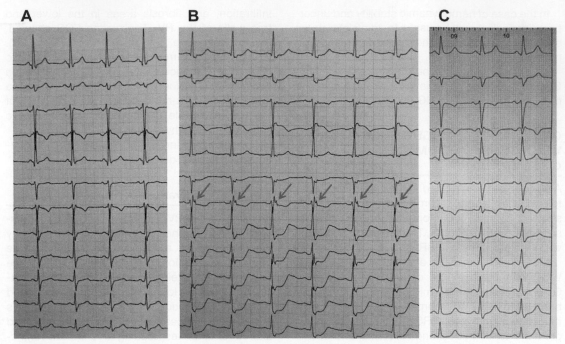

Fig. 2. Case 1. ECG 3 months before the cardiac arrest is within normal limits (*A*) as is the ECG recorded 3 days after cardiac arrest (*C*). ECG post defibrillation shows sinus rhythm (*B*), with epsilon wave (*blue arrows*).

in the RV but also in the left ventricle [LV]) caused by fibrous and/or fibro-fatty replacement of myocardium; its presence is considered a major diagnostic criterion.

Although the ECG is normal in up to 40% of patients at the initial stage of the disease, during the follow-up characteristic and progressive ECG changes will occur, suggestive of disease progression.[12] Diagnostic electrocardiographic features of inherited channelopathies are frequently transient, being present in 1 ECG and absent in the subsequent tracings; this characteristic, well described in Brugada syndrome,[13] was also evident in our patient (**Fig. 2**A, C).

The epsilon wave, as a manifestation of delayed conduction, may be accentuated by other channelopathies associated with the desmosomal defect.

Several studies have demonstrated that the desmosomal protein PKP2 coprecipitates with Nav1.5, and that loss of PKP2 expression alters the amplitude and kinetics of the sodium current (INa).[14,15]

In this patient, a cardioversion shock could have induced an increase of intracellular Ca^{2+} concentration, invreasing diastolic transmembrane V, reducing Na^+ channel availability, and decreasing velocity of conduction. The appearance of the diagnostic epsilon wave would have been a manifestation of the slowing of impulse propagation. The evidence of the epsilon wave only in the

ECG recorded after defibrillation could therefore have been due to a "defibrillation revealing effect."

CASE 2. VENTRICULAR TACHYCARDIA ORIGINATING FROM THE RIGHT BUNDLE BRANCH NEAR THE HIS BUNDLE
Case Presentation

A 76-year-old man without structural heart disease was evaluated for palpitation of 48 hours duration.

The ECG during palpitations shows a well-tolerated wide QRS tachycardia, with QRS duration of 120 milliseconds and cycle length of 280 milliseconds (**Fig. 3**).

Administration of adenosine 12 mg interrupted the tachycardia.

During a subsequent electrophysiologic study (EPS) an arrhythmia was induced in the clinic, with ventricular stimulation and isoproterenol infusion (**Fig. 4**A).

Mapping of the arrhythmia identified the earliest activation at the septal region of the RV. Ablation in this area resulted in tachycardia termination (**Fig. 4**B) and, on SR, resumption with a right bundle branch block (RBBB) (**Fig. 5**).

Electrocardiogram Interpretation

Fig. 3 shows a regular tachycardia with cycle length of 300 milliseconds, LBBB morphology with normal QRS axis, and QRS duration of

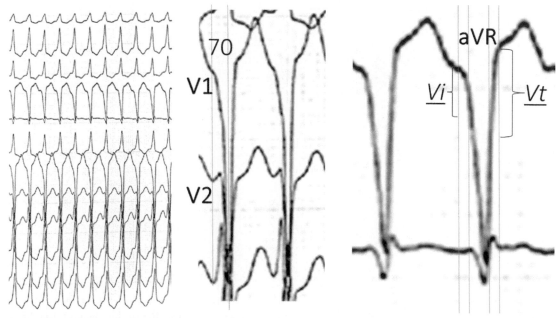

Fig. 3. Case 2. ECG recording during WCT with LBBB morphology. See text for figure explanation.

120 milliseconds. Differential diagnosis of the arrhythmia suggests VT based on a ratio of first and last 40 ms less than 1 in the aVr lead (Vereckei criteria, see **Box 1**), and an intrinsicoid deflection of greater than 60 milliseconds in V1-V2 (Kindwall criteria, see **Box 1**).

Administration of adenosine results in SR restoration.

Clinical Considerations

The differential diagnosis in this case of WCT is between VT and aberrancy. In the absence of major criteria excluding SVT (AV dissociation or fusion) the criteria used are based on QRS morphology.[1] Despite the consistency of the criteria in keeping with VT, in the presence of a borderline QRS duration

A   **B**

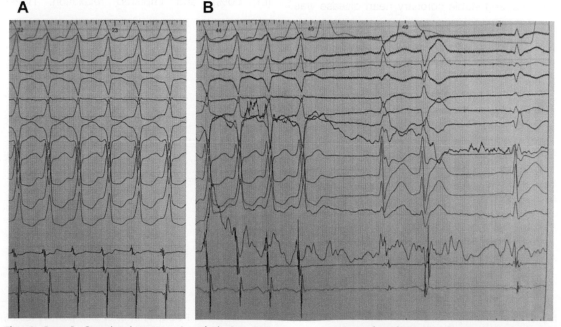

Fig. 4. Case 2. Sustained WCT induced during EPS (*A*). Interruption of tachycardia during radiofrequency ablation (*B*).

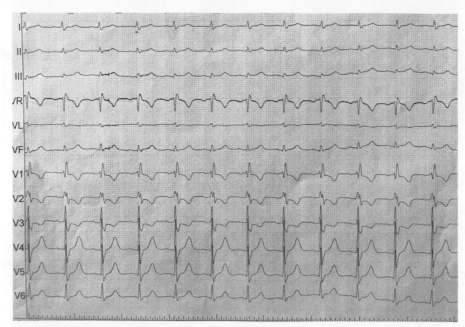

Fig. 5. Case 2. SR with RBBB. The ablation of the site of tachycardia origin, near the His bundle produced RBBB.

adenosine was infused to reach a more certain diagnosis. This test surprisingly terminated the tachycardia, in keeping with triggered activity based on cAMP-dependent delayed afterdepolarizations.[16]

CASE 3. OUTFLOW TRACT PREMATURE VENTRICULAR COMPLEXES WITH V3 PRECORDIAL TRANSITION
Case Presentation

A 68-year-old man with a history of hypertension, diabetes, and stable coronary heart disease was referred for worsening symptomatic palpitation and dyspnea despite β-blocker (metoprolol 50 mg bid) and amiodarone treatment.

The ECG shown in **Fig. 6** shows SR with RBBB and left anterior fascicular block, premature ventricular complex (PVC) with inferior axis, positive lead I, and precordial transition in lead V3 (see **Fig. 6**).

Echocardiography showed mild concentric remodeling of the LV, preserved systolic function (EF 60%), and impaired relaxation. Holter

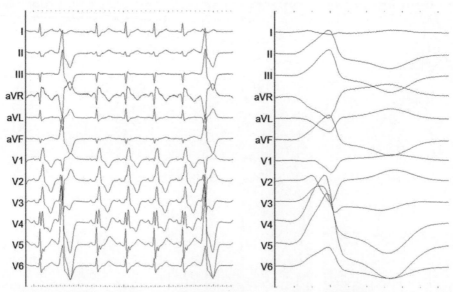

Fig. 6. Case 3. Left panel, SR with RBBB and left anterior fascicular block, PVC with inferior axis, positive lead I, precordial transition in lead V3 (25 mm/s); right panel, V1/V2 duration index = 0.35, V1/V2 amplitude index = 0.2, V2S/V3R ratio = 1.91, V2 S amplitude = 1.54 mV, V3 duration index = 0.65 (200 mm/s).

monitoring showed 28,000 PVCs in 24 hours. The patient underwent EPS with possible radiofrequency ablation of the arrhythmogenic focus.

Electrocardiogram Interpretation

Both RV and LV outflow tracts (OTs) were mapped with the CARTO 3 system (Biosense Webster, Diamond Barr, CA, USA). During RV reconstruction, catheter manipulation caused RBBB, with normal HV interval. Voltage bipolar mapping showed no scar. Guided by activation mapping, the RV OT posterior septal region showed good pace mapping (95% match) and a presystolic potential (−20 ms). Radiofrequency ablation led only to transient suppression of the PVC. Mapping the aortic sinus cusp region, below the right coronary cusp, showed a better pace mapping (98%) and presystolic potential (−38 ms). Radiofrequency ablation in this region led to complete suppression of the VA. **Fig. 7** shows electroanatomic reconstruction of the RV OT and aortic sinus cusp region and ablation sites.

Clinical Considerations

This case shows the difficulty of localizing precisely the earliest breakthrough of VT. Confirming the anatomic location is more than just an ECG challenge because it can help in deciding an ablative approach to treating the arrhythmia. Precordial transition is the criterion used to distinguish between the RV or LV sites of origin (SOO); its

sensitivity and specificity becomes weaker when the transition zone is midline at V3, and the breakthrough is within RV or LV OTs. Several more-detailed criteria have been put forward, some incorporating variables determining the transition, other based on clinical observations.

Recently, Betensky and colleagues[17] developed a criterion that corrects the QRS morphology of the VA with respect to SR, thus taking into account variations in body habitus, cardiac rotation, respiratory variation, and ECG lead positioning. Using the formula [R/(R + S)]PVC ÷ [R/(R + S)]RS in lead V2, a value ≥0.6 predicts an LV OT origin with good sensitivity and positive predictive value (PPV) of 95% and 100%, respectively, whereas specificity and negative predictive value (NPV) have been decreased to 44.8% to 61% and 48.4% to 64%, respectively, in subsequent works.[18,19] Yoshida and colleagues[18] observed that the R wave in lead V3 and the S wave in lead V2 are the morphologic variables with the best ability to discriminate between LV and RV OT-Vas, and a V2S/V3R amplitude ratio ≤1.5 predicts an LV OT origin with a sensitivity, specificity, PPV, and NPV of 94%, 78%, 79%, and 94%, respectively. Recently, we developed our own algorithm to discriminate the SOO of OT-VAs with an LBBB morphology and a transition zone in V3: using a sequential approach, a V2 S wave amplitude ≤1.2 mV established diagnosis of LV OT-VA (sensitivity 73.3%, specificity 100%, PPV 100%, NPV 78.9%, P = .000, area under the curve [AUC] = 0.924); if V2 S wave is >1.2 mV, a V3 duration index <50% establishes a certain diagnosis of origin at RV OT (sensitivity 100%, specificity 88.2%, PPV 100%, NPV 88.2%, P = .000, AUC = 0.893). Ventricular arrhythmias with a V2 S wave >1.2 mV and V3 duration index ≥50% may originate from LV OT (VPP 88.2%), and a study of both ventricles is recommended (overall accuracy, 94.73%).

In our clinical case, as described above, PVCs originating in posteroseptal RV OT and the right coronary cusp share a V3 precordial transition, with a broad R wave in V2 and lead I. Current ECG diagnostic criteria would have classified the SOO at the RV OT. On the contrary, using the broad V3 R wave criteria, our criterion would have correctly identified the location of the PVC in the LV OT.

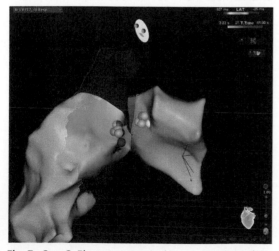

Fig. 7. Case 3. Electroanatomical reconstruction of the RV OT (*left*) and aortic sinus cusps region (*right*) with CARTO 3 system in anteroposterior view. The aorta is represented as a pink tube and the pulmonary artery as a blue tube. The different colored points (*light pink, dark pink, red,* and *white*) are ablation site on RV and their different color represents integration of variables such as power, contact force, and time.

CASE 4. TYPICAL ATRIAL FLUTTER WITH 1:1 ABERRANT ATRIOVENTRICULAR CONDUCTION ON IC ANTIARRHYTHMIC DRUG
Case Presentation

A 69-year-old man arrived at the emergency room because of palpitations. His arterial

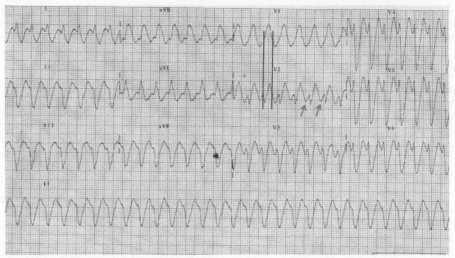

Fig. 8. Case 4. ECG demonstrates a wide QRS tachycardia with cycle length of 330 milliseconds, QRS duration of 230 milliseconds with RBBB morphology. The red lines mark the beginning and the end of QRS complex. The green arrows indicate atrial activity.

pressure was 100/60 mm Hg. ECG showed a WCT with fast ventricular rate (**Fig. 8**). The echocardiogram excluded structural heart disease. The patient was on flecainide 100 mg twice a day for paroxysmal atrial fibrillation (AF). He had taken 1 more pill of flecainide due to palpitations.

Adenosine 12 mg was administered to define the AV relationship (**Fig. 9**).

Ablation of the cavotricuspid isthmus was performed, which returned the patient to SR.

Electrocardiogram Interpretation

In the initial ECG, QRS complexes were very wide and did not appear clearly distinguishable from ventricular repolarization (see **Fig. 8**). Identifying the exact beginning and the end of the QRS is very important in these patients to avoid misinterpreting atrial activity as a delayed beginning of QRS complex (see **Fig. 8**). In V1 a distinct QRS is identifiable with a positive monophasic complex.

According to the Brugada algorithm, a duration of QRS more than 140 milliseconds, a monophasic

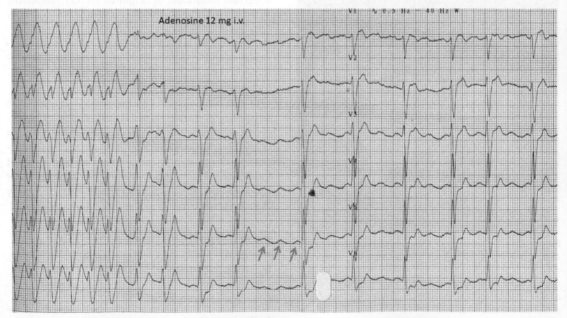

Fig. 9. Case 4. Following adenosine infusion the QRS duration narrows to 160 milliseconds with a nonspecific morphology. Flutter waves with variable conduction are evident (*green arrows*).

QRS complex in lead V1, and the presence of an R/S ratio less than 1 in V6 suggest a VT (Wellens criteria, see **Box 1**). Also, a q wave duration of greater than 40 milliseconds in aVR (Vereckei criteria, see **Box 1**) suggests VT.

The administration of adenosine was diagnostic, demonstrating atrial flutter with 1:1 conduction and wide QRS complex secondary to flecainide administration (see **Fig. 9**).

Clinical Considerations

Atrial flutter can present with a 1:1 atrioventricular conduction either in patients with accessory pathway and antidromic conduction, or in patients receiving class I AADs. IC AADs often reorganize AF into an atrial flutter because of a depressant effect on atrial conduction velocity and a moderate effect on prolongation of myocardial refractoriness. By slowing arrhythmia cycle length, without an effect on the AV node, these drugs facilitate 1:1 AV conduction.[7]

The slowing of AV conduction after adenosine administration excludes the presence of an accessory pathway as the mechanism underlying the arrhythmia. The rapid ventricular rate response leads to QRS widening because of use dependency, and an ECG mimicking VT.[20]

CASE 5. CONCURRENT VENTRICULAR AND ATRIAL TACHYCARDIA
Case Presentation

A 57-year-old man was admitted because of syncope. One year earlier, the patient had received an ICD for primary prevention.

Electrocardiogram Interpretation

Close observation of leads II and III shows P waves. The P-P interval seems to be regular and P morphology seems to be upright in lead III, the cycle length of atrial activity is 270 milliseconds. Also, ventricular activity is regular with a cycle length of 440 milliseconds. There is no obvious P-QRS relationship (**Fig. 10**). Interestingly, there are QRS morphologic variations suggestive of some degree of fusion.

QRS morphology can be assessed after identifying its beginning and end on the 12 leads (see **Fig. 10**). From this analysis it seems that the QRS width is 170 ms and, in lead V1, the R-S interval is 110 milliseconds, fulfilling 1 of the Brugada and Kindwall criteria for VT (see **Fig. 10**).

Interrogation of the ICD demonstrates 2 concurrent arrythmias (**Fig. 11**).

The endocavitary electrograms during arrhythmia obtained with the interrogation of the defibrillator confirm the ventricular origin of the arrhythmia.

The A and V channels show 2 ongoing tachycardias. Atrial tachycardia is a regular tachycardia with a cycle length of 270 ms. The VT cycle length is 440 ms. There is no appreciable relationship between A and V, and no variations in the VT cycle length, confirming AV dissociation. Subtle morphologic changes are observable in the far-field channel (see **Fig. 11**)

Clinical Considerations

The simultaneous presence of ventricular and atrial tachycardias makes surface ECG interpretation difficult. QRS width and morphology are in keeping with VT diagnosis.

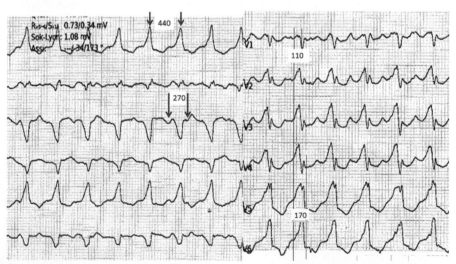

Fig. 10. Case 5. Admission ECG shows a wide complex tachycardia with constant LBBB morphology and irregular baseline. See text for figure explanation. The *red arrows* in lead DI show the interval between QRS complexes; the *red arrows* in lead DIII show the interval between P waves.

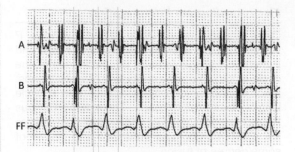

Fig. 11. Case 5. Endocavitary electrogram obtained interrogating the ICD during tachycardia. The first line is atrial channel (A). The second line is ventricular channel (B). The third line is far-field channel (FF).

Dissociated atrial activity with unclear morphology, but with cycle length shorter than VT, should make the observer suspicious of 2 ongoing arrhythmias. Interrogation of the ICD was, in this case, diagnostic.

CASE 6. WOLF-PARKINSON-WHITE SYNDROME WITH OTHODROMIC ATRIOVENTRICULAR RE-ENTRANT TACHYCARDIA AND PRE-EXCITED ATRIAL FIBRILLATION

Case Presentation

A 57-year-old woman with normal cardiac function was admitted to the intensive care unit for chest pain and palpitation. The ECG showed a regular WCT (**Fig. 12**A). The patient was hemodynamically unstable, so defibrillation was performed. The ECG in SR was normal (**Fig. 12**B).

During hospital monitoring, a second narrow complex tachycardia with a similar cycle length of 240 milliseconds was recorded (**Fig. 12**C).

The patient underwent an EPS.

Electrocardiogram Interpretation

The initial ECG (see **Fig. 12**A) shows a WCT with cycle length of 240 milliseconds, clinically poorly tolerated in a patient with normal cardiovascular system. Ventricular tachycardia is suggested by the positivity of aVR (Vereckei criteria, see **Box 1**) and monophasic R in V1 (Wellens criteria, see **Box 1**). The sudden transition of polarity in V6 is unusual. The narrow complex tachycardia has the same cycle length as the presenting arrhythmia; furthermore, a retrograde P wave is clearly visible following the QRS in the inferior leads and V1 (see **Fig. 12**C), with an R-P interval of 120 ms. Haemodynamically unstable pre-excited AF was induced during EPS by atrial burst stimulation and it was interrupted by DC-shock (**Fig. 12**D). A diagnosis of VT is suggested by the clinical presentation and the combination of criteria previously examined. On the contrary, the identical cycle length in both tachycardias is suggestive of a common circuit with a different direction of propagation, as is the case in accessory pathway-mediated tachycardias.

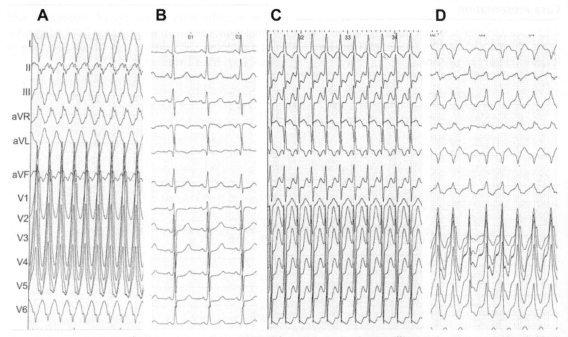

Fig. 12. Case 6. ECG on admission (*A*). It shows WCT with cycle length of 240 milliseconds. SR restored by defibrillation (*B*). Narrow complex tachycardia (*C*). Hemodynamically unstable atrial fibrillation during EPS interrupted by DC shock (*D*).

The long R-P and the unusually negative V6, the morphology of which could be related to the left lateral location of the accessory pathway, is also in keeping with this possibility. This latter hypothesis is confirmed during an EPS, in which the clinical arrhythmia demonstrated a left lateral accessory pathway sustaining an orthodromic tachycardia (**Fig. 13**A), with periods of pre-excitation during induced AF (**Fig. 13**B). The absence of manifest pre-excitation during SR is likely to be due to the distant location of the accessory pathway and the fast conduction through the AVN.

Clinical Consideration

This clinical case shows that, in the presence of an accessory pathway, we can have more types of arrhythmias. During tachycardia with wide QRS complexes the differential diagnosis between supraventricular and ventricular origin of arrhythmia is insidious because ventricular activation via the accessory pathway does not meet the morphologic criteria of SV.

Most manifestations of Wolf-Parkinson-White syndrome are different types of arrhythmia: orthodromic atrioventricular re-entrant tachycardia (AVRT), antidromic AVRT, and pre-excited AF.

The orthodromic AVRT occurs via anterograde conduction through the atrioventricular node, followed by retrograde conduction through the bundle of Kent, producing a tachycardia with narrow QRS morphology. Wide QRS tachycardia can occur in patients with antidromic AVRT, when anterograde conduction through the accessory pathway is followed by retrograde conduction through the AV node,[21] and also during pre-excited AF.

A left lateral accessory pathway was successfully ablated in this patient.

CASE 7. SLOW-FAST ATRIOVENTRICULAR NODAL RE-ENTRY TACHYCARDIA WITH ABERRANT ATRIOVENTRICULAR CONDUCTION
Case Presentation

A 50-year-old man was admitted at the emergency room for palpitations. He was hemodynamically stable. ECG showed wide QRS tachycardia (**Fig. 14**A).

The administration of adenosine 6 mg restored SR (**Fig. 14**B).

The patient underwent EPS, which excluded the presence of an accessory pathway. Programmed

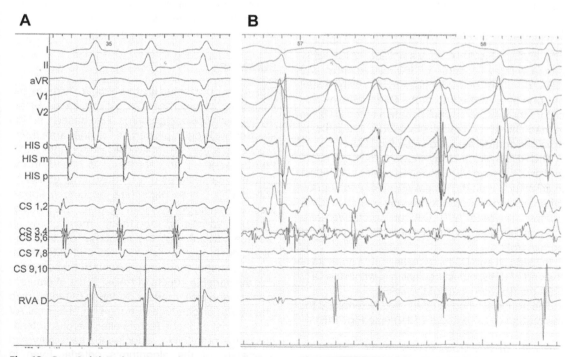

A **B**

Fig. 13. Case 6. (*A*) Endocavitary electrograms during narrow complex tachycardia. The signals recorded by catheter localized in coronary sinus (CS) shows regular atrial activity with first activation of CS 1 or 2 (lateral part of mitral ring). I, II, aVR, V1, V2, ECG leads. His d, distal His. His m, middle His. His p, proximal His. CS 1 to 10, coronary sinus catheter mapping p the mitral ring from lateral wall (CS 1, 2) to coronary sinus os (CS 9, 10). RVA D, right ventricular catheter. (*B*) Endocavitary electrograms during atrial fibrillation. The signals recorded by the catheter localized in CS shows totally disorganized atrial electrical activity.

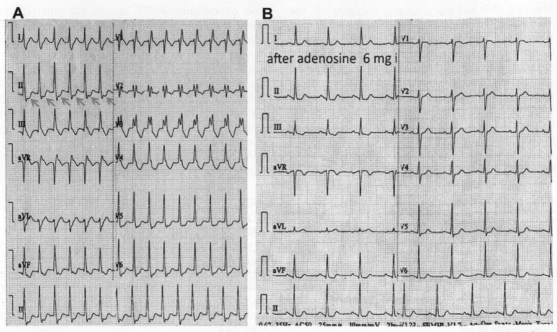

Fig. 14. Case 7. ECG during tachycardia (*A*); the green arrows indicate P waves. ECG in SR after adenosine administration (*B*).

atrial pacing induced a slow-fast atrioventricular nodal re-entry tachycardia. Slow nodal pathway ablation was performed.

Electrocardiogram Interpretation

The ECG in **Fig. 14**A shows a wide QRS tachycardia with cycle length of 360 milliseconds, and QRS duration of 120 milliseconds with RBBB morphology. At the end of the QRS complex and before the T wave, a small negative notch is visible in lead DII, which is attributable to a P wave with atrial retrograde activation (see **Fig. 14**A).

The RBBB morphology shows an rsR′ in lead V1 and an rR′ in lead V2, with the R′ peak being higher in amplitude than the R peak (Sandler and Marriott criteria), and the predominantly negative QRS complex in lead aVR without notch (Vereckei criteria), suggests a supraventricular origin of the tachycardia.

In leads DI and DII the terminal notch appears at the end of QRS, but its beginning is within the QRS (<80 ms from the start of the QRS).

The administration of adenosine determined the restoration of SR without RBBB (see **Fig. 14**B).

Clinical Considerations

Arrhythmia interruption after adenosine administration and morphologic aspects of tachycardia with regular cycle length are suggestive of slow-fast atrioventricular nodal re-entry tachycardia with aberration of conduction. Although it is not possible to rule out orthodromic atrioventricular re-entrant tachycardia, the short R-P interval makes it very unlikely.[22] This possibility was subsequently excluded during the EPS, which did not showed an accessory pathway.

SUMMARY

The cases presented in this article illustrate the limitations of algorithms in the diagnosis of arrhythmias. When algorithms are based on the electrophysiologic properties of the arrhythmia mechanism they are often diagnostic. Differentiation between VT and aberrancy is based on the fundamental features of VT or SVT with abnormal conduction. These algorithms assume a known electrophysiologic behavior in response to predictable variations; aberrancy may occur in diseased tissue, but the response of abnormal His-Purkinje system fibers is well understood. On the other hand, there is no algorithm that can predict the variable effects of AADs, scars of different location and size, marked dilatation of the cardiac chambers, or conduction trough an abnormal AV connection, as these factors alter the characteristics of the arrhythmia, reducing the sensitivity and specificity of the algorithm's criteria. Even in normal hearts, ECG identification of the SOO of VT originating in regions anatomically complex and morphologically variable becomes less reliable. RV and LV OTs with adjacent aortic, aortomitral continuity, pulmonary valves, and coronary sinus constitute a common SOO of sporadic or sustained VT. Their anatomic complexity and close relationship reduce the predictive accuracy of the most common algorithms, particularly when the arrhythmia SOO is in the cardiac midline (V3 precordial transition). Because pre-ablation localization saves procedural time and improves results, many more specific algorithms have been put forward, some based on clinical observations other incorporating variables such as body habitus, cardiac rotation, and respiratory variations. The difficulty of reaching a commonly accepted algorithm in these situations stems, as previously mentioned, from the unpredictable nature of these variables, which can never be precisely assessed.

Therefore, the first step in the analysis of any arrhythmia, but specifically of WCT, is the review of the patient's clinical status and history including medications. An evaluation of cardiac status, including an educated guess on chamber size, presence of known or suspected scars, and pre-existing conduction defects should be integral parts of any ECG analysis. With that knowledge, one can proceed to the determination of the wide QRS tachycardia mechanism. Algorithms differentiating between VT and aberrancy are based on sound clinical and experimental data, and are very helpful with regard to the limitations previously described. More in-depth analysis, including SOO of VT or explanation of QRS variations during WCT, can become exceedingly difficult, and there is no algorithm that can predictably be used to reach the final diagnosis. Experience, extensive knowledge of cardiac electrophysiologic behavior, and clinical skills, are all required to comfortably evaluate these more challenging tracings. This review presents methods of ECG analysis with reasoned examples of difficult tracings, indicating the limitations of electrocardiographic tracings.

REFERENCES

1. De Ponti R, Bagliani G, Padeletti L, et al. General approach to wide QRS complex. Card Electrophysiol Clin 2017;9:461–85.
2. Sandler IA, Marriott HJ. The differential morphology of anomalous ventricular complexes of RBBB type in lead V5: ventricular ectopy versus aberration. Circulation 1965;31:551–6.
3. Wellens HJ, Bar FW, Lie KI. The value of the electrocardiogram in the differential diagnosis of a tachycardia with a widened QRS complex. Am J Med 1978;64:27–33.
4. Kindwall KE, Brown J, Josephson ME. Electrocardiographic criteria for ventricular tachycardia in wide complex left bundle branch block morphology tachycardia. Am J Cardiol 1988;61:1279–83.
5. Brugada P, Brugada J, Mont L, et al. A new approach to the differential diagnosis of a regular tachycardia with a wide QRS complex. Circulation 1991;83:1649–59.
6. Vereckei A, Duray G, Szenasi G, et al. New algorithm using only lead aVR for differential diagnosis of wide QRS complex tachycardia. Heart Rhythm 2008;5: 89–98.
7. De Ponti R, Marazzato G, Bagliani G, et al. Peculiar electrocardiographic aspects of wide QRS complex tachycardia: when differential diagnosis is difficult. Card Electrophysiol Clin 2018;10: 317–32.
8. Crijns HJGM. Changes of intracardiac conduction induced by antiarrhythmic drugs. Importance of the use and reverse use dependence. Groningen (the Netherlands): Academic Thesis. University of Groningen; 1993. ISBN 90.61.48.007.8.
9. Alzand BS, Crijns HJ. Diagnostic criteria of broad QRS complex tachycardia: decades of evolution. Europace 2011;13:465–72.
10. Sharma AD, Klein GJ, Yee R. Intravenous adenosine triphosphate during wide QRS complex tachycardia: safety, therapeutic efficacy, and diagnostic utility. Am J Med 1990;88:337.
11. Priori SG, Blomström-Lundqvist C, Mazzanti A, et al. ESC guidelines for the management of patients with ventricular arrhythmias and the prevention of sudden cardiac death: the task force for the management of patients with ventricular arrhythmias and the prevention of sudden cardiac death of the European Society of Cardiology (ESC). Eur Heart J 2015; 36:2793–867.
12. Jaoude SA, Leclercq JF, Coumel P. Progressive ECG changes in arrhythmogenic right ventricular disease. Evidence for an evolving disease. Eur Heart J 1996;17(11):1717–22.
13. Veltmann C, Schimpf R, Echternach C, et al. A prospective study on spontaneous fluctuations between diagnostic and non-diagnostic ECGs in Brugada syndrome: implications for correct phenotyping and risk stratification. Eur Heart J 2006;27: 2544–52.
14. Cerrone M, Noorman M, Lin X, et al. Sodium current deficit and arrhythmogenesis in a murine model of plakophilin-2 haploinsufficiency. Cardiovasc Res 2012;95:460–8.
15. Sato PY, Coombs W, Lin X, et al. Interactions between ankyrin-g, plakophilin-2, and connexin43 at the cardiac intercalated disc. Circ Res 2011;109: 193–201.
16. Lerman BB, Stein KM, Markowitz SM. Adenosine-sensitive ventricular tachycardia: a conceptual approach. J Cardiovasc Electrophysiol 1996;7: 559–69.

17. Betensky BP, Park RE, Marchlinski FE, et al. The V(2) transition ratio: a new electrocardiographic criterion for distinguishing left from right ventricular outflow tract tachycardia origin. J Am Coll Cardiol 2011;57: 2255–62.

18. Yoshida N, Yamada T, McElderry HT, et al. A novel electrocardiographic criterion for differentiating a left from right ventricular outflow tract tachycardia origin: the V2S/V3R index. J Cardiovasc Electrophysiol 2014;25(7):747–53.

19. Ludwik B, Deutsch K, Mazij M, et al. Electrocardiographic algorithms to guide the management strategy of idiopathic outflow tract ventricular arrhythmias. Pol Arch Intern Med 2017;127(11): 749–57.

20. Brembilla-Perrot B, Houriez P, Beurrier D, et al. Predictors of atrial flutter with 1:1 conduction in patients treated with class I antiarrhythmic drugs for atrial tachyarrhythmias. Int J Cardiol 2001;80: 7–15.

21. Silverman A, Taneja S, Benchetrit L, et al. Atrial fibrillation in a patient with an accessory pathway. J Investig Med High Impact Case Rep 2018;6:1–4.

22. Di Biase L, Gianni C, Bagliani G, et al. Arrhythmias involving the atrioventricular junction. Card Electrophysiol Clin 2017;9:435–52.

QRS Variations During Arrhythmias
Mechanisms and Substrates. Toward a Precision Electrocardiology

Giuseppe Bagliani, MD[a,b,*], Josep Brugada, MD[c],
Roberto De Ponti, MD, FHRS[d], Graziana Viola, MD[e],
Paola Berne, MD[e], Fabio M. Leonelli, MD[f]

KEYWORDS

• Wide QRS complex • Cardiac arrhythmias • QRS variations • Ventricular tachycardia

KEY POINTS

• The mechanism of QRS widening is often problematic, and 4 possibilities must be considered: a ventricular origin, intraventricular conduction delay, ventricular preexcitations, and artificial pacing.
• In the differential diagnosis it is important to consider the presence of the classical criteria (ventriculoatrial dissociation and particular QRS patterns).
• When in the course of an arrhythmia the QRS complex changes, the correct electrocardiogram interpretation can offer the key to understand the arrhythmia mechanism.
• The QRS variations therefore become a parameter to be identified and interpreted as all the other.

INTRODUCTION

Electrocardiographic interpretation of an arrhythmia consists of understanding the mechanism causing the generation and maintenance of the abnormal rhythm.[1]

Concomitantly with this analysis come the observations on QRS morphology variations due to differences of ventricular activation. Changes in QRS are obvious and immediately attract the observer's attention albeit their understanding may be often incomplete. **Fig. 1** clearly shows that changes of QRS can involve its duration, morphology, or both.

QRS duration is the time lasting from the first to the last activation of the ventricles and is a reliable parameter of global synchronization of the ventricles at all.[2] The cut-off of 110 ms is able to differentiate a normal-narrow from a wide-abnormal QRS.

QRS morphology is a parameter that, independently from the QRS duration, reflects the spatial activation of the ventricles. Conventionally lead V1 represents the referring lead (**Fig. 2**) and a wide QRS can be defined as follows:
Right bundle branch (RBB) morphology when in V1 the positive component is predominant

No relevant conflicts to disclose.
[a] Arrhythmology Unit, Cardiology Department, Foligno General Hospital, Via Massimo Arcamone, Foligno, Perugia 06034, Italy; [b] Cardiovascular Disease Department, University of Perugia, Piazza Menghini 1, Perugia 06129, Italy; [c] Hospital Clinic, University of Barcelona, Calle Villarroel, 170, Barcelona 08036, Spain; [d] Department of Heart and Vessels, Ospedale di Circolo and Macchi Foundation, University of Insubria, Viale Borri, 57, Varese 21100, Italy; [e] Cardiology Department, Nuoro General Hospital, via Mannironi 1, Nuoro 08100, Italy; [f] Cardiology Department, James A. Haley Veterans' Hospital, University of South Florida, 13000 Bruce B Down Boulevard, Tampa, FL 33612, USA
* Corresponding author. Arrhythmology Unit, Cardiology Department, Foligno General Hospital, Via Massimo Arcamone, Foligno, Perugia 06034, Italy.
E-mail address: giuseppe.bagliani@tim.it

Card Electrophysiol Clin 11 (2019) 315–331
https://doi.org/10.1016/j.ccep.2019.02.006
1877-9182/19/© 2019 Elsevier Inc. All rights reserved.

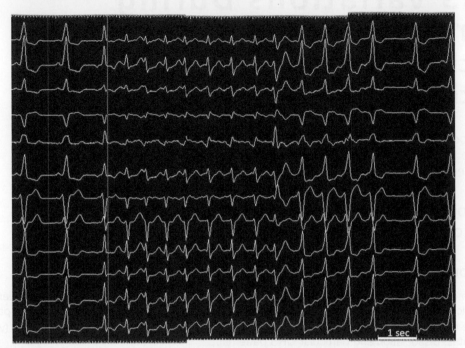

Fig. 1. Typical QRS variation: evident changes in heart rate and QRS morphology. See **Figs. 3** and **10** for further explanations (same case).

Left bundle branch (LBB) morphology when in V1 the QRS is negative

In this context, to better analyze the QRS variations, one should analyze independently the duration and the morphology of the QRS! Goal of this chapter is to demonstrate how to identify correctly the relevant findings in the analysis of QRS variations (duration/morphology) leading to

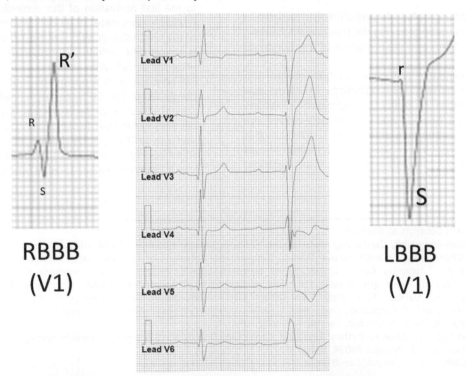

Fig. 2. Right bundle branch block and left bundle branch block: typical patter in lead V1.

the understanding of the electrophysiologic (EP) mechanisms behind these variations. Several clinical cases will supplement the theoretic approach to demonstrate the EP principles presented.

QRS COMPLEX: DEFINITION OF NARROW AND WIDE VARIATIONS

Analyzing QRS duration, a QRS can be defined as narrow or wide:

A narrow QRS has a duration of up to 110 ms and, within this normal limit, some variations can be due to delay of activation of small ventricular areas (hemiblocks and incomplete bundle branch blocks [BBBs]).

A wide QRS has a duration of more than 110 ms; this delay represents asynchronous electrical propagation of larger portions of one or both ventricles and can have many reasons (delay of activation, ectopic activation, preexcitation, or artificial stimulation)[3]

The challenge of defining variations:

Definition: during an arrhythmia, the generic concept of variations defines any change in the pattern of QRS, both morphology and/or duration, from a reference QRS. A QRS variation can be related to a change of the mechanism of the arrhythmia or can be a bystanding effect of the same arrhythmia.

Methodological approach to a QRS variation

Fig. 3 explains a rational approach to an arrhythmia presenting QRS variations. It is, therefore, a fundamental step in this analysis to obtain a QRS representing usual conduction. To explain the mechanism of the observed variations, it is necessary to use a schematic approach based on the identification of a Basic, Dominant, and Variant ECG (see **Fig. 3**) defined as follows:

Basic QRS: QRS recorded during spontaneous ventricular activation; a basic ECG can be normal or can demonstrate some conduction abnormalities. The analysis of basic QRS represents the "corner-stone" of the patient's conduction and can be obtained during sinus rhythm outside the arrhythmias or at the beginning of the arrhythmia itself.

Dominant QRS: is the ECG representing the initial and main ventricular activation during the arrhythmia? Comparing this ECG with basal ECG can demonstrate complete similarity or differences of ventricular activation.

Variant QRS: once the dominant QRS has been identified, any changes of ventricular activation during the arrhythmias represent a "variant QRS."

The gold standard of the analytical process is the identification of the 3 ventricular activations (Basic/Dominant/Variant) and the relationship between them constitutes the subject of this article.

Searching for these variations requires an attentive comparison of ECGs acquired at different times both during normal sinus rhythm and during different periods of arrhythmias. It is important to apply a logic deductive method of analysis in this comparison and avoid personal bias or sudden personal intuitions.

ELECTROPHYSIOLOGIC MECHANISMS POTENTIALLY SUSTAINING QRS VARIATIONS

Behind variations of QRS morphology are alterations of cardiac channels, cellular connections or properties, and overall tissue histology. These pathologies lead to alterations of EP mechanisms, which can be summarized as follows[3]:

Delay and block of conduction: electrical conduction delay or block in one of the His-Purkinje system (HPS) divisions is responsible for a hindered activation of a portion or the entire chamber of one of the ventricles leading

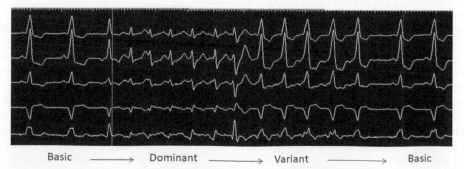

Basic ⟶ Dominant ⟶ Variant ⟶ Basic

Fig. 3. QRS variation and definition of the BASIC-DOMINANT-VARIANT morphologies.

to a prolonged duration of a segment or the whole QRS. The delay/block can be permanent, in the case of stable anatomic alteration of the conduction system, temporary, or varying of degree from beat to beat, depending on the momentary EP status of the HPS's fibers. Functional aberrancy refers to the latter situation and can be due to failure of adaptation of a fascicle or branch of the HPS exposed to a fast rate of stimulation (phase 3 aberrancy). More rarely, a transient instability of transmembrane V leads to a drift toward more positive values of this parameter with inactivation of Na channels. A depolarizing wavefront will generate in the stimulated cells an action potential with decreased velocity of depolarization likely to block or delay impulse propagation (phase 4 aberrancy).

Saltatory conduction or muscle-to-muscle conduction: impulse propagation, spreading by muscle-to-muscle connections outside the conduction system, is characterized by unpredictable and slow propagation. This situation is observed in 3 clinical scenarios:

Electrical activation originating within the V muscle, either because of focal activity or because of larger reentrant circuits, will spread by saltatory conduction, characterized by unpredictable and slow propagation. This wavefront of depolarization will, at some stage, reenter the HPS terminal arborizations propagating more rapidly to the remainder of the ventricles. For this schematic mechanism the wide-QRS of ectopic origin is a fusion complex with a first delayed component and a second fast component.

A similar situation is observed also in Wolff-Parkinson-White (WPW) syndrome where a group of muscle fibers (the AP) will conduct part of the atrial impulse using a direct connection into V muscle. In this case, retrograde conduction within the HP is usually prevented by the simultaneous engagement of the system by an antegrade wavefront traveling via the atrioventricular node (AVN)-HPS.

Artificial ventricular stimulation by an artificial pacemaker is characterized by a wide QRS preceded by an electrical artifact. Fusion between this activation wavefront and a normal V activation induced by normal AVN-HPS ventricular capture (pseudofusion) is frequently observed particularly to assess the correct function of the artificial pacemaker.

The generic concept of "fusion"

As previously mentioned, parallel to the ectopic origin and the consequent salutatory-conduction of the ventricular activation front, there is the concept of fusion between a slow and a fast activation front. The definition of "fused QRS" refers to a QRS generated by 2 different activation fronts resulting in a QRS morphology intermediary between the QRS of each activation fronts. Common examples of fusion are recorded (**Fig. 4**) in the setting of

Ventricular arrhythmias (A)
WPW (B)
Artificial pacemakers (C).

The fusion phenomenon, by itself nonpathognomonic of a particular EP situation, becomes fundamental in specific diagnostic contexts. This is the situation of QRS narrowing during VT due to supraventricular beats: this observation confirms the ventricular origin of the rhythm. Similarly, during artificial cardiac pacemaker stimulation, QRS morphologic variations define a change in the pattern of V capture and are of great importance in the analysis of pacemaker function. This is particularly true during biventricular stimulation where 3 possible wavefronts of V activation are possible (right pacing, left pacing, and normal His-Purkinje activation): in paced ECG, a QRS variation may be due to normal or abnormal pacemaker function.

QRS VARIATIONS: METHODOLOGICAL APPROACH

Focus on present scenario. Keep in mind the big picture and the basic questions:

How many different QRS morphologies can we detect?
Is the basic ECG known?
Which is the basic and variant ECG?

Each observed ECG will need to be defined in terms of morphology and duration, and later a laddergram will be constructed linking atrial and ventricular events.

QRS duration variations: while the definition of normal QRS width is a based on a specific measurement, variations of this waveform can be very subtle with duration of this waveform remaining within normal limits. A change from normal QRS to BBB is obvious, but minor variations due to appearance or disappearance of subtle conduction delays or competitive rhythms causing fusion require a more attentive analysis because they are likely to be relevant.

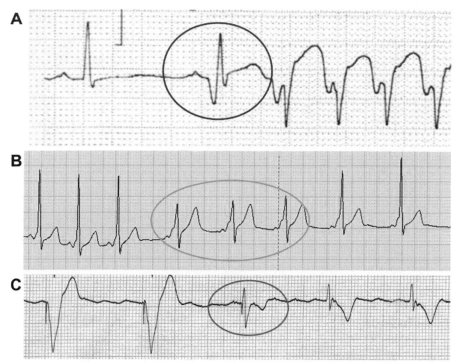

Fig. 4. Morphologic changes of QRS due to "ventricular fusion" in 3 different situations: (*A*) red circle, a fusion at the beginning of a ventricular tachycardia; (*B*) green circle: increase degree of ventricular preexcitation during sinus rhythm; (*C*) blue circle: a fusion of electrical activity between a paced rhythm and a spontaneous rhythm.

QRS morphology variations: This parameter provides important information on the origin and progression of the activation waveform; it is based on the analysis of QRS spatial location derived from limb leads and waveform components from examination of single leads, in particular lead V1 and aVr.This analysis compares a reference QRS (the normal or the dominant) and an "abnormal" QRS carrying the variation in question. Reference QRS does not imply normality as subtle variations of axis or of a small portion of the QRS and can occur in a QRS already altered by preexisting anomalies of conduction.

CONSTRUCTING THE LADDERGRAM AFTER THE ANALYSIS OF QRS

A laddergram is the graphic representation of atrial and ventricular events with their correlations represented by different lines (color or slope) (**Fig. 5**). A fundamental aspect of this analysis is the exact time representation of each interval. This approach can greatly aid the formulation of differential diagnosis even if, in the case of WCT, the construction of a laddergram may be problematic.

The QRSs: from a practical point of view, to begin a laddergram it is necessary to accurately identify, for each case, every QRS morphology available during sinus rhythm (SR) and tachycardia. In WCT a fundamental step is to observe lead V1 and aVr to detect all the features aiding the differential diagnosis between VT and aberrancy.[4,5]

The RR intervals: the next step is to identify all QRS variations and correlate them with preceeding, accompanying, or following R-R intervals. For example, similar QRS variations, as the same BBB, will have different EP explanations depending on the shortening or lengthening of the preceeding R-R. The logical construction of an all inclusive laddergram will allow the generation of several differential diagnosis, among which one will be selected with the aid of more advanced analysis and the use of diagnostic keys (see following sections).

The P waves: detailed analysis of 12 lead P wave will differentiate between[6] sinus P wave, ectopic P wave, and retrograde P wave and diagnose characteristic morphologies such as atrial flutter or atrial fibrillation (AF).

The search for P waves needs to include QRS-ST deflections and when undetected their

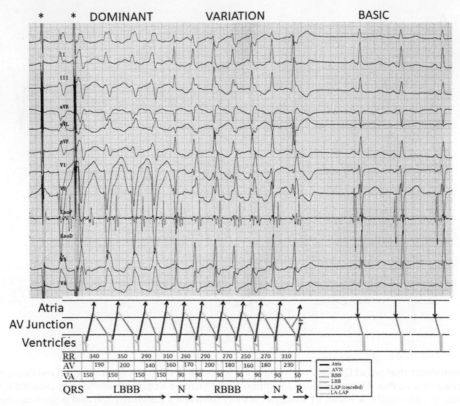

Fig. 5. Laddergram construction during a wide complex tachycardia. After 2 premature atrial stimulations (*asterisk*), a nonsustained wide complex tachycardia develops. A well evident change of QRS morphology (dominant, variation, and basic) is evident.

presence hypothesized, when logically suspected. At times, vagal maneuvers can, by slowing V rate, identify hidden P waves.

   Atrioventricular relationship: this is the more expert phase in the construction of the laddergram. Deep EP phenomenon can be involved in the process as explained in the following clinical cases.

QRS MORPHOLOGY VARIATIONS: FROM LADDERGRAM TO ADVANCED ELECTROPHYSIOLOGIC CONCEPTS

Experience in ECG analysis and knowledge of EP principles are fundamental in the interpretation of complex arrhythmias such as variations in ECG morphology. Nevertheless, formulation of differential diagnosis and identification of diagnostic findings are truly the most important aspects of this analysis. Having constructed a laddergram, its analysis is directed to find, based on deductive reasoning, evidence of general findings to construct a differential diagnosis.

Scenarios and Mechanisms of QRS Morphology Variations

A QRS variation will depend on 4 different scenarios identified using the reasoning previously described.

QRS morphology variations during supraventricular trachycardia

During supraventricular trachycardia (SVT) aberrant conduction can be initiated by a long/short sequence (Ashman phenomenon) and continue due to "linking," which is the concealed retrograde conduction in the blocked His bundle branch (**Fig. 6** and clinical case 1). In this case, aberrancy will cause a wide QRS with typical features in V1 and aVr. In the absence of an identifiable P wave, as in AF, evidence of long/short cycle in the preceeding R-R intervals is particularly useful to diagnose a similar mechanism of aberrancy. With a similar EP mechanism, when a short/long sequence occurs (reverse Ashman phenomenon), the intraventricular activation delay disappears and QRS normalizes. Ashman phenomenon also explains aberrancy in the very rare situation of His alternans during atrioventricular nodal

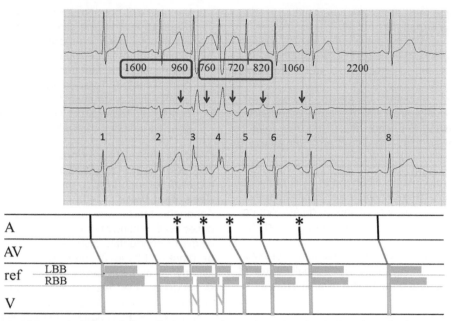

Fig. 6. Case 1: QRS morphology variations during SVT. Aberrant conduction can be initiated by a long/short (1600/960) sequence (Ashman phenomenon).

reentrant tachycardia (AVNRT) manifesting itself with a 2:1 AV block. Normalization of antegrade conduction will double V rate and may be accompanied by aberrancy (**Fig. 7** and clinical case 2).

In WPW, SR will activate the ventricles with a double wavefront. The initial portion of the QRS, due to AP activation of the V, will be wide due to the slow saltatory propagation of the electrical impulse. The terminal part of the QRS will narrow due to the physiologic activation via the HPS of the remainder of the V. This may also occur in SVTs (AF, AT, and AVNRT) using the AP as a passive

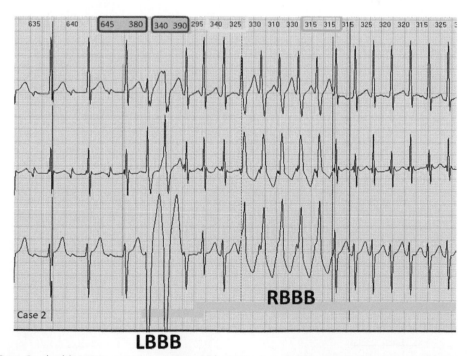

Fig. 7. Case 2: double QRS variation: LBBB and RBBB due to the same aberrant mechanism (Ashman phenomenon).

conduit for antegrade conduction resulting in QRS morphology variations.

Most commonly the presence of an AP, manifest or occult, will constitute part of the macro reentry circuit observed in orthodromic and more rarely antidromic SVT.

QRS morphology variations during AP-mediated tachycardia can be, as in other SVTs, due to Ashman phenomenon and rate-related BBB. Specific to AP-mediated arrhythmias are 3 situations:

- R-R prolongation observed in BBB homolateral to AP (**Figs. 8** and **9** and clinical case 3)
- Possible emergence of antegrade AP conduction as passive by standard (**Fig. 10** and clinical case 4).
- Antidromic tachycardia (maximum of preexcitation) reversing to SR with a small degree of preexcitation (**Fig. 11** and clinical case 5)

QRS morphology variations in common and uncommon ventricular tachycardia

Common causes of QRS variation during VTs can be observed due to the following:

- Fusion and/or capture of ventricular activity by a sinus beat (**Fig. 12** and clinical case 6)

- Variable exit point in course of stable reentry (**Figs. 13** and **14** and clinical case 7)
- A particular electrocardiographic morphology, expression of a specific substrate is the Catecolaminergic Bidirectional VT (**Fig. 15** and clinical case 8). Torsade de Point and ventricular fibrillation represent 2 typical polymorphic ventricular tachycardia and are described in specific sections of this book.

QRS morphology variations during bradycardias: BB resumption, normalization of a bundle branch blocks, and bradycardia-dependent block

Although there are terminologies in some cases confounding about the electrogenic mechanisms of conductive disorders of the HPS (delay or block? "Phase 3" and "phase 4" block as synonyms of tachycardia-dependent or pause-dependent), the electrocardiographic aspects concerning ventricular conductive pathology refer to well-defined ECG pattern (BBB) (see **Fig. 2**; and **Fig. 16**). QRS morphology variations during bradycardia are due to reversible block in one of the bundles of the HPS; the mechanism is different from Ashman phenomenon, which can be considered physiologic responses to premature stimulation (or failure of adaptation). In bradycardia the

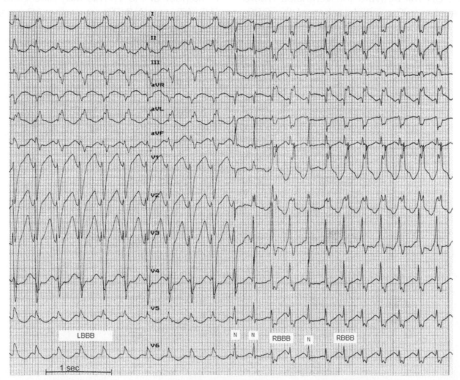

Fig. 8. Case 3: a very concealed accessory pathway: 2 wide-QRS none preexcited. ECG shows an initial LBBB regular tachycardia normalizing for 2 beats followed by a sequence of RBBB-normal-RBBB.

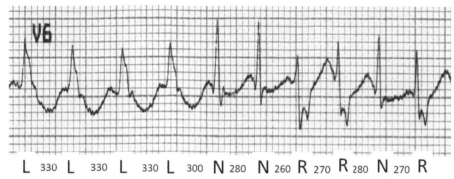

L 330 L 330 L 330 L 300 N 280 N 260 R 270 R 280 N 270 R

Fig. 9. Case 3: a very concealed accessory pathway: 2 wide-QRS none preexcited. QRS changes in relation to R-R interval. LBBB is associated with R-R = 330 ms, narrow QRS with R-R = 300 ms, and RBBB follows long/short sequence (280/260 ms).

block is due to spontaneous depolarization of the His fibers until its inexcitability and the result is a BBB. In the concept of trifascicular activation, the fascicles can impair its conduction individually (hemiblock). Combining the information derived from QRS morphology and AV conduction (PQ interval), it is possible to define the site and the mechanisms of the delay/block: the construction of a precise laddergram is very important for a correct diagnosis (clinical case 9).

QRS morphology in patients with cardiac pacemakers

In patients with pacemaker, the electrical activity of the myocardium is determined in parallel by both the natural excitation-conduction system and the implantable device. This latter detects the presence of spontaneous rhythm and in condition of reduced spontaneous activation stimulates the ventricles; based on this scenario the ventricular electrical activity can be spontaneous, paced or fused (**Fig. 17**). Each of these situations is associated to a particular QRS morphology. The knowledge of these complex properties is crucial to properly recognize the pacemaker functioning and avoid mistaken diagnosis of malfunctions (**Fig. 18**); this situation (pacing and/or sensing impairment) can be evident on further particular ECG features (**Fig. 19** and clinical case 10).

DIAGNOSTIC KEYS FROM ELECTROPHYSIOLOGIC CLINICAL CASES

The following clinical cases illustrate a method to guide the reader to data collection and

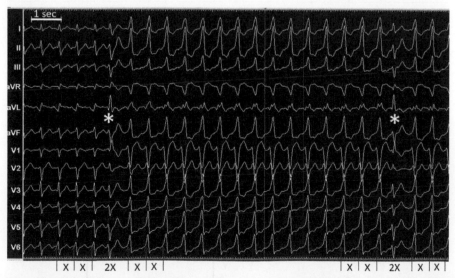

Fig. 10. Case 4: an on and off bystanding accessory pathway: a reentrant arrhythmia clarified by a ventricular premature complex (VPC). WPW syndrome (same case of **Figs. 1** and **3**). A narrow complex tachycardia cycle length (CL) 620 ms. A VPC (*asterisk*) changes the QRS morphology into a preexcited tachycardia without changing the basic CL. Also a second VPC during preexcited tachycardia (*asterisk*) does not change QRS morphology.

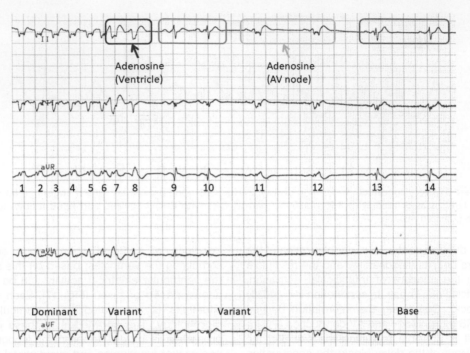

Fig. 11. Case 5: adenosine-induced QRS variations during antidromic AVRT (beats 1–6). Sinus rhythm is restored (beats 9–14) after 2 ectopic beats (7–8). See text for detailed analysis.

interpretation to reach a diagnosis of the arrhythmia mechanism.

Ashman Phenomenon: The Simplest QRS Variation

During Holter monitoring (see **Fig. 6**) an episode of nonsustained atrial tachycardia is recorded (*red arrows and asterisks*). Conduction during the arrhythmia is 1:1, the first 2 aberrantly due to the Ashman phenomenon; aberrant conduction, in this case, is due to a functional block of conduction most commonly affecting the RB, observed during a variation of the R-R interval (short R-R preceded by long R-R; *red square*).

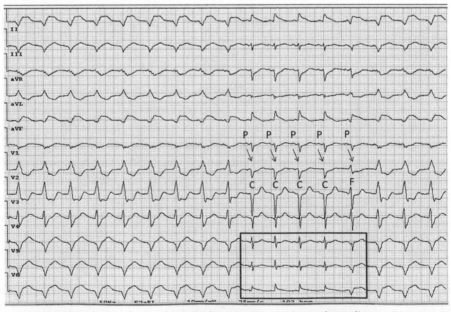

Fig. 12. Case 6: capture and fusion during WCT. During a wide complex tachycardia a sudden narrowing of the QRS (*red box*) is due to ventricular capture (C) and fusion (F) by a sinus P wave.

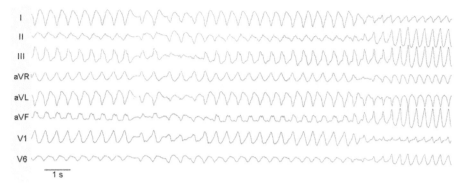

Fig. 13. Case 7: a polymorphic incessant VT. Peripheral and precordial (V1 and V6) leads during incessant VT with variations of the morphology of the QRS complex.

Normalization of conduction occurs following a relative prolongation of the R-R interval (*blue square*).

The laddergram shows the mechanisms of Ashman phenomenon, perpetuation of the aberrancy, and normalization of conduction.

The third QRS occurs prematurely at an interval of 960 ms compared with a basic cycle length of 1600 ms finding the RB still refractory; conduction blocks in this bundle cause the Ashman phenomenon.

The following QRS happens at an interval of 760 ms and despite the similarity to the previous R-R (960 and 760 ms) continues to show an RBBB morphology. Persistence of aberrancy in this case is due to the phenomenon of "linking."

Physiologic conduction of RB in the previous beat is blocked because of prematurity; the RB will be activated with some delay (approx. 60–80 ms) via concealed transseptal conduction from the LB foreshortening the RBB to RBB

interval. The fifth QRS is normal as the action potential duration of the RB is now shorter having accommodated to the increased rate of stimulation.

Diagnostic key: QRS 3 and 4 in lead V1 develop an rsR′ morphology following a long/short cycle.

Double QRS Variation: Aberrant R and LBBB Due to the Same Mechanism

During a sustained episode of AVNRT, ventricular rate doubles (see **Fig. 7**) due to a change of AV conduction from 2:1 to 1:1. This phenomenon is not uncommon, albeit often unrecognized as it is limited to short sequences, and it is due to His alternans. R-R doubling creates a long-short interval (CL change from 645 to 380 ms; *red square*) triggering LB aberrancy via Ashman phenomenon. Aberrancy is maintained for 2 beats until R-R interval prolongs from 340 to 390 ms (blue square) restoring normal conduction. Three beats later a

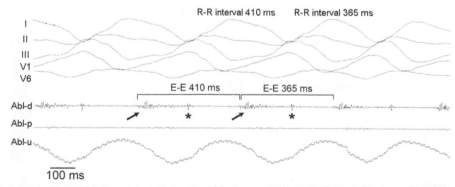

Fig. 14. Case 7: a polymorphic incessant VT. Cardiac ablation procedure. Surface and intracavitary bipolar recordings from the distal (Abl-d) and proximal (Abl-p) electrode pairs of the ablation catheter and unipolar recording from the distal electrode of the same catheter. In Abl-d, a mid-to-end diastolic low-voltage fragmented electrogram (*arrow*) is observed and consistent with slow conduction over a channel possibly related to the VT; an accompanying systolic electrogram (*asterisk*) is also recorded. Beat-to-beat variation in the interval between the intracavitary signals (E-E) precedes the variation of the R-R interval, suggesting that this is an area critical for reentry.

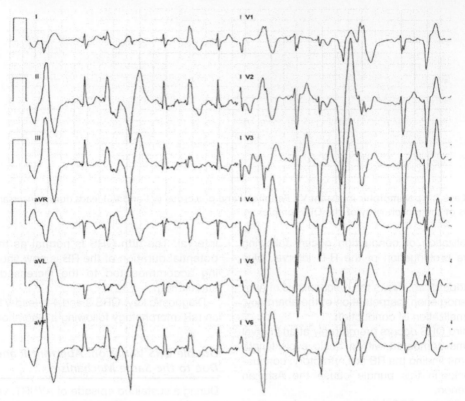

Fig. 15. Case 8: catecholaminergic VT. ECG during submaximal stress test shows increasingly complex polymorphous ventricular arrhythmia as heart rate increases. See text for further discussion.

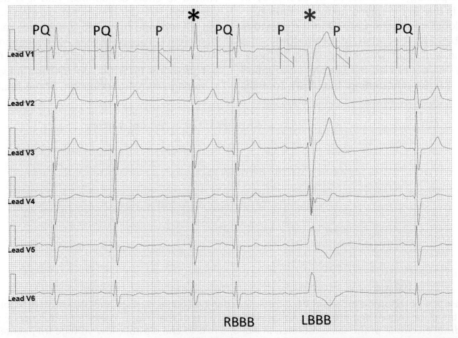

Fig. 16. Case 9: nonconducted P waves with double morphology escaping beats (RBBB and LBBB). Three nonconsecutive P wave (red P) are nonconducted to the ventricles. Two escaping beats emerge: an RBBB morphology identical to the basic one (*black asterisk*) as for junctional origin and an LBBB (*red asterisk*) morphology as for an origin from the right side of the conducting system.

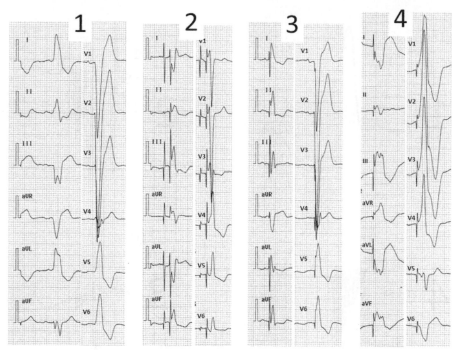

Fig. 17. Case 10: variable QRS in a patient with biventricular pacemaker. (1) Baseline ECG before implant: LBBB with QRS duration of 180 ms. (2) DDD pacing: QRS duration 120 ms, "Qr" in leads I and aVl, and an initial r in V1 and V2. (3) VDD pacing: QRS duration 100 ms with incomplete LBBB morphology, loss of Q wave in I and aVL, and loss of r in V1 and V2. (4) VVI pacing: RBBB morphology with a QRS duration of 180 ms.

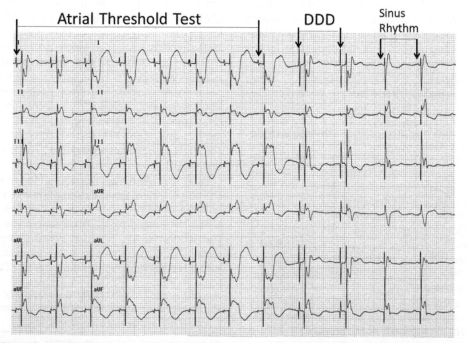

Fig. 18. Case 10: variable QRS in a patient with biventricular pacemaker. Atrial threshold test: well evident changes in QRS morphology related to presence or absence of effective atrial pacing. See text for further explanations.

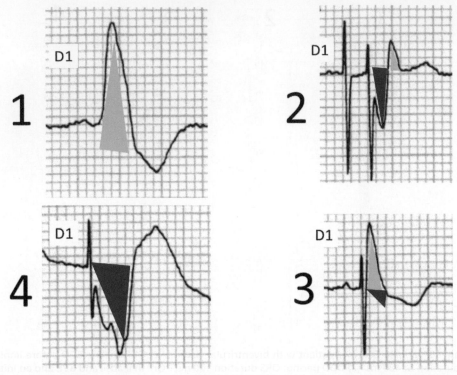

Fig. 19. Case 10: variable QRS in a patient with biventricular pacemaker. (ECG 1, 2, 3, 4) Same modalities of pacing as in **Fig. 17**. The component of ventricular activation due to normal conduction system (*green*). The component of ventricular activation due to pacing system (*red*) (isolated left ventricular activation due to the malfunction of right ventricular lead). (1) Ventricular activation of the ventricles completely spontaneous. (2 and 3): 2 different patterns of fused ventricular activation. (4) Ventricular activation due to isolated left ventricular pacing.

new long-short R-R (from 340 to 320 ms; *yellow square*) induces RB aberrancy, which continues until rate-dependent gradual shortening of RB refractory period allows normal conduction (*green square*).

Diagnostic key: R and LB aberrancy during same tachycardia preceded by a similar R-R variation.

A Very Concealed Accessory Pathway: 2 Wide-QRS None Preexcited

ECG of a 21-year-old with recurrent palpitations (see **Fig. 8**) shows an initial LBBB for the first 6 beats of a regular tachycardia normalizing for 2 beats followed by a sequence of RBBB-normal-RBBB. Considering QRS changes in relation to R-R interval (see **Fig. 9**), it seems that LBBB is associated with R-R of 330 ms, narrow QRS with R-R of 300 ms, and RBBB follows long/short sequence (280/260 ms).

RBBB persists with R-R of 280 ms. During EP study the arrhythmia mechanism was demonstrated to be AVNRT using a left lateral concealed pathway without antegrade conduction. RF was curative.

Diagnostic key: LBBB is associated to a prolongation of tachycardia CL (300 ms) because the macro-reentrant circuit involves a left side AP; LBBB prolongs the circuit length and so the RR interval. The normalization of the conduction in the LBB shortens the circuit length and consequently R-R interval (330→300); a further shortening of RR interval (280>260), probably due an improvement in AV node conduction, promotes RBBB aberrancy via Ashman phenomenon. Subtle changes of R-R interval impinge on RB refractory period and can either normalize or reinduce RBBB. R-R equal or shorter than 270 ms will maintain RBBB.

Note that the AP participates in the mechanism of the tachycardia as the retrograde arm of the circuit but does not contribute the widening of the QRS. This would presuppose antegrade conduction along the AP, which is never demonstrated during SR. Its conduction is therefore concealed and does not manifest on the 12 lead ECG.

An On and Off Bystanding Accessory Pathway: a Reentrant Arrhythmia Clarified by a Ventricular Premature Complex

A patient presented with WPW syndrome, well evident during SR (see **Fig. 10**, same case of **Figs. 1** and **2**), and recurrent palpitations. The tracing shows a narrow complex tachycardia. A VPC (*asterisk*) changes the QRS morphology into a preexcited tachycardia (the morphology of the QS is the same as that shown during SR) without changing the basic cycle length (x + x = 2x). This represents a shift in antegrade conduction from AVN to AP induced by VPC, which by blocking retrogradely into the AVN allows the emergence of antegrade conduction on an AP. The shift is favored by the septal location of the AP. A second VPC does not change QRS morphology and a basic cycle length of the tachycardia.

Diagnostic key: the mechanism of the arrhythmia is clarified by the VPCs, which do not affect the CL of the tachycardia. This observation excludes the presence of an AP as part of the reentrant circuit as premature capture of the V should have reset for one beat the entire arrhythmia CL. A reentrant arrhythmia, which is unaffected by a VPC, can only be an AVNRT that does not depend on V activation. In this case, the AP played only a by-stander role.

Adenosine-Induced QRS Variations During Antidromic Atrioventricular Nodal Reentrant Tachycardia: Considering Its Pharmacologic Effects

ECG is recorded in the emergency room following intravenous infusion of 6 mg of adenosine to treat a wide complex tachycardia. Sinus rhythm is restored. At the end of the infusion there are a significant QRS variation compared with the dominant morphology of presentation. Ameticulous analysis of the rhythm is necessary in particular rhythm/morphology of all the QRSs that include

- *Dominant morphology*: the initial 6 beats represent the wide complex tachycardia of presentation; R-R shortening a little between the last 2.
- *Variant morphologies*: the following 6 beats show significant irregular R-R interval and different QRS morphologies. The seventh beat is a premature ventricular beat and also the eighth beat probably represents a VPC. The following 4 beats (9–12) are sinus beats:ninth and 10th beats are consistent with SR and some degree of preexcitation, 11th and 12th beats are sinus rhythm with more marked preexcitation.
- Base morphology
  The final beats (13–14) show a mild degree of preexcitation and represent the basic QRS morphology during normal sinus rhythm.
  The ECG sequences reported in this case raise the question of the mechanism of the tachycardia unlock. Usually adenosine

action is at level of AVN, generating transient AV block and so interrupting all the tachycardia in which circuit involves AVN. But in this case a careful analysis of the ECG gives us many information on the electrophysiology of the tachycardia and its interruption.

- Diagnostic keys: the end of the tachycardia is due to the effect of the ventricular beat on the circuit reentry; this ECG clearly shows the different effect of the adenosine on the heart, first increasing ventricular automaticity and generating the VPCs (*red arrow*) and second, a delayed effect blocking AVN conduction and maximizing ventricular preexcitation (*green arrow*).
- The QRS morphology during tachycardia (beats 1–6) is identical to that of SR and maximal preexcitation (11–12), confirming the hypothesis of an antidromic macro reentrant tachycardia.

Capture and Fusion During WCT

During a wide complex tachycardia (see **Fig. 12**) a sudden narrowing of the QRS is noted (*red box*), due to antegrade capture (C) and fusion (F) between ventricular and supraventricular capture.

Diagnostic keys: capture and fusion during WCT are diagnostic of ventricular tachycardia.

A Polymorphic Incessant Ventricular Tachycardia

A 68-year-old man with prior anterior myocardial infarction was admitted to the hospital with palpitations and hypotension. The ECG shows a VT with a variable QRS complex morphology and cycle length (see **Fig. 13**). Specifically, although V1 shows constantly a positive QRS complex consistent with an RBBB morphology, the polarity of the QRS complex varies over time from negative to positive in leads II and V6 and from positive to negative in aVR. Accordingly, the tachycardia cycle length varies from 450 to 310 ms. The mechanism underlying this polymorphous VT is unclear and cannot be determined from surface ECG. It can be hypothesized that this arrhythmia is related to the scar of the previous myocardial infarction, but, if a reentry mechanism is involved, it could be a complex form. Alternatively, a multifocal mechanism could be involved. For the iterative presentation, the patient underwent an electrophysiology procedure.

Diagnostic key: during the procedure, in a phase with stable tachycardia morphology (RBBB morphology and inferior axis deviation) the ablation catheter positioned in the lateral region of the left ventricular (LV) apex recorded (see **Fig. 14**) a mid- to end-diastolic, low-voltage, fractioned electrogram with an accompanying systolic electrogram and a variable tachycardia cycle length from 410 to 365 ms. Interestingly, the beat-to-beat variations of the cycle length observed in the local electrogram preceded the variations in the R-R interval on surface ECG, suggesting that the ablation catheter was positioned in a slow conduction channel critical for reentry. Therefore, ablation was decided in this site with no further pacing maneuver, such as reset or entrainment, which could have been nondiagnostic in the presence of a variable arrhythmia cycle length. A single radiofrequency energy application not only interrupted the tachycardia after cycle length prolongation but also completely suppressed arrhythmia inducibility, which was reproducible before. However, the procedure was completed with further ablation in the surrounding areas showing late and fragmented potentials in sinus rhythm. The patient had an uneventful follow-up. In this case, these findings suggest the presence of a common central pathway of slow conduction, which was involved partially (shorter cycle length) or entirely (longer cycle length) in the reentry, with different exit points responsible for the variations in morphology of the QRS complex. In this case, limited ablation in the arrhythmia-related channel close to the exit point identified by the mid- to end-diastolic potential suppressed the slow conduction critical for reentry maintenance.

Catecholaminergic Ventricular Tachycardia

A 34-year-old male patient presented for an athletic cardiac screening. He had a history of a single exercise–related syncope (age 7 years) and no family history of sudden cardiac death. Basal 12 lead ECG was normal.

The ECG during submaximal stress test (see **Fig. 15**) shows increasingly complex polymorphous ventricular arrhythmia as heart rate increases:

Isolated polymorphic ventricular ectopic beats at 139 bpm
Ventricular bigeminy at 142 bpm
Ventricular couplets at 145 bpm
Nonsustained polymorphic VT started at 147 bpm

Diagnostic key: clinical presentation and exercise-related polymorphous ventricular arrhythmias are typical of catecholaminergic VT. Patient's genetic analysis revealed a heterozygous missense mutation in *CASQ2* gene (CPVT-2).

Nonconducted P Waves with Escaping Beats

During a long sequence of regular SR 3 nonconsecutive P wave are nonconducted to the ventricles. Two different escaping beats emerge: the first one (*black asterisk*) has an RBBB morphology identical to the basic one (junctional origin); differently, the second (*red asterisk*) has an LBBB morphology as for an origin from the right side of the conducting system.

Variable QRS in a Patient with Biventricular Pacemaker

ECG analysis is an important tool in the evaluation of pacemaker function particularly in the presence of a biventricular device where narrowing of QRS can be used as indication of effective resynchronization.

The following ECG (see **Fig. 17**) belongs to a patient with dilated CMP who received a biventricular implantable cardioverter defibrillator 3 years before with good clinical response. Baseline ECG before implant shows an LBBB with QRS duration of 180 ms (see **Fig. 17**.1). Paced ECG shows 3 distinct QRS morphologies:

- During DDD pacing QRS duration 120 ms, with "Qr" in leads I and aVl and an initial r in V1 and V2 (see **Fig. 17**.2)
- During VDD pacing QRS duration 100 ms with incomplete LBBB morphology, loss of Q wave in I and aVL and loss of r in V1 and V2 (see **Fig. 17**.3)
- During VVI pacing an RBBB morphology with a QRS duration of 180 ms (see **Fig. 17**.4)

Diagnostic key: the observation of changes in QRS morphology related to presence or absence of atrial pacing (see **Fig. 18**), well evident during atrial threshold test. The ventricular vectors generated by atrial pacing versus spontaneous SR should be similar as both travel via the same HPS. The difference is the time lag between origin of the atrial depolarization and engagement of the conduction system. A paced rhythm activates the atria from the RAA generating a wavefront further away from the normal conduction axis if compared with atrial depolarization from a sinus beat. The longer the intraatrial conduction lag, the lesser the amount of the V depolarized before the arrival of the wavefront generated by the LV pacing. Observing the 3 different ECGs during pacing (ECG 2, 3, 4 of **Figs. 17** and **19**) it is possible to identify the degree of fusion between these 2 wavefronts and infer the effect of intraatrial delay by observing the presence or absence of atrial pacing:

- During atrial pacing (ECG 2 of **Figs. 17** and **19**), the initial depolarizing vector is carried by LV pacing wavefront with a left to right vector (see **Fig. 19** ECG 2, red component and negative deflections in lead I and aVL, r in V1 and V2); the late activation from the HPS will become evident later with an R to L vector (green component in **Fig. 19**.2 and late positive component of I and aVL in **Fig. 17**.2).

- During SR (ECG 3 in **Fig. 17** and in **Fig. 19**), the V activation originating from sinus node will become manifest at the beginning of the QRS and depolarize most of the ventricles (green component). The QRS will resemble an incomplete LBBB and its shorter duration is due to the fusion with the LV pacing wavefront (red component), which is evident in the later portion of the QRS.
- During VVI ventricular pacing (ECG 4 in **Figs. 17** and **19**), noticeable is the lack of RV pacing in any of these tracings: the ventricles are activated exclusively in L to R direction (red component). The malfunction of RV lead was documented by interrogating the pacemaker.
- An interesting point in this case is the patient's good clinical response despite apparent loss of pacing synchrony due to RV lead failure. This probably was due to the fusion between physiologic conduction via the HPS and LV pacing.

SUMMARY

Interpretation of the causes of QRS widening has always represented a major difficulty. This problem is rendered even more problematic during WCTs where identification of P waves and AV relationship becomes problematic. When the number of leads available for examination is limited, as during porlonged monitoring, the problem may become unsurmountable. Because of these problems, it is necessary to use every information available in an ECG tracing. The goal of this article is to focus on the reasons for QRS variations occurring during a tachycardia. Correct interpretation of these data can offer the key to understand the arrhythmia mechanism. QRS variations therefore become a parameter to be identified and interpreted as all the other more conventional parameters (ie, morphology patterns in V1 and aVr, AV dissociation, fusion etc.) used in the analysis of WCTs.

The examples presented in this article describe the electrophysiologic mechanisms causing QRS widening (aberrancy, V origin, preexcitation, and pacing) aiming to establish the foundations for a diagnostic level, which can be defined as "precision electrocardiology."

According to this approach it should be possible starting from a careful analysis of the ECG "phenotype" to proceed to unravel the electrophysiological "genotype."

By this term the authors intend the complex interplay of anatomic structure, channel distribution and function as well as autonomic effects behind any arrhythmia's mechanism.

REFERENCES

1. Luigi Padeletti L, Bagliani G. General Introduction, classification and Electrocardiographic diagnosis of cardiac arrhythmias. Card Electrophysiol Clin 2017; 9:345–63.

2. Bagliani G, De Ponti R, Gianni C, et al. The QRS complex: normal activation of the ventricles. Card Electrophysiol Clin 2017;9:453–60.

3. De Ponti R, Bagliani G, Padeletti L, et al. General approach to a wide QRS. Card Electrophysiol Clin 2017;9:461–85.

4. Brugada P, Brugada J, Mont L, et al. A new approach to the differential diagnosis of a regular tachycardia with a wide QRS complex. Circulation 1991;83(5): 1649–59.

5. Vereckei A, Duray G, Szénási G, et al. New algorithm using only lead aVR for differential diagnosis of wide QRS complex tachycardia. Heart Rhythm 2008;5(1): 89–98.

6. Bagliani G, Leonelli F, Padeletti L. P wave and the substrates of arrhythmias originating in the atria. Card Electrophysiol Clin 2017;9:365–82.

Polymorphic Wide QRS Complex Tachycardia
Differential Diagnosis

Zeynab Jebberi, MD[a], Jacopo Marazzato, MD[b],
Roberto De Ponti, MD, FHRS[b], Giuseppe Bagliani, MD[c,d],
Fabio M. Leonelli, MD[e], Serge Boveda, MD, PhD[a,*]

KEYWORDS

- Polymorphic ventricular tachycardia • Torsade de pointes • Bidirectional ventricular tachycardia
- Ventricular fibrillation • Afterdepolarizations • Phase 2 reentry • Preexcited atrial fibrillation

KEY POINTS

- Polymorphic ventricular tachycardia can be subclassified into 2 arrhythmia patterns: a specific one, which includes both torsade de pointes and bidirectional ventricular tachycardia, and a nonspecific one with multimorphic QRS complexes characterized by irregular morphology and R-R intervals.
- Polymorphic ventricular tachycardia shares many features with ventricular fibrillation, such as clinical symptoms and causing syndromes and in some cases degenerates into ventricular fibrillation.
- Preexcited atrial fibrillation over multiple accessory pathways results in a polymorphic wide QRS complex tachycardia, which is rarely encountered and represents a challenging diagnosis. Similar to polymorphic ventricular tachycardia, it is associated with high risk for sudden cardiac death.

INTRODUCTION

In patients presenting with polymorphic wide QRS complex tachycardia, a ventricular mechanism should be first considered, especially in the emergent clinical setting.[1,2] Very fast and usually irregular polymorphic ventricular tachycardia (PMVT) could potentially lead to recurrent syncope or, in worst cases, sudden cardiac death. On the other hand, worrisome consequences could be expected also in case of preexcited atrial fibrillation with fast atrioventricular conduction over multiple accessory pathways. In fact, under certain circumstances, a preexcited atrial fibrillation could mimic the clinical and electrocardiographic presentation of a PMVT and may degenerate into ventricular fibrillation (VF). The urgent clinical circumstances usually associated with the presentation of these arrhythmias require a fast, straightforward, and accurate electrocardiographic analysis for correct patient management.

In **Box 1**, a classification of both supraventricular and ventricular polymorphic wide QRS complex tachycardias is proposed. Q-T interval prolongation represents the mainstay of PMVT classification, but, apart from torsades de pointes (TdP), Q-T interval assessment might be of little use in common clinical practice, because most

Disclosure Statement: No conflicts to disclose.
[a] Cardiac Arrhythmia Management Department, Clinique Pasteur, BP 27617, 45 Avenue de Lombez, Toulouse 31076, France; [b] Department of Heart and Vessels, Ospedale di Circolo and Macchi Foundation, University of Insubria, Viale Borri, 57, Varese 21100, Italy; [c] Cardiology Department, Arrhythmology Unit, Foligno General Hospital, Foligno, Via Massimo Arcamone, Foligno, Perugia 06034, Italy; [d] Cardiovascular Diseases Department, University of Perugia, Piazza Menghini 1, Perugia 06129, Italy; [e] Cardiology Department, James A. Haley Veterans' Hospital, University of South Florida, 13000 Bruce B Down Boulevard, Tampa, FL 33612, USA
* Corresponding author.
E-mail address: sboveda@clinique-pasteur.com

Card Electrophysiol Clin 11 (2019) 333–344
https://doi.org/10.1016/j.ccep.2019.02.004

PMVTs occur with normal Q-T interval. Therefore, a pathogenetic classification related to the triggering mechanism of these tachycardias could be much more useful in this challenging clinical scenario.

In the following sections, some of the most common polymorphic tachycardias will be presented based on clinical cases and briefly discussed.

CASE-BASED PRESENTATION OF POLYMORPHIC WIDE QRS COMPLEX TACHYCARDIA
Case 1: Torsade de Pointes

An 85-year-old man with prior history of ischemic heart disease, mitral regurgitation, and previous episodes of atrial flutter was admitted to the emergency department for dizziness. On admittance, the electrocardiogram (ECG) showed sinus rhythm with complete atrioventricular block (**Fig. 1**). Because no clear reversible cause of the block was identified, the patient underwent a dual-chamber pacemaker implantation (Medtronic ASTRA DR) and the Managed Ventricular Pacing (MVP) algorithm was activated with the intention to minimize unnecessary right ventricular stimulation. After a few hours, the patient had syncope with evidence of a polymorphic and wide QRS complex tachycardia on ECG monitoring. As shown in **Fig. 2**, the arrhythmia presented with a progressive change and twisting pattern in the morphology of the QRS complexes, followed by an almost disorganized activity rapidly leading to VF. All these elements are in favor of TdP with quick degeneration into VF. Careful evaluation of the ECG before the event revealed a short-long-short (SLS) ventricular sequence initiating the TdP (**Fig. 3**). In fact, the short-coupled premature ventricular complex occurs after a long pause facilitated by the MVP pacing mode, which usually

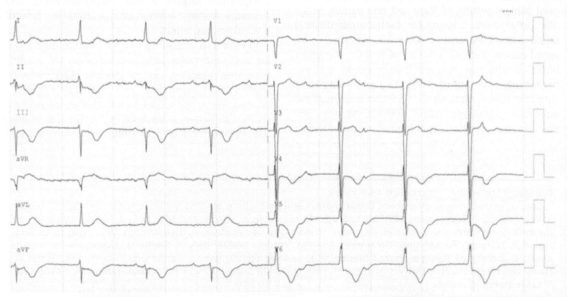

Fig. 1. Case 1. Sinus rhythm with complete atrioventricular block and slow rate subjunctional rhythm with relatively narrow QRS complex.

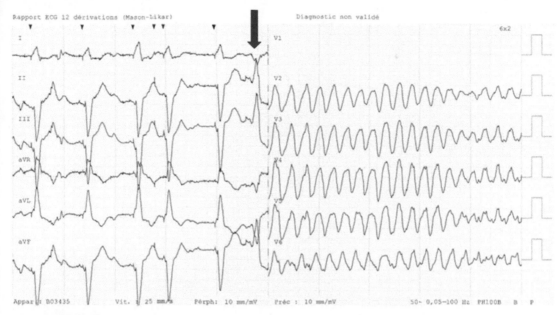

Fig. 2. Case 1. Initiation of a polymorphic ventricular tachycardia by a premature ventricular complex (*red arrow*) observed in the peripheral leads. Subsequently, in the precordial leads, a short sequence of QRS complexes with a pattern twisting from positive to negative is observed, which complies with the definition of torsade de pointes. In this patient, this arrhythmia quickly degenerated into VF.

allows longer and irregular R-R intervals in order to facilitate the native conduction. In this patient affected by significant structural heart disease, this pause caused dispersion of repolarization with longer Q-T interval in the last paced beat, which favored TdP. After successful defibrillation and pacemaker reprogramming in permanent DDD mode, the ventricular arrhythmia did not recur any longer during follow-up (**Fig. 4**).

Bidirectional Ventricular Tachycardia

Case 2: bidirectional ventricular tachycardia occurring in catecholaminergic polymorphic ventricular tachycardia syndrome

A 15-year-old girl with no prior significant clinical history was referred for outpatient evaluation because of recurrent exercise-related syncope. The ECG of a first-degree relative was available and showed a regularly irregular wide QRS

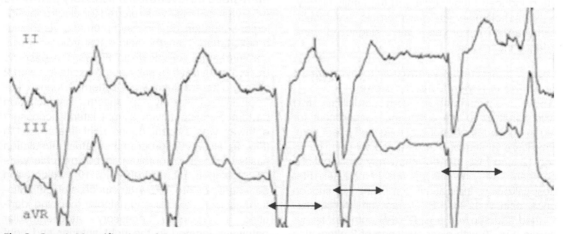

Fig. 3. Case 1. Magnification of the short-long-short sequence of QRS complexes observed in the previous figure. A Q-T interval dispersion is evident (*red horizontal arrows* show the Q-T interval durations) favored by the pacing modality. The shortest Q-T interval is observed after the first short R-R interval, whereas the longest occurs after the long pause and the subsequent premature ventricular complex generates a short R-R interval and initiates a pause-dependent torsade de point.

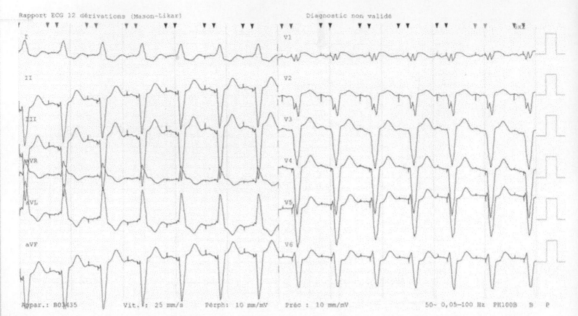

Fig. 4. Case 1. Pacemaker reprogramming in DDD mode allows stable 1:1 atrioventricular conduction, avoids pauses, and eliminates short-long-short sequences with Q-T interval normalization.

complex tachycardia with 2 alternating morphologies of the QRS complex and 2 different R-R intervals (**Fig. 5**), which can be diagnosed as bidirectional ventricular tachycardia (BVT). The 12-lead ECG of this young patient was normal at rest, and the echocardiogram did not show any structural heart disease. A 24-hour Holter monitoring showed an effort-induced ventricular bigeminal rhythm rapidly degenerating into a self-limiting episode of polymorphic ventricular tachycardia (**Fig. 6**). In consideration of the effort-induced tachycardia and the family history, a catecholaminergic polymorphic ventricular tachycardia syndrome was diagnosed and adequately treated.

Case 3: bidirectional ventricular tachycardia occurring in ischemic heart disease

A 56-year-old man with an old myocardial infarction was admitted to the emergency department for recent episodes of brief dizziness and chest pain. Physical examination was unremarkable, and baseline 12-lead ECG did not show any modifications compared with previous tracings. Immediately after hospitalization, the patient complained of sudden chest pain. A 12-lead ECG was immediately performed and showed a wide QRS complex tachycardia (**Fig. 7**) with clear evidence of 2 alternating morphologies of the QRS complex and, in lead II, also alternating polarity of the QRS complex. Moreover, the R-R intervals were regularly irregular with a sequence of shorter (280 ms) and longer (320 ms)

intervals. The tachycardia self-terminated within 2 minutes. The patient underwent a coronary angiogram with no evidence of significant coronary artery disease and no increase in the cardiac biomarkers was observed. All these clinical and electrocardiographic elements suggest BVT in the context of chronic ischemic heart disease.

Preexcited Atrial Fibrillation

Case 4: preexcited atrial fibrillation over 2 right-sided atrioventricular accessory pathways

A 51-year-old man was referred for electrophysiologic evaluation due to asymptomatic ventricular preexcitation. Transthoracic echocardiogram was unremarkable. As shown in **Fig. 8**, the baseline ECG in sinus rhythm showed preexcitation with 2 slightly different delta-wave patterns. During electrophysiologic study, a uniform preexcitation pattern consistent with a right lateral accessory pathway was evident during right lateral pacing (**Fig. 9**). However, programmed atrial stimulation easily induced a nontolerated polymorphic wide QRS complex tachycardia (**Fig. 10**), which soon degenerated into VF. After successful defibrillation, accurate bipolar and unipolar mapping identified 2 distinct accessory atrioventricular pathways located in the right anterior and right posteroseptal regions, which were successfully ablated during the same session. In this case, the polymorphic tachycardia was actually a preexcited atrial fibrillation with alternating antegrade

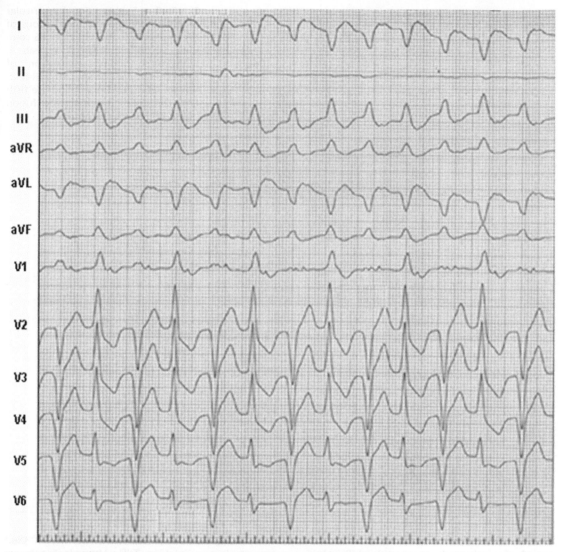

Fig. 5. Case 2. Bidirectional ventricular tachycardia with 2 morphologies of QRS complex and 2 R-R intervals alternating in a regular way. The R-R interval between the negative QRS complex in V2-V6 is constantly shorter than the subsequent R-R interval between the positive and negative QRS complex.

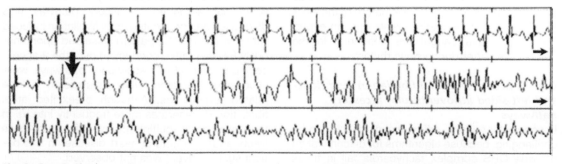

Fig. 6. Case 2. Single continuous ECG tracing during Holter monitoring in a patient with circumstantial evidence of catecholaminergic polymorphic ventricular tachycardia. In the second line during effort-related sinus tachycardia, initiation of a sequence (*vertical arrow*) of ventricular premature complexes with short-long-short R-R intervals eventually inducing a polymorphic ventricular tachycardia is shown. This arrhythmia will convert to sinus rhythm after 2 minutes (not shown) (*Horizontal arrows*) mean that tracing is continuing in the 3 panels (from the superior panel to the inferior one...).

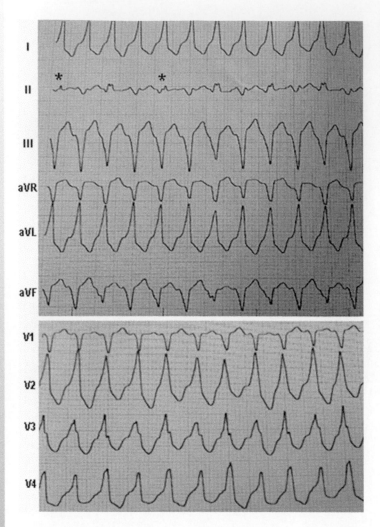

Fig. 7. Case 3. Bidirectional ventricular tachycardia with regular variations of the axis and duration of the QRS complex, particularly evident in lead II, with corresponding alternation of short (280 ms) and long (320 ms) R-R intervals. Of note, the first and the fifth QRS complexes (*asterisks*) are fusion beasts with sinus rhythm.

conduction over these 2 accessory pathways. In **Fig. 10**, the antegrade conduction shift between the 2 accessory pathways is evident as a change in QRS complex polarity in the inferior leads. In this setting, a clear differential diagnosis can be easily made due to the invasive nature of the electrophysiologic investigation, while only an expert eye might have caught the difference in the delta-wave patter during sinus rhythm.

Case 5: preexcited atrial fibrillation over right- and left-sided atrioventricular accessory pathways

In some other cases, differential diagnosis can be challenging, because algorithms for discrimination of wide QRS complex tachycardia fail in these cases. In fact, **Fig. 11** shows the ECG of a 21-year-old male patient with hypertrophic cardiomyopathy who presented to the emergency department with well-tolerated palpitations. Although limited to 3 tracings, this ECG clearly shows an alternating pattern of the QRS complex morphology mimicking TdP. After electrical cardioversion, only the right-sided ventricular preexcitation was manifest in sinus rhythm. However, during electrophysiologic study, a second atrioventricular left-sided accessory pathway was diagnosed and preexcited atrial fibrillation induced with the same ECG pattern observed spontaneously for alternative conduction over the 2 accessory pathways. Both accessory pathways were successfully ablated with suppression of the related arrhythmias. Although preexcited atrial fibrillation degenerates more frequently into VF in the presence of multiple atrioventricular by-pass tracts and/or structural heart disease, in this patient such an event was not observed.

These cases are paradigmatic of the fact that, although rare, preexcited atrial fibrillation over 2 accessory pathways may mimic a PMVT and it should always be considered in the differential diagnosis.

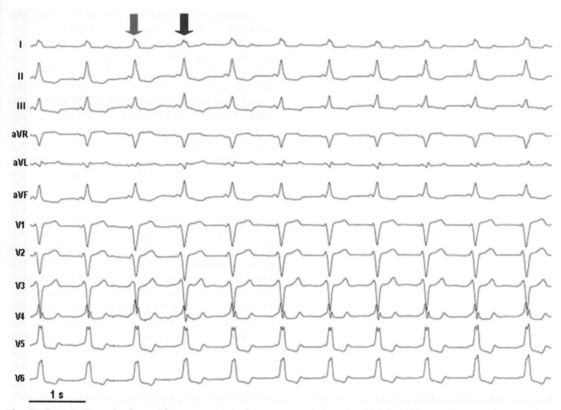

Fig. 8. Case 4. Sinus rhythm with overt ventricular preexcitation and 2 slightly different patterns (blue and red *arrows*), more evident in leads I, aVL, and V4.

DISCUSSION

PMVT is defined as a ventricular tachyarrhythmia with a changing QRS complex morphology and axis on a beat-to-beat basis, often with irregular R-R intervals in any ECG lead.[3] As commonly observed in clinical practice, PMVT is usually a fast arrhythmia, but slower polymorphic tachycardias with manifest changing QRS complex morphologies have been also described.[4] Despite being closely related to VF, PMVT should be kept nosologically distinct.[2] In fact, during VF episodes, QRS complexes are not consistently identifiable on ECG due to the completely chaotic electrical activation occurring in the ventricles and, differently from VF, PMVT has tendency to self-termination.[2]

In the following sections, the pathogenetic mechanisms triggering PMVT and giving rise to specific and nonspecific electrocardiographic patterns are briefly presented and discussed.

Torsades de Pointes

First described by Dessertenne in 1966,[5] TdP (literally "twisting of the points") is regarded as a distinct PMVT usually presenting with a peculiar ECG pattern showing a progressive undulating variability in the QRS complex morphology, amplitude, and polarity, creating a peculiar twisting aspect of the arrhythmia. TdP generally occur in the setting of a prolonged Q-T interval.[2,6] Normally, Q-T interval is the expression of myocardial action potential duration determined by the balance between positive outward (repolarizing) currents, mediated by potassium delayed rectifier channels (IKs and IKr), and positive inward calcium ions.[7] A variation of action potential duration between epicardial myocytes and midendocardial cells has been described[8] with the longest effective refractory period occurring in the midendocardial cells, which mostly influence both total Q-T interval duration and transmural dispersion of repolarization. Therefore, a genetically determined or acquired prolongation of the Q-T interval enhances a nonuniform prolongation of repolarization among myocytes, worsening the transmural dispersion of repolarization and facilitating early afterdepolarization (EAD)-triggered activity and reentry.[9] This pathogenetic mechanism underpins the SLS sequence on ECG often preceding initiation of "pause-dependent" TdP, observed in most patients with acquired or congenital long Q-T interval.[10,11] In this setting, a long ventricular

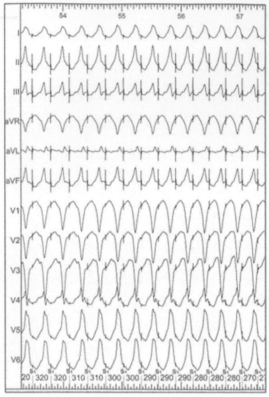

Fig. 9. Case 4. At electrophysiologic study, the preexcitation pattern becomes uniform during incremental right lateral atrial pacing. Numbers in the bottom line indicate the pacing cycle length.

pause induces phase-3 EAD-triggered activity generating a ventricular extra beat with a quite short coupling interval, generally less than 600 ms.[11] The ventricular premature complex then propagates in areas with highly heterogeneous action potential prolongation, maintaining TdP through a reentrant mechanism.[9] Pause-dependent TdP episodes occurring in patients implanted with cardiac devices have been also reported.[12,13] Sweeney and colleagues[12] reported 139 such cases from the PainFREE RxII and EnTRUST studies. As in the first case presented, specific pacing modalities might induce SLS sequences and right ventricular pacing might increase dispersion in ventricular activation times, creating vulnerable windows for reentry[14] and favoring the occurrence of PMVTs.

In a minority of cases, TdP episodes may occur in the setting of a pause-independent mechanism.[11,15] "Pause-independent" TdP usually develop in young patients affected by severe forms of congenital long Q-T syndromes, in whom sinus tachycardia per se may be sufficient

to generate short-coupled premature ventricular contractions ensued from phase-2 EAD.[10,11]

Finally, a short-coupled variant of TdP (scTdP) has been reported[16–18] usually occurring in the setting of absence of structural heart disease and normal Q-T interval with an extremely short (<300 ms) coupling interval of the first tachycardia beat. Different pathogenetic mechanisms have been advocated, but the verapamil sensitivity of this polymorphic arrhythmia would suggest a triggered activity mediated by EAD or delayed afterdepolarizations (DAD).[16,17] In the scTdP case presented by Shiga and colleagues,[17] the electrophysiologic study showed a clear heterogeneity of ventricular refractoriness together with the shortest ventricular effective refractory period measured at the right ventricular inflow site, where the paced QRS complex had an identical morphology compared with the one initiating scTdP. In the seminal work by Haïssaguerre and colleagues,[19] twenty-seven cases resuscitated from idiopathic VF undergoing electrophysiologic evaluation had similar clinical and electrocardiographic presentation compared with the patients affected by scTdP reported in previous works.[16,17] However, the triggering premature ventricular beats mainly originated from the peripheral Purkinje conducting system and ablation of these foci resulted in a high success rate in term of clinical outcome. Therefore, a clear distinction between scTdP and idiopathic VF is lacking and until the pathogenesis is further specified, scTdP should be regarded as a subgroup of idiopathic VF.[20]

Bidirectional Ventricular Tachycardia

As shown in **Box 2**, a variety of acquired and congenital conditions[21–28] are associated with BVT. Actually, diagnosis of this ventricular arrhythmia is merely clinical based on the ECG pattern. BVT is defined as a regularly irregular PMVT with the typical electrocardiographic expression of 2 distinct QRS complex morphologies with alternating axis of opposite polarities.[29] Although a QRS complex with a right bundle branch block morphology and alternating axis on bipolar leads is the most frequently encountered electrocardiographic pattern,[30] other ECG presentations have been described, such as alternating right and left bundle branch block patterns or narrower QRS complexes with alternating axis.[31] Different pathogenetic molecular explanations have been advocated for BVT, but DAD-triggered activity ensued from intracellular calcium overload is now considered the main underlying mechanism.[32] Whatever the cause of exaggerated calcium release from sarcoplasmic reticulum, the

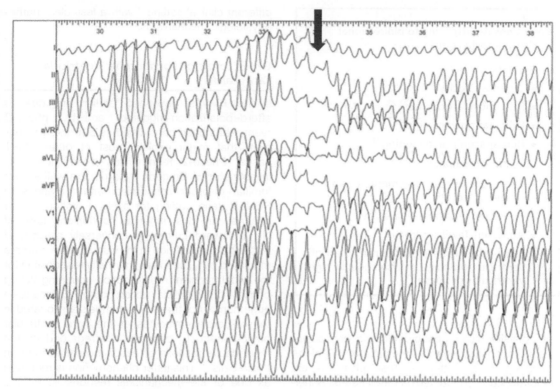

Fig. 10. Case 4. Twelve-lead ECG of the polymorphic tachycardia induced during electrophysiologic study. The arrhythmia quickly degenerates into ventricular flutter/fibrillation (from *red arrow* on). On the left hand side of the figure, although precordial leads show invariably a left bundle branch block morphology, in the inferior leads 2 alternating morphologies of the QRS complex are identified with negative and positive complexes, which suggests antegrade conduction over 2 distinct right-sided accessory pathways.

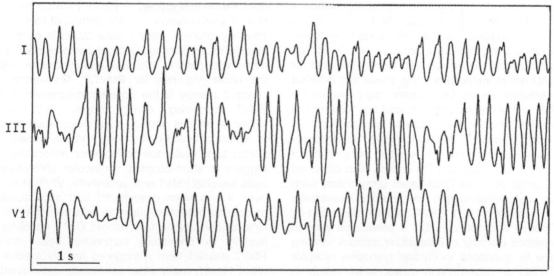

Fig. 11. Case 5. Leads I, III, and V1 of the ECG of a patient presenting with palpitations. The patient had a diagnosis of hypertrophic cardiomyopathy and Wolff-Parkinson-White syndrome with right-sided ventricular preexcitation. In this ECG, an almost regular alternation of 2 QRS complex morphologies is observed, which configures a pattern of polymorphic tachycardia, related in this case to preexcited atrial fibrillation over 2 accessory pathways. Although the first pattern has positive complexes in lead I and negative in III and V1 consistent with a right-sided posterolateral accessory pathway, the second shows negative complexes in I and positive in III and V1, due to conduction over a second left lateral accessory pathway, not evident during sinus rhythm.

Box 2
Conditions predisposing to bidirectional ventricular tachycardia

1. Acquired:
   - Digitalis toxicity[21]
   - Ischemic heart disease[22,23]
   - Fulminant myocarditis[24]
   - Herbal aconitine poisoning[25]

2. Idiopathic/familial:
   - Catecholaminergic polymorphic ventricular tachycardia[30]
   - Hypokalemic periodic paralysis[26]
   - Andersen-Tawil syndrome[27]
   - Fibro-fatty tissue infiltration in the right ventricle (possibly arrhythmogenic right ventricular dysplasia)[28]

pathophysiologic process by which triggered activity spontaneously generates the peculiar BVT electrocardiographic pattern is less clear. In an elaborate study conducted on rabbit hearts, Baher and colleagues[29] proposed a "ping-pong" model for the mechanism of BVT. According to this study, different heart rate thresholds for DAD exist in specific regions of the heart, probably located in the distal His-Purkinje system.[33] Therefore, a fast sinus rhythm initially provokes a premature ventricular beat from myocardial areas with lower threshold for DAD-triggered activity originating a bigeminal ventricular rhythm. As a consequence, heart rate doubles and new areas with higher threshold for DAD are recruited producing a new and different premature ventricular complex; this maintains the BVT with a mechanism activated in a "ping-pong" fashion. This model could also explain PMVT. In fact, if more than 2 foci with triggered activity properties are recruited, the resulting arrhythmia will have a pleomorphic ECG aspect, also observed in some of these DAD-based arrhythmias, such as catecholaminergic polymorphic ventricular tachycardia (CPVT). CPVT, originally described by Coumel and colleagues,[34] is associated with an inherited disorder of intracellular calcium handling due to mutations in cardiac ryanodine receptor (RYR2) or calsequestrin genes, which results in stress-induced bidirectional or polymorphic ventricular arrhythmias potentially degenerating into VF.[35] Finally, although rare, BVT has also been reported in ischemic heart disease as in the clinical case presented earlier and could occur during acute myocardial infarction[22] or in a completely

different clinical setting[23] with a less clear pathophysiologic mechanisms.

Other Forms of Polymorphic Ventricular Tachycardia

If the PMVTs described earlier are due to afterdepolarization-triggered activity, phase-2 reentry has been considered as a further mechanism that might explain most of other PMVT cases. Phase-2 reentry has been thoroughly investigated in Brugada syndrome, a well-known familial disorder associated with mutations in SCN5A gene coding for a Na + voltage-gated channel. In this inherited condition, loss of Na + inward current is conversely associated with a gain of function in the outward K+ currents mediated by I_{to} channels, normally responsible for the initial transient repolarization occurring during phase 1 of the cellular action potential. Because a huge number of these K+ channels are located in the epicardial myocytes of the right ventricular outflow tract, I_{to} channels are regarded as the main cause for loss of action potential dome in these cells.[36] This latter phenomenon is regarded as one of the mechanisms responsible for the development of PMVTs, observed in many cases affected by this syndrome, in which the epicardial action potential dome spreads from sites where it is maintained to sites where it is lost. This causes a phase-2 short-coupled premature ventricular complex, which triggers a PMVT initiated by an R-on-T phenomenon.[36] In the setting of these J-wave syndromes, early repolarization is considered to share common pathophysiologic mechanisms with patients with Brugada syndrome and the underlying risk for PMVT.[37] Furthermore, phase-2 reentry is the potential mechanism for PMVT occurring during acute myocardial ischemia. In this setting, a heterogeneous loss of action potential dome occurs in the ischemic border zone where the nonischemic myocardium triggers a short-coupled ventricular premature beat, causing PMVT and, potentially, VF.[38] Moreover, it has been described[39] that after acute myocardial infarction, surviving cells from the Purkinje system might have altered Ca^{++} handling, leading to premature ventricular beats and PMVT ensued from a triggered activity mechanism. Finally, many other genetically determined abnormalities predispose to PMVT with different potential explanations. For instance, in the short Q-T syndrome, the gain of function in the outward repolarization currents increases the transmural dispersion of refractoriness, provoking life-threatening arrhythmias in these patients[40] with a mechanism similar to the one previously described in long Q-T patients.

SUMMARY

The electrocardiographic presentation of a polymorphic wide QRS complex tachycardia is in most cases associated with a ventricular origin. Considering the wide spectrum of causes and the emergent clinical setting in which it usually occurs, diagnosis is challenging and correct patient management difficult. The arrhythmogenetic mechanism of PMVT can be variable and includes afterdepolarization as a triggering mechanism and "ping-pong" reciprocating bigeminal activity or reentry as perpetuating mechanisms. These phenomena may lead to specific and sometimes pathognomonic ECG patterns, such as TdP or BVT. Rarely, but not exceptionally, preexcited atrial fibrillation over multiple accessories can mimic a PMVT. Although this supraventricular arrhythmia carries a similar risk for sudden death considering the presence of multiple accessory pathways, it requires a completely different management.

REFERENCES

1. Passmann R, Kadish A. Polymorphic ventricular tachycardia, long Q-T syndrome, and torsades de pointes. Med Clin North Am 2001;85:321–41.
2. Choudhuri I, Pinninti M, Marwali MR, et al. Polymorphic ventricular tachycardia-part I: structural heart disease and acquired causes. Curr Probl Cardiol 2013;38:463–96.
3. Waldo AL, Akhtar M, Brugada P, et al. The minimally appropriate electrophysiologic study for the initial assessment of patients with documented sustained monomorphic ventricular tachycardia. J Am Coll Cardiol 1985;6:1174–7.
4. Nguyen PT, Scheinman MM, Seger J. Polymorphous ventricular tachycardia: clinical characterization, therapy, and the QT interval. Circulation 1986;74: 340–9.
5. Dessertenne F. Ventricular tachycardia with 2 variable opposing foci. Arch Mal Coeur Vaiss 1966;59: 263–72 [in French].
6. Choudhuri I, Pinninti M, Marwali MR, et al. Polymorphic ventricular tachycardia–part II: the channelopathies. Curr Probl Cardiol 2013;38:503–48.
7. Chen L, Sampson KJ, Kass RS. Cardiac delayed rectifier potassium channels in health and disease. Card Electrophysiol Clin 2016;8:307–22.
8. Yan GX, Antzelevitch C. Cellular basis for the normal T-wave and the electrocardiographic manifestation of the long-QT syndrome. Circulation 1998;98: 1928–36.
9. Anztelevich C, Shimizu W. Cellular mechanism underlying the long QT syndrome. Curr Opin Cardiol 2002;17:43–51.
10. Roden DM, Anderson ME. The pause that refreshes, or does it? Mechanisms in Torsade de Pointes. Heart 2000;84:235–7.
11. Noda T, Shimizu W, Satomi K. Classification and mechanism in Torsade de Pointes initiation in patients with congenital long QT syndrome. Eur Heart J 2004;25:2149–54.
12. Sweeney MO, Ruetz LL, Belk P, et al. Bradycardia pacing-induced short-long-short sequences at the onset of ventricular tachyarrhythmias. A possible mechanism of proarrhythmia? J Am Coll Cardiol 2007;50:614–22.
13. Vavasis C, Slotwiner DJ, Goldner BG, et al. Frequent recurrent polymorphic ventricular tachycardia during sleep due to managed ventricular pacing. Pacing Clin Electrophysiol 2010;33:641–4.
14. Kuo CS, Amlie JP, Munakata K, et al. Dispersion of monophasic action potential durations and activation times during atrial pacing, ventricular pacing, and ventricular premature stimulation in canine ventricles. Cardiovasc Res 1983;17:152–61.
15. Viskin S, Fish R, Zeltser D, et al. Arrhythmias in congenital LongQT syndrome: how often is Torsade de Pointes pause dependent? Heart 2000;83: 661–6.
16. Leenhardt A, Glaser E, Burguera M, et al. Short-coupled variant of torsade de pointes: a new electrocardiographic entity in the spectrum of idiopathic ventricular tachyarrhythmias. Circulation 1994;89: 206–15.
17. Shiga T, Shoda M, Matsuda N, et al. Electrophysiological characteristic of a patient exhibiting the short-coupled variant of torsade de pointes. J Electrocardiol 2001;34:271–5.
18. Chokr MO, Darrieux FC, Hardy CA, et al. Short-coupled variant of "torsades de pointes" and polymorphic ventricular tachycardia. Arq Bras Cardiol 2014;102:e60–4.
19. Haïssaguerre M, Shoda M, Jaïs P, et al. Mapping and ablation of idiopathic ventricular fibrillation. Circulation 2002;106:962–7.
20. Visser M, Van der Heijden JF, Doevendans PA, et al. Idiopathic ventricular fibrillation; the struggle for definition, diagnosis, and follow-up. Circ Arrhythm Electrophysiol 2016;9:e003817.
21. Valent S, Kelly P. Digoxin-induced bidirectional ventricular tachycardia. N Engl J Med 1997;336: 550.
22. Sonmez O, Gul EE, Duman C, et al. Type II bidirectional ventricular tachycardia in a patient with myocardial infarction. J Electrocardiol 2009;42: 631–2.
23. Wase A, Masood AM, Garikipati NV, et al. Bidirectional ventricular tachycardia with myocardial

infarction: a case report with insight on mechanism and treatment. Indian Heart J 2014;66:466–9.

24. Berte B, Eyskens B, Meyfroidt G, et al. Bidirectional ventricular tachycardia in fulminant myocarditis. Europace 2008;10:767–8.

25. Smith SW, Shah RR, Hunt JL, et al. Bidirectional ventricular tachycardia resulting from herbal aconitine poisoning. Ann Emerg Med 2005;45:100.

26. Stubbs WA. Bidirectional ventricular tachycardia in familial hypokalemic periodic paralysis. Proc R Soc Med 1976;69:223–4.

27. Morita H, Zipes DP, Morita ST, et al. Mechanism of U wave and polymorphic ventricular tachycardia in a canine tissue model of Andersen-Tawil syndrome. Cardiovasc Res 2007;75:510–8.

28. Ueda-Tatsumoto A, Sakurada H, Nishizaki M, et al. Bidirectional ventricular tachycardia caused by a reentrant mechanism with left bundle branch block configuration on electrocardiography. Circ J 2008; 72:1373–7.

29. Baher AA, Uy M, Xie F, et al. Bidirectional ventricular tachycardia: ping-pong in the his-purkinje system. Heart Rhythm 2011;8:599–605.

30. Leenhardt A, Luvet V, Denjoy I, et al. Catecholaminergic polymorphic ventricular tachycardia in children: a 7-year follow-up of 21 patients. Circulation 1995;91:1512–9.

31. Rothfeld EL. Bidirectional tachycardia with normal QRS duration. Am Heart J 1976;92:231–3.

32. Sumitomo N. Current topics in catecholaminergic polymorphic ventricular tachycardia. J Arrhythm 2016;32:344–51.

33. Cerrone M, Colombi B, Santoro M, et al. Bidirectional ventricular tachycardia and fibrillation elicited in knock-in mouse model carrier of a mutation in the cardiac ryanodine receptor. Circ Res 2005;96: e77–82.

34. Coumel P, Fidelle J, Lucet V, et al. Catecholaminergic-induced severe ventricular arrhythmias with Adams-Stokes syndrome in children: report of four cases. Br Heart J 1978;40:28–37.

35. Sumitomo M, Harada K, Nagashima M, et al. Catecholaminergic polymorphic ventricular tachycardia: electrocardiographic characteristics and optimal therapeutic strategies to prevent sudden death. Heart 2003;89:66–70.

36. Antzelevich C. The Brugada syndrome: ionic basis and arrhythmia mechanism. J Cardiovasc Electrophysiol 2001;12:268–72.

37. Koncz I, Gurabi Z, Patocskai B, et al. Mechanisms underlying the development of the electrocardiographic and arrhythmic manifestations of early repolarization syndrome. J Mol Cell Cardiol 2014;68: 20–8.

38. Yan GX, Joshi A, Guo D, et al. Phase 2 reentry as a trigger to initiate ventricular fibrillation during early acute myocardial ischemia. Circulation 2004;110: 1036–41.

39. Haissaguerre M, Vigmond E, Stuyvers B, et al. Ventricular arrhythmias and the His-Purkinje system. Nat Rev Cardiol 2016;13:155–6.

40. Extramiana F, Antzelevitch C. Amplified transmural dispersion of repolarization as the basis for arrhythmogenesis in a canine ventricular-wedge model of short-QT syndrome. Circulation 2004; 110:3661–6.

Arrhythmias due to Inherited and Acquired Abnormalities of Ventricular Repolarization

Emanuela T. Locati, MD, PhD[a,b,]*, Giuseppe Bagliani, MD[c,d],
Franco Cecchi, MD[h,e,f], Helou Johny, MD[c],
Maurizio Lunati, MD[g], Carlo Pappone, MD[a]

KEYWORDS

- Ventricular repolarization • QT interval • Ventricular arrhythmias • Ventricular fibrillation
- Sudden death • T-wave alternans • Long QT syndrome • Short QT Syndrome

KEY POINTS

- Several cardiac and noncardiac drugs and disease conditions, including mutations of genes encoding ion channels, may affect the ventricular repolarization process and favor arrhythmogenesis.
- Congenital and acquired ventricular repolarization abnormalities can be reflected on the surface electrocardiogram as prolonged or shortened QT interval, early repolarization, and abnormal T-wave configuration.
- Multiple mechanisms, including abnormal automaticity, afterdepolarization-induced triggered activity, and functional or structural reentry circuits, can provoke ventricular arrhythmias in congenital or acquired conditions of abnormal ventricular repolarization.
- Ventricular arrhythmias associated with abnormalities of ventricular repolarization typically are rapid, usually polymorphic, ventricular tachycardia or torsades de pointes, often degenerating into ventricular fibrillation.

INTRODUCTION

Genetic channelopathies have been recognized as a heterogeneous group of diseases, associated with mutations in genes encoding cardiac ionic channels that conduct sodium, potassium, and/or calcium ions, often linked to abnormal patterns of ventricular repolarization predisposing to life-threatening cardiac arrhythmias.[1–3]

For many years, prolongation of ventricular repolarization was recognized as associated with the genesis of life-threatening ventricular arrhythmias, both in acquired and in congenital conditions. Congenital long QT syndromes (LQTSs), due to several different mutations in genes encoding sodium and potassium channels, are characterized by prolonged QT interval and

[a] Department of Arryhmology, IRCCS San Donato Hospital, Piazza Edmondo Malan 2, 20097 San Donato Milanese, Milano, Italy; [b] Studio Cardiologico Locati, Viale Beatrice d'Este, 20, Milano 20122, Italy; [c] Cardiology Department, Arrhythmology Unit, Foligno General Hospital, Via Massimo Arcamore 5, Foligno 06034, Italy; [d] Cardiovascular Diseases Department, University of Perugia, Piazza Universita 1, Perugia 06123, Italy; [e] Heart and Vessels Department, University of Florence, Piazza San Marco 4, 50121 Florence, Italy; [f] IRCCS Auxologico, Milano, Cardiovascular San Luca Hospital, Piazzale Brescia 1, 20100 Milan, Italy; [g] Cardiothoracovascular Department, Electrophysiology Unit, Niguarda Hospital, Piazza Ospedale Maggiore 1, 20162 Milano, Italy
* Corresponding author. Studio Cardiologico Locati, Viale Beatrice d'Este, 20, Milano 20122, Italy.
E-mail address: emlocati@studiocardiologicolocati.it

Card Electrophysiol Clin 11 (2019) 345–362
https://doi.org/10.1016/j.ccep.2019.02.009

abnormal T-wave configuration and increased susceptibility to polymorphic ventricular tachycardia (VT), often defined as torsades de pointes (TdP).[4–6]

More recently, there has been major focus on arrhythmogenesis associated with abnormalities of the early phase of ventricular repolarization, defined as *early repolarization syndromes (ERSs)* or *J-wave syndromes*, among which the best known is the Brugada syndrome (BrS).[7,8] The last disorder of ventricular repolarization associated with ventricular tachyarrhythmias is the short QT syndrome (SQTS), a rare genetically inherited cardiac channelopathy on the same spectrum as other familial arrhythmogenic diseases.[9]

PHYSIOPATHOLOGIC BASIS OF ABNORMAL REPOLARIZATION

Even in normal conditions, ventricular repolarization is more heterogeneous than ventricular depolarization. The presence of progressive shorter repolarization in areas of later activation tends to synchronize ventricular repolarization, and it may be an important physiologic mechanism in the prevention of arrhythmias. A variety of congenital and acquired conditions (including genetic abnormalities of cardiac ion channels or different inherited and acquired cardiomyopathies, cardiac ischemia, bundle branch block, pre-excitation, and exposure to cardiac and non-cardiac drugs) can alter the repolarization process, favoring the arrhythmogenesis.[2]

The physiology of the repolarization process has been reviewed in detail elsewhere.[10] In synthesis, although the ventricular activation, reflected by the QRS complex on the surface ECG, corresponds to the fast spreading of the depolarization through the ventricular muscle, the ventricular repolarization, reflected by the ST segment and T wave, represents the recovery period of the ventricles. Thus, the QT interval on the surface ECG represents the sum of depolarization and repolarization process of the ventricles.

Although ventricular depolarization is based mainly on fast inward sodium-dependent currents, ventricular repolarization depends mainly on the transmembrane outward transport of potassium ions, to reestablish the endocellular electronegativity.[1,10] The stability of cardiac electrical activity, particularly in the plateau and recovery phase the plateau phase, is secured by some degree of redundancy in combination with the tight voltage-gated dependence regulation of ion channels. The various potassium channels involved in repolarization of the action potential represent a good example of such redundancy, and this phenomenon has been described as the *repolarization reserve*.[1,3,4,11] Outward potassium channels represent a heterogeneous family of ionic carriers, whose global kinetics is modulated by heart rate and sympathetic nervous activity and affected by several cardiac and noncardiac drugs and disease conditions and by gene mutations determining distinct channelopathies.[2,3,11]

MECHANISMS OF ARRHYTHMOGENESIS AND ABNORMALITIES OF VENTRICULAR REPOLARIZATION

The mechanisms responsible for cardiac arrhythmias are generally divided into 2 major categories: enhanced or abnormal impulse formation (due to abnormal automaticity or to triggered activity) and conduction disturbances supporting structural or functional reentry mechanisms.[2,11]

Abnormal Automaticity

In normal conditions, atrial or ventricular myocardial cells do not display automaticity (ie, spontaneous diastolic depolarization) but can develop this characteristic when depolarized, a phenomenon defined as *depolarization-induced automaticity*.[2] Like normal automaticity, enhanced automaticity is favored by catecholamines and by reduction of external potassium.

Any acquired or congenital disease condition leading to a reduced deactivation of sodium inward currents or to a reduced activation of potassium outward currents or of potassium inward rectifying currents, that mainly determine the shift from depolarization to repolarization, can lead to abnormal depolarization and to the development of enhanced or abnormal automaticity, particularly in Purkinje pacemakers. Like normal automaticity, enhanced automaticity is favored by catecholamines and by reduction of external potassium.

After Depolarization and Triggered Activity

Depolarizations that occur during or after the cardiac action potential are defined as afterdepolarization, divided in 2 subclasses: early afterdepolarization (EADs) and delayed afterdepolarizations (DADs). EAD interrupts or retards repolarization during phase 2 and/or phase 3 of the cardiac action potential, whereas DAD occurs after full repolarization. When EAD or DAD amplitude suffices to bring the membrane to its threshold potential, a spontaneous action potential, referred to as a *triggered response*, can result, and these triggered events give rise to extrasystoles, which can precipitate tachyarrhythmias.[2,10,11]

EADs develop when the balance of currents active during phase 2 and/or phase 3 of the action potential shifts in the inward direction. Several pharmacologic interventions or pathophysiological conditions, such as LQTS channelopathies, are associated with EAD development and triggered activity. The main mechanisms are linked either to a reduction of repolarizing potassium currents (IKr, IKs, or IK1) or to an increase in the availability of calcium currents (facilitated by catecholamines), sodium-calcium exchange currents (INCx), or late sodium currents (late INa). Combinations of several factors (ie, channelopathies leading to impaired ionic channel functions, calcium loading, hypokalemia, catecholamines, and drug actions) can act synergistically to facilitate the development of EADs and triggered activity[2]

DADs generally are observed under conditions that augment intracellular calcium, such as after exposure to toxic levels of digitalis or catecholamines. A typical example of DAD-induced arrhythmia is the catecholaminergic polymorphic VT (CPVT). DADs also can manifest in hypertrophied and failing hearts and in Purkinje fibers surviving myocardial infarction. In contrast to EADs, often shown to be bradycardia or pause dependent, DADs always are induced at relatively rapid rates.[2]

Reentry Mechanisms

Circus movement reentry occurs when an activation wavefront propagates around an anatomic or functional obstacle or core and re-excites the site of origin. Reentry also can be classified as anatomic and functional, although there is a gray zone in which both functional and anatomic factors are important in determining the characteristics of reentrant excitation. Transmural dispersion of repolarization due to presence of cell types with different repolarization properties within the ventricular wall plays an essential role in the development of transmural functional reentry responsible for the maintenance of VT.

Reentry also can occur without structural circus movement, as in reflection reentry and phase 2 reentry, which has been proposed as the mechanism responsible for the closely coupled extrasystole that precipitates VT or ventricular fibrillation (VF) associated with BrS and ERSs.[2,8]

Functional reentry and spatial heterogeneity may occur because ventricular myocardium is electrically heterogeneous and composed of 3 distinct cell types, epicardial cells, M cells, and endocardial cells, which differ with respect to phase 1 and phase 3 repolarization characteristics.[2] Specifically, ventricular epicardial cells and M cells, but not endocardial cells, generally display a prominent phase 1, due to large transient outward current (Ito), giving the action potential a

spike and dome or notched configuration. Amplification of transmural heterogeneities normally presents in the early and late phases of the action potential due to inherited channelopathies, including BrS, LQTSs and SQTSs, and catecholaminergic VT can lead to the development of a variety of tachyarrhythmias.[2,8]

TORSADES DE POINTES: RAPID POLYMORPHIC VENTRICULAR TACHYCARDIA ASSOCIATED WITH PROLONGED VENTRICULAR REPOLARIZATION

TdP is a rapid polymorphic VT with a distinctive, twisting configuration, typically associated with prolonged repolarization, either congenital or acquired.[4] TdP is variable in duration and often stops spontaneously, although longer runs may degenerate into VF, thus provoking sudden cardiac death. A diagnosis of TdP has great clinical implications because treatment differs from that of other forms of sustained VT.[4]

The electrophysiologic mechanisms involved in the genesis of TdP have not been conclusively established, and both reentry from dispersion of repolarization and triggered activity associated with EAD have been proposed.[2,4] Either hypothesis could explain some of the features typically observed in TdP, such as the long coupling interval of the initial extrasystole, the facilitation by slow heart rate, and the presence of a pause determining a typical initiating pattern, often referred to as long-short sequence. The prodromal pause, often associated with further prolongation of ventricular repolarization in the following beat, supports the definition of TdP as a typical example of bradycardia-dependent arrhythmias[2,12] (Fig. 1).

Atrial fibrillation or paroxysmal atrioventricular block, or even single premature supraventricular or ventricular beats, in conditions of abnormally prolonged ventricular repolarization, can precipitate TdP by generating the spontaneous occurrence of short-long-short sequences, favoring the onset of EAD-dependent triggered activity[12,24] (Fig. 2).

ACQUIRED CONDITIONS FAVORING ABNORMAL VENTRICULAR REPOLARIZATION AND ARRHYTHMOGENESIS

Ventricular repolarization is affected by several congenital or acquired conditions, including abnormalities in ionic and hormonal levels, several cardiac and noncardiac drugs, and multiple cardiac diseases, such as cardiac ischemia, cardiomyopathies, and channelopathies due to cardiac

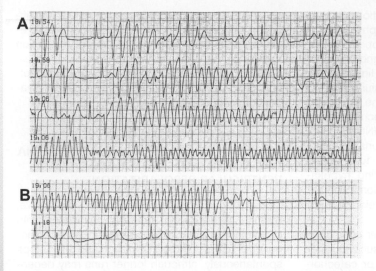

Fig. 1. TdP preceded by short-long short sequence in an LQTS patient (female, 16 years old, genotype unknown). (*A*) Several unstained runs of TdP, preceded by short-long-short pattern, followed by a sustained TdP run; (*B*) sustained TdP run self-terminating after approximately 90 seconds.

ionic gene mutations, and by many noncardiac diseases. Additional age-gender and gene-environment interactions often determine the occurrence of repolarization disturbances and arrhythmogenesis.[1–4]

Electrolyte Disturbances

Electrolyte or metabolic disturbances, including hyperkalemia and hypokalemia, hypercalcemia or hypocalcemia, and hypomagnesemia, due to renal or gastrointestinal or hormonal diseases or

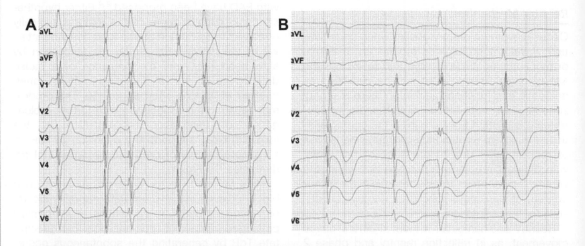

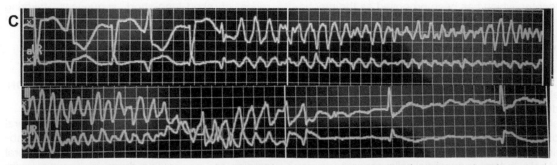

Fig. 2. QT prolongation and TdP during atrioventricular block. A female patient (age 64 years) with permanent atrial fibrillation (*A*) developed atrioventricular block, QT prolongation with wide negative T wave (*B*), and a self-terminating polymorphic VT (TdP) (*C*).

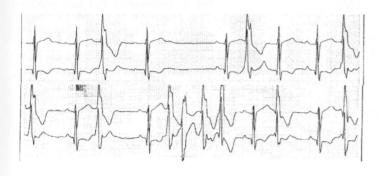

Fig. 3. QT prolongation with notched T wave, isolated ventricular beats and unsustained run of polymorphic VT arising from the later components of the T wave in a patient with Bartter syndrome and severe hypokalemia (male, age 17 years old, K^+ 2.9 mEq/L).

to the use of diuretics, are the most common causes of perturbation of ventricular repolarization, provoking QT interval and in T-wave morphology changes. The specific effects of ionic disturbances on the action potential provoking changes in T-wave morphology and QT interval duration are reviewed in detailed elsewhere.[10]

The ionic disturbance associated more frequently with arrhythmogenesis is hypokalemia, due to any acquired or congenital condition, leading to a reduced activity of iK1, that can favor the development of enhanced or abnormal automaticity, particularly in Purkinje pacemakers. Because IK1 channels are sensitive to extracellular potassium concentration, congenital and acquired conditions provoking severe hypokalemia can lead to major reduction in IK1, giving rise to abnormal arrhythmogenicity (**Fig. 3**).

A reduction in IK1 also can occur secondary to a mutation in KCNJ2, the gene that encodes for this channel, leading to increased automaticity and extrasystolic activity, presumably arising from the Purkinje system. Loss of function KCNJ2 mutation gives rise to Andersen-Tawil syndrome, which is characterized among other things by a marked increase in extrasystolic activity.[2,11]

Cardiac and Noncardiac and Drugs

Many different cardiac drugs (mainly antiarrhythmic class 1a and class 3 drugs) and noncardiac drugs (including antihistaminic, antispsycothic, antidepressant, antibiotic, antimalaric, gastrointestinal, and anesthetic agents) have been implicated in the prolongation of the ventricular repolarization and proarrhythmias. Virtually all QT-prolonging drugs act by the blocking potassium channels, mainly the rapid component of the delayed rectifier potassium channel (I_{kr}) encoded by the human ether-a-go-go–related gene (hERG).[2] The electrophysiologic and electrocardiograph changes on ventricular repolarization induced by these drugs are reviewed in detail elsewhere.[4,10]

The list of specific drugs that prolong the QT interval can be found at www.qtdrugs.org. Some of these drugs either have been restricted or withdrawn from the market due to the increased incidence of TdP. Approximately 5% to 20% of patients with drug-induced TdP have mutations in genes that cause LQTS. These patients have normal to borderline QTc interval at baseline but can develop QT prolongation and TdP, when exposed to Ikr-blocking drugs.[4,13]

Cardiac drugs

Antiarrhythmic agents are the leading cause of drug-induced QT prolongation and proarrhythmias. The risk of proarrhythmic effect is higher in women and in patients with structural heart disease, heart failure, and electrolyte disturbance, due to use of diuretics or to renal or gastrointestinal diseases.

Class IA agents (quinidine, procainamide, and disopyramide) block both Na and K channels (mainly I_{kr}). TdP can occur either at theravpeutic or subtherapeutic doses and are precipitated by concomitant hypokalemia or hypomagnesaemia.

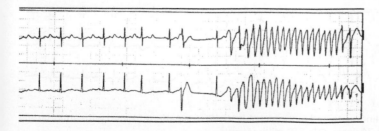

Fig. 4. Quinidine-induced QT prolongation and TdP run with onset preceded by typical short-long sequence, initially triggered by an isolated supraventricular beat (female, age 54 years).

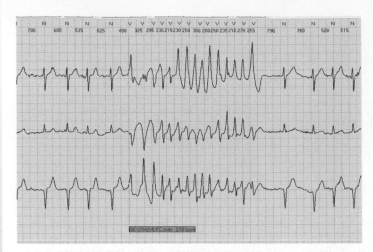

Fig. 5. Unsustained fast polymorphic VT in a patient with ischemic cardiomyopathy and chronic atrial fibrillation treated with sotalol (male, age 69 years, EF 50%). The patient was not inducible at EP test and was then treated with β-blockers (bisoprolol), but he died suddenly 3 years later. EP, electrophysiologic study.

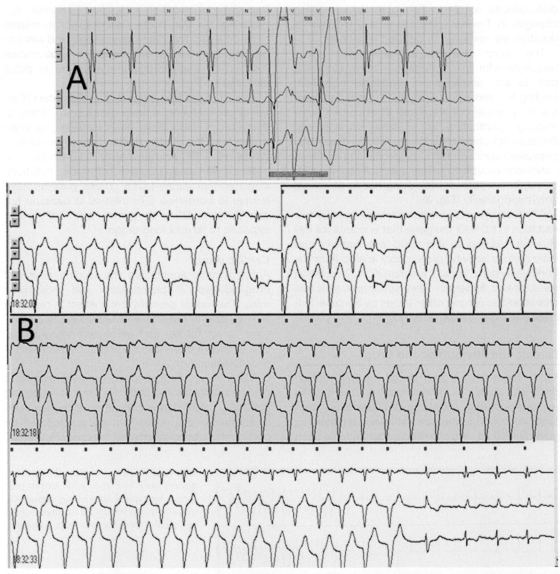

Fig. 6. Unsustained polymorphic VT (*A*) and sustained monomorphic VT (*B*) in a patient treated with amiodarone with major QT prolongation (male, age 74 years, QTc 550 milliseconds).

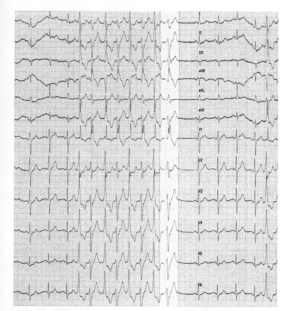

Fig. 7. Bidirectional unsustained VT observed in a patient with digitalis intoxication (female, age 75 years, history of paroxysmal atrial fibrillation).

Quinidine, a selective I_{kr} blocker, mainly prolongs action potential duration (APD) at lower heart rates, an effect defined as reverse use-dependence and may be linked to the occurrence of bradycardia-induced EAD[2,4,12,13] (**Fig. 4**).

Class III agents are potent I_{Kr} blockers and prolong QT interval in a dose-dependent manner. The potassium-blocking effect is maximum at low heart rate due to reverse use dependency feature. Dofetilide, ibutilide, and sotalol carry the highest risk for TdP, whereas amiodarone rarely causes TdP despite its evident QT-prolonging effect (**Fig. 5**). The rare proarrhythmic effect of amiodarone can be explained by some of its unique features, such as lack of reverse use-dependency, decreased QT dispersion across ventricular myocardium, L-type calcium blocking effects, and B-blocking effect.[2,4,13,14] Proarrhythmias may be favored by concomitant factors, such as female gender, electrolyte imbalance, bradycardia, atrial fibrillation or reduced left ventricular function, and the concomitant use of other QT-prolonging drugs. Although TdP is the most common arrhythmia observed as proarrhythmic effect of amiodarone, monomorphic VT also can be observed (**Fig. 6**).

Digitalis also can have proarrhythmic effects, mainly premature ventricular contractions and bidirectional VT, due to DAD-related triggered automaticity. The molecular target of digoxin is the sodium-potassium ATPase pump and the downstream pathways, including the sodium-calcium exchanger and other systems involved in intracellular calcium homeostasis. Therefore, candidate genes that can modulate digoxin effects include those encoding sodium-potassium-ATPase, the sodium-calcium exchanger, and ones regulating intracellular calcium homeostasis. Accordingly, it is possible that congenital arrhythmia syndromes altering intracellular calcium control, such as CPVT or the ankyrin-B–related form of the congenital LQTS, predispose to digoxin toxicity[2] (**Fig. 7**).

Noncardiac drugs A growing number of drugs have been described to alter ventricular repolarization and favor arrhythmogenesis, by blocking the potassium channels, mainly the rapid component of the delayed rectifier potassium channel (I_{kr}). Drug-to-drug interactions have been described, because several of these drugs are metabolized by the cytochrome P450 enzymes, CYP3A4 or CYP2D6. Patients with liver

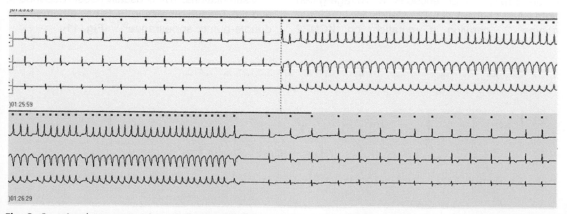

Fig. 8. Sustained monomorphic VT (lasting 30 s) in a patient with ischemic cardiomyopathy and chronic atrial fibrillation treated with paroxetine (female, age 75 years, EF 50%).

dysfunction or coadministration of other drugs or food that inhibit the CYP3A4 orCYP2D6 can result in higher drug levels and favor proarrhythmic effects.[4,13,14]

Gene-drug interactions probably also exist at different levels: rare ion-channel mutations that increase the risk of QT prolongation by drug use, common genetic variants that potentiate the QT-prolonging effect of drugs, variation within drug metabolizing and transporting proteins that influence drug pharmacokinetics, and simultaneous use of multiple QT-prolonging drugs may favor the potential proarrhythmic effect of drugs[4,14] (**Figs. 8** and **9**).

GENETIC CHANNELOPATHIES AND ARRHYTHMOGENESIS

Mutations of the genes that encode the cardiac ionic channels result in congenital channelopathies that can cause sudden death by causing rapid, polymorphic VT or TdP degenerating into VF. The mechanisms of arrhythmogenesis can be triggered activity (due to afterdepolarization, as in LQTS and CPVT) or reentry, due to adjacent areas of the myocardium having different electrophysiologic characteristics, such as the right ventricular outflow tract in BrS. In general, loss of function of potassium conductance leads to action potential prolongation as in LQTS; vice versa, gain of function results in shortening APD as in SQTS or BrS.

Long QT Syndromes

More than 11 different types of congenital LQTS have been recognized, and LQT1, LQT2, and LQT3 account for a majority of the cases.[5,6] The 3 most common genotypes (LQT1, LQT2, and LQT3) "LQT1" stands for LQTS genotype 1, carrying a mutation on KCNQ1, a gene on chromosome 11p15.5 that encodes a voltage-gated potassium channel. "LQT2" stands for LQTS genotype 2, carrying a mutation on KCNH2

(previously also defined as hERG), a gene on chromosome 7q36.1 that encodes an alpha subunit of voltage-gated, potassium channels. "LQT3" stands for LQTS genotype 3, carrying a mutation on SCN5A, a gene on chromosome 3p21 that encodes an integral membrane protein and tetrodotoxin-resistant voltage-gated sodium channel alpha subunit tend to have genotype-specific syncope triggers for cardiac events, have characteristic T-wave morphologies, and have age and gender–correlated features of high risk.[6,15,16] Subjects with LQT1 and LQT2 tend to have several warning syncopal episodes before a sudden death, whereas in LQT3 the first presentation is commonly sudden death. In all genotypes, the strongest predictors for high risk are previous cardiac arrest or syncope and a QTc interval recorded at any time during follow-up of more than 500 ms.[17]

LQT1 accounts for 40% to 55% of cases of the LQTS, and it is caused by mutations in the KVLQT1 (also called KCNQ1) gene, encoding Iks. LQT1 patients typically show a prolonged QT interval and a broad-based T wave on the resting ECG, and children and adolescents, predominantly male, are at highest risk, especially during exercise, in particular swimming[15,16] (**Fig. 10**).

LQT2 accounts for 35% to 45% of cases of congenital LQTS, and it is caused by a variety of mutations in the hERG (also known as KCNH2) potassium channel gene, located on chromosome 7, encoding Ikr. The mutations may involve the pore or the nonpore region of the hERG channel. Pore mutations carry high risk for cardiac events and may affect young patients whereas nonpore mutations often lead to TdP in the presence of hypokalemia [1–3, 6]. In LQT2, adult women, particularly up to 9 months postpartum, are at highest risk. Ventricular arrhythmias in LQT2 typically are observed during sleep or during emotional or auditory stimulations. TdP is usually pause-dependent, and the T-wave on resting ECG has a notched, or double-bump, appearance[6,15] (**Fig. 11**).

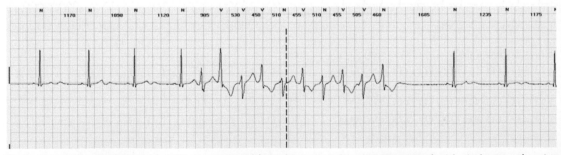

Fig. 9. Unsustained polymorphic VT in a patient without known cardiac disease treated with citalopram showing QT prolongation and camel hump T wave (female, age 49 years, QTc 520 milliseconds).

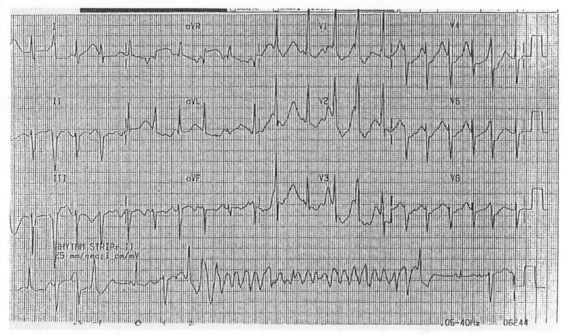

Fig. 10. Unsustained fast polymorphic VT (TdP) preceded by short-long-short pattern in a patient with LQT1 (male, age 12 years). "LQT1" stands for LQTS genotype 1, carrying a mutation on KCNQ1, a gene on chromosome 11p15.5 that encodes a voltage-gated potassium channel.

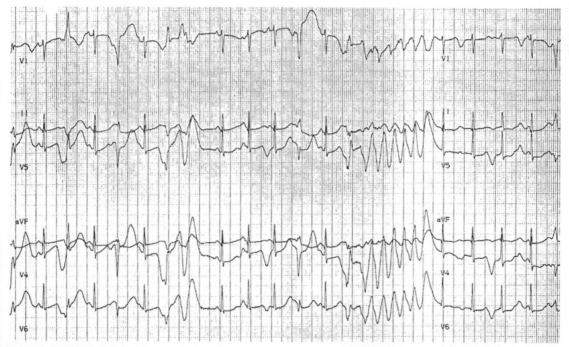

Fig. 11. Unsustained fast polymorphic VT (TdP) preceded by T-wave alternans in a patient with LQT2 (female, age 24 years). "LQT2" stands for LQTS genotype 2, carrying a mutation on KCNH2 (previously also defined as hERG), a gene on chromosome 7q36.1 that encodes an alpha subunit of voltage-gated, potassium channels.

LQT3 is caused by mutations in the sodium channel gene (SCN5A) located on chromosome 3 at location 21-24, and it is characterized by events occurring at rest or during sleep. LQT3 is due to perturbation of Na$^+$-channel inactivation that can prolong the cellular action potential and alter cellular excitability, and it has the higher frequency of fatal cardiac events.[6] In LQT3 patients, gene carriers are often bradycardic with very prolonged QT interval and late-onset T waves on resting ECG; typical T-wave alternans can be observed before the occurrence of TdP (**Figs. 12** and **13**).

Short QT Syndrome (SQTS)

SQTS is much rarer than LQTS and it has been related to several mutations affecting the function of ion channels responsible for the currents

that generate the cardiac action potential that may cause either hyperfunction of the delayed rectifier potassium current or hypofunction of the calcium current. Mutations in 5 genes have been associated with SQTS: *KCNH2, KCNJ2, KCNQ1, CACNA1c,* and *CACNB2.*[1,2] Mutations in these genes cause either a gain of function in outward potassium channel currents (IKr, IKs, and IK1) or a loss of function in inward calcium channel current (ICa).[9] These result in a shortening of the repolarization period and an increase in transmural dispersion of repolarization, which explain the main features of this syndrome: short QT interval, short atrial and ventricular effective refractory periods, and, as a result of them, susceptibility to atrial fibrillation and VF.[9] The abbreviation of the action potential in SQTS may be heterogeneous with preferential

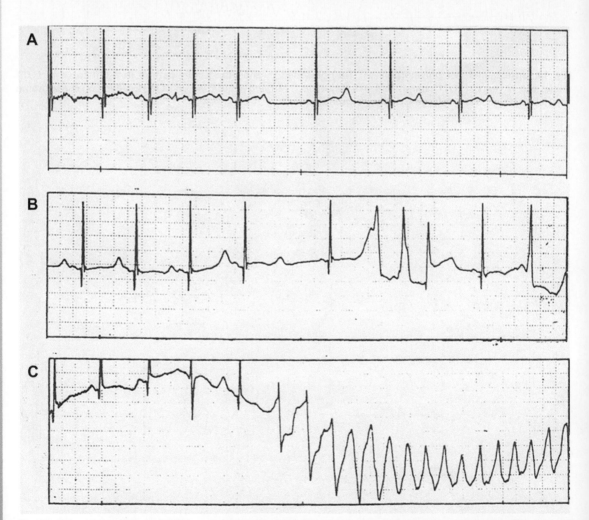

Fig. 12. QT prolongation and TdP in a patient with LQT3 (male, age 13 years): (*A*) late component of the T-wave enhanced in the beat preceded by a pause; (*B*) 2:1 T-wave alternans followed by a pause and unsustained VT arising from the late component of the T wave; and (*C*) sustained TdP preceded by relative sinus tachycardia with T-wave alternans.

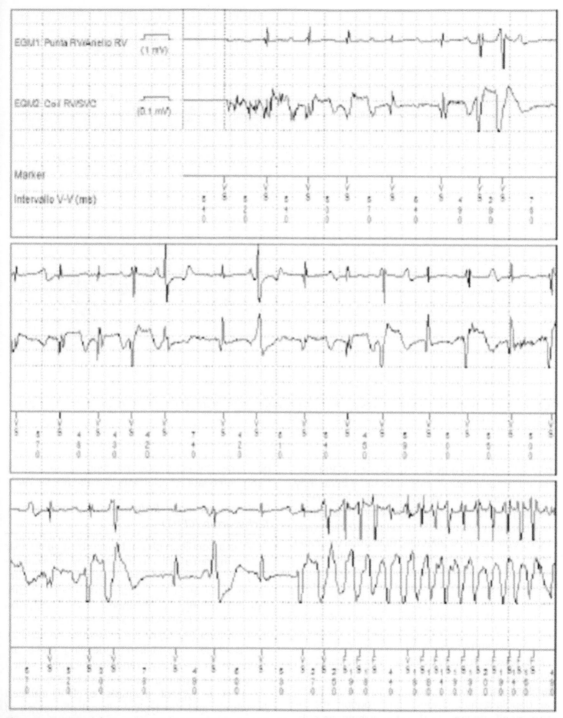

Fig. 13. Sustained fast polymorphic VT (TdP) preceded by short-long-short pattern in a patient with LQT3 implanted with ICD (female, age 18 years), detected by intracardiac recording.

abbreviation of either ventricular epicardium or endocardium, giving rise to an increase in temporal dispersion in ventricular repolarizations that may create the substrates for reentry arrhythmias (**Fig. 14**).

J Wave Syndromes: Brugada Syndrome (BrS) and Early Repolarization Syndrome (ERS)

The J-wave syndromes, both BrS and ERSs, may be due to a gain of function of Ito, the transient outward potassium current, which is the main current

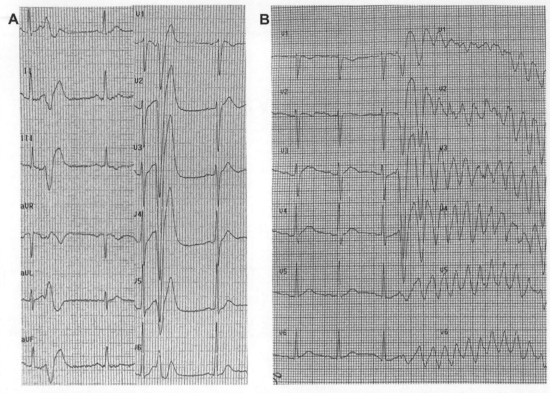

Fig. 14. Patient with SQTS (male, 40 years, history of syncope) with short QT interval (320 milliseconds), ventricular ectopic beats (*A*), and spontaneous onset of VF (*B*).

contributing to the repolarizing phase 1 of the cardiac action potential. A gain of function of Ito may be due to a loss-of-function mutation in SCN5A, resulting in a reduction in INa. The principal difference between BrS and ERS is related to the region of the ventricle most affected. Epicardial mapping studies in BrS patients report accentuated J waves and fragmented and/or late potentials in the epicardial region of the right ventricular outflow tract, whereas in ERS only accentuated J waves, particularly in the inferior wall of left ventricle, are observed.[7,8] The effect of sodium channel blockers on surface ECG have differential effects in BrS, where they predominantly accentuate the repolarization defects and increase the J-wave manifestation, whereas in ERS they accentuate the depolarization defects and reduce the J-wave manifestation.[8] In BrS, the arrhythmic substrate is located in the epicardial surface of the right ventricular outflow tract. In a few patients, the spontaneous Brugada pattern can be detected by recording the V1-V3 precordial leads in upper intercostal locations (**Fig. 15**). Also, the typical modifications induced by ajmaline can be detected specifically in the area corresponding to the right ventricular outflow tract, and they can

be shown by epicardial mapping as an area of fragmented late components of wider amplitude.[18]

Cathecolaminergic Polymorphic Ventricular Tachycardia (CPVT)

CPVT is a condition characterized by a ventricular tachyarrhythmia typically triggered by physical activity or emotional stress. Episodes of VT can cause syncope and unexpected sudden death, typically arising in childhood. CPVT may be caused by the mutation of either the type 2 ryanodine receptor (RyR2) or the calsequestrin (CSQ2). The principal mechanism underlying these arrhythmias is the leaky ryanodine receptor, which is aggravated during catecholamine stimulation. CVPT is a typical example of DAD-induced arrhythmia and the typical clinical phenotype of CPVT is bidirectional VT. Typical ECG pattern and ventricular arrhythmias of CPVT are reviewed in detail elsewhere.

STRUCTURAL CARDIAC DISEASES

Abnormalities of ventricular repolarization, including prolonged QT interval and increased QT dispersion, have been described in several

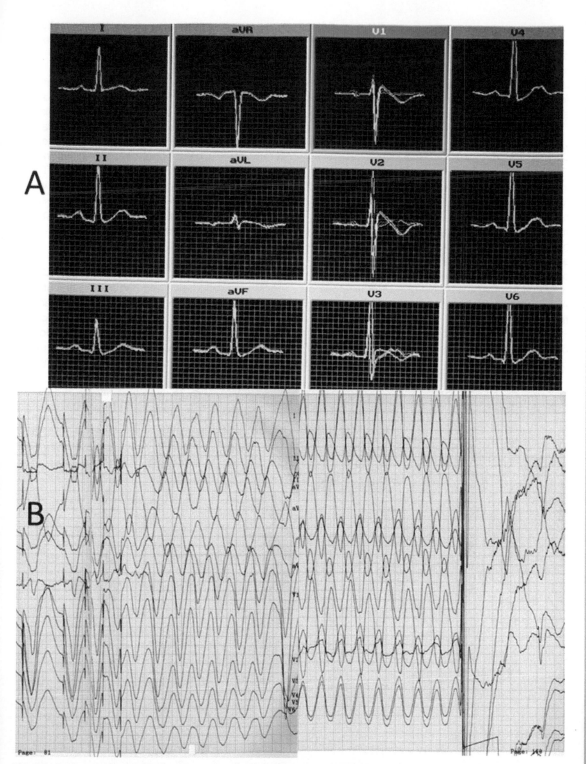

Fig. 15. Patient with BrS (male, 15 years, whose father died suddenly at 35 years) the spontaneous Brugada pattern was be detected by recording the V1-V3 precordial leads in upper intercostal locations. (*A*) ECG 12-lead recording, with superimposed precordial recording taken at standard and upper location: only at V1-V3 taken at upper locations the spontaneous coved type 1 Brugada pattern was observed. (*B*) VF was induced during electrophysiologic testing that was performed due to the familial history of sudden death.

acquired or idiopathic cardiomyopathies, including ischemic cardiomyopathy and hypertrophic cardiomyopathies (HCMs), both primary and secondary due to arterial hypertension, but the true prognostic significance of these parameters for predicting malignant ventricular arrhythmias and sudden cardiac death remains unclear.[1,19–22]

Ischemic Cardiomyopathy

Coronary artery disease (CAD) and myocardial infarction are well known to prolong QT interval, and the rate-adjusted QT-interval (QTc) is prognostic of sudden death in myocardial infarction patients.[19] QT prolongation may predict coronary heart disease and sudden death even in apparently healthy adult men. In addition to QT prolongation, QT wave dispersion also has been described in CAD, possibly due to differences of APD among different myocardial areas, or within the ventricular walls.

The heterogeneity of ventricular repolarization due to myocardial ischemia and infarction may account for the genesis of spiral waves (rotors) around an anatomic obstacle, typically an ischemic scar, supporting the main role of reentry mechanisms of ventricular arrhythmias in CAD. Spiral wave activity (or rotors) also has been used to explain the electrocardiographic patterns observed during monomorphic and polymorphic cardiac arrhythmias as well as during fibrillation. Monomorphic VT results when the spiral wave is stable within the ventricular myocardium, because it may occur in case of ischemic scars. In contrast, drifting spiral waves cause polymorphic VT and VF-like activity. VT often precedes VF, which may develop when a single spiral wave responsible for VT breaks up, leading to the development of multiple chaotic spirals[2] (**Fig. 16**).

Hypertrophic Cardiomyopathy (HCM)

HCM is a well-known and common cause of sudden arrhythmic death in children and young adults, characterized by an unexplained thickening (hypertrophy) of the left ventricle, and occasionally of the right, with predominant involvement of the interventricular septum. The ECG features of

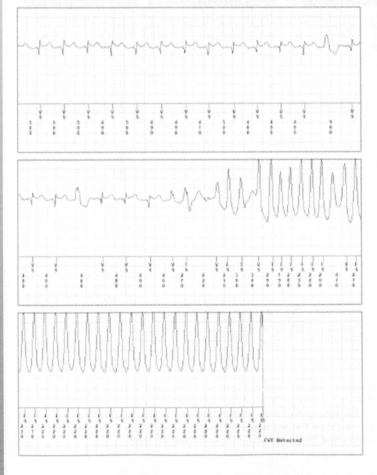

Fig. 16. Sustained fast VT in a patient with ischemic cardiomyopathy (male, age 55 years, EF 45%) detected by implantable loop recorder (possible ST elevation preceding the onset of VT, later degenerating into VF).

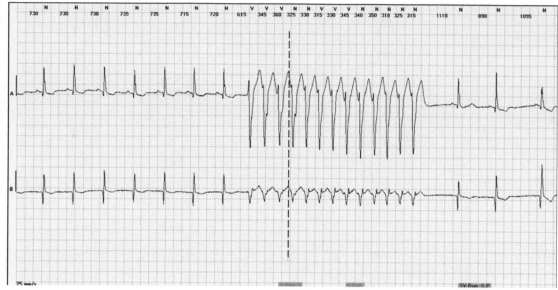

Fig. 17. Unsustained fast monomorphic VT in a patient with HCM (female, age 18 years), recorded by external loop recorder.

HCM are variable, and often the abnormalities of ventricular repolarization are not revealed on surface ECG, and when present they have a low predictive power for occurrence of life-threatening arrhythmias.[19,23] The most typical ECG features are increased precordial voltages in QRS complex and nonspecific ST segment and giant T-wave inversion in the precordial leads, more frequent in apical HCM is giant T-wave inversion in the precordial leads. Understanding of the mechanism

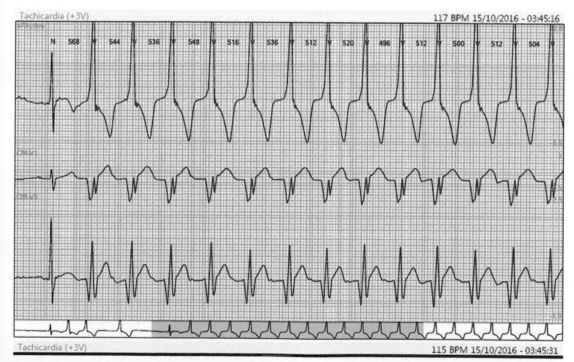

Fig. 18. Sustained fast monomorphic VT in a patient with HCM (male, age 20 years, history of palpitation on effort), recorded by prolonged Holter monitoring at sixth day of monitoring.

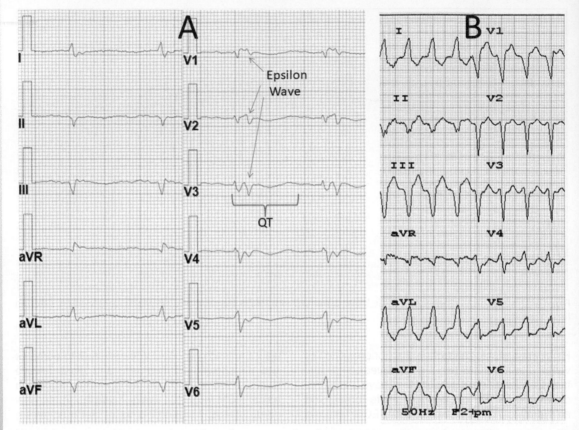

Fig. 19. Fragmented QRS complex with epsilon wave and prolonged QT interval on 12-lead ECG in a patient with arrhythmogenic right ventricular cardiomyopathy (male, age 70 years). Monomorphic VT with left bundle branch block–like morphology also was observed in this patient.

of arrhythmogenesis in HCM is still lacking, and both increased inward and reduced outward currents have been advocated, but their role in promoting repolarization abnormalities remains unknown. Recent experimental studies suggested that, at a difference with the ionic remodeling associated with heart failure, HCM cardiomyocytes exhibited a significant overexpression of the L-type Ca^{2+} current (ICaL), which together with an increase in the late Na^+ (INaL) and a reduction in K^+ repolarizing currents, contributes to a prolonged AP and Ca^{2+} transient. Experimental recordings also provide evidence that HCM may facilitate the occurrence of EADs from hypertrophied left ventricular wall, acting as triggers for ventricular arrhythmias, because EADs could be associated with R on T extrasystoles, initiating polymorphic VT. Reentry mechanisms may

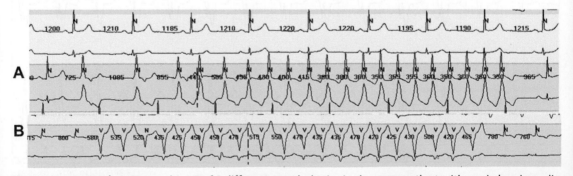

Fig. 20. Unsustained monomorphic VT of 2 different morphologies in the same patient with nonischemic cardiomyopathy due to sarcoidosis (male, age 57 years, EF 40%): (*A*) left bundle branch block–like VT; (*B*) right bundle branch block–like VT (both recordings obtained during prolonged monitoring by external loop recorder).

occur within the hypertrophic ventricular wall, explaining why in HCM monomorphic VT rather that polymorphic VT are often encountered[2,19] (**Figs. 17** and **18**).

Non Ischemic Cardiomyopathy (NICM)

Nonischemic cardiomyopathies are a heterogenous group of disorders, including idiopathic dilated cardiomyopathy and arrhythmogenic right ventricular cardiomyopathy, that have been shown highly associated with SCD and ventricular arrhythmias. Identification of the arrhythmogenic substrate and the electrophysiologic substrate underlying ventricular arrhythmias is still debated. The arrhythmogenic substrate in nonischemic cardiomyopathies is characterized by patchy, layered fibrosis and irregular myocyte disarray usually in a perivalvular distribution with a propensity for the midmyocardial and epicardial layers. The epicardial electroanatomic mapping often shows the presence of fat or fibrosis in the perivalvular region as well as in the interventricular septum that could mimic scar that can be the substrate for VT in Non ischemic cardiomyopathies (NICM) favoring reentry by creating areas of delayed conduction and intramural heterogeneity.[2,22,23]

Typically, patients with NICD show fragmented QRS complex, whereas with respect to repolarization abnormalities, QT dispersion, T-wave alternans, and early repolarization on the surface ECG have been reported as potential risk factors for ventricular life-threatening arrhythmias (**Fig. 19**). The relationship between these markers and susceptibility to tachyarrhythmias, however, is not clearly established.[2,22] The surface ECG morphology of VT can be helpful for localizing the likely source and planning the ablation procedure. Multiple VT morphologies when identified a priori often predict more extensive distribution of the underlying substrate (**Fig. 20**).

SUMMARY

Abnormal ventricular repolarization, with abnormal T-wave configuration, prolonged or markedly shortened QT interval, early repolarization, and increased dispersion of QT interval duration, has been associated with an increased risk of ventricular arrhythmias in congenital and acquired conditions that may affect the ventricular repolarization and increase the susceptibility to ventricular arrhythmias. The ventricular recovery process mainly depends on the transmembrane outward transport of potassium ions to reestablish the endocellular electronegativity. Outward potassium channels represent a heterogeneous family of ionic carriers, modulated by heart rate and autonomic nervous activity, and impaired outward K currents reduce the repolarization reserve, favoring arrhythmogenesis. Also, sodium and calcium inward channel abnormalities may predispose to ventricular arrhythmias, because when inward currents are increased, voltage depolarizations can occur during the repolarization phase of the action potential, giving rise to abnormal afterdepolarization (EAD or DAD) and triggered activity. Cardiac channelopathies, due to gene mutations modifying cardiac ionic channels that regulate ventricular repolarization, may develop sudden death induced by rapid, usually polymorphic VT (or TdP) or VF. Genetic background and acquired disorders may interplay, creating conditions that may precipitate life-threatening arrhythmias.

REFERENCES

1. Priori SG, Wilde AA, Horie M, et al. HRS/EHRA/APHRS expert consensus statement on the diagnosis and management of patients with inherited primary arrhythmia syndrome. Heart Rhythm 2013;10: 287–94.
2. Antzelevitch C, Burashnikov A. Overview of basic mechanisms of cardiac arrhythmia. Card Electrophysiol Clin 2011;3:23–45.
3. Skinner JR, Winbo A, Abrams D, et al. Channelopathies that lead to sudden cardiac death: clinical and genetic aspects. Heart Lung Circ 2019;28:22–30.
4. Roden D. The long QT syndrome and torsades de pointes: basic and clinical aspects. In: El-Sherif N, Samet P, editors. Cardiac pacing and electrophysiology. Philadelphia: WB Saunders; 1991. p. 265–83.
5. Moss AJ, Schwartz PJ, Crampton RS, et al. The long QT syndrome. Prospective longitudinal study of 328 families. Circulation 1991;84:1136–44.
6. Schwartz PJ, Crotti L, Insolia R. Long QT syndrome: from genetics to management. Circ Arrhythm Electrophysiol 2012;5:868–77.
7. Brugada P, Brugada J. Right bundle branch block, persistent ST segment elevation and sudden cardiac death: a distinct clinical entity and electrocardiographic syndrome A multicentric report. J Am Coll Cardiol 1992;20:1391–6.
8. Antzelevitch C, Yan GX, Ackerman M, et al. J-Wave syndromes expert consensus conference report: Emerging concepts and gaps in knowledge. J Arrhythm 2016;32:315–39.
9. Patel C, Yan GX, Antzelevitch C. Short QT syndrome: from bench to bedside. Circ Arrhythmia Electrophysiol 2010;3:401–8.
10. Locati ET, Bagliani G, Padeletti L. Normal ventricular repolarization and QT interval: ionic background, modifiers, and measurements. Card Electrophysiol Clin 2017;9:487–513.

11. Bastiaenen R. Behr ER Sudden death and ion channel disease: pathophysiology and implications for management. Heart 2011;97:1365–72.

12. Locati EH, Maison-Blanche P, Dejode P, et al. Spontaneous sequences of onset of torsade de pointes in patients with acquired prolonged repolarization: quantitative analysis of Holter recordings. J Am Coll Cardiol 1995;25:1564–75.

13. Schwartz, Task Force of the Working Group on Arrhythmias of the European Society of Cardiology: the Sicilian Gambit. A new approach to the classification of antiarrhythmic drugs based on their actions on arrhythmogenic mechanisms. Circulation 1991;84:1835–51.

14. Arunachalam K, Lakshmanan S, Maan A, et al. Impact of drug induced long QT syndrome: a systematic review. J Clin Med Res 2018;10:384–90.

15. Moss AJ, Zareba W, Benhorin J, et al. ECG T wave patterns in genetically distinct forms of the hereditary long QT syndrome. Circulation 1995;92:2929–34.

16. Schwartz PJ, Priori SG, Locati EH, et al. Long QT syndrome patients with mutations on the SCN5A and HERG genes have differential responses to Na+ channel blockade and to increase in heart rate. Implications for gene-specific therapy. Circulation 1995;92:3381–6.

17. Locati ET QT interval duration remains a major risk factor in long QT syndrome patients. J Am Coll Cardiol 2006;48:1053–5.

18. Pappone C, Ciconte G, Manguso F, et al. Assessing the malignant ventriuclar arrhythmic substrate in patients with the Brugada syndrome. J Am Coll Cardiol 2018;71:1631–46.

19. Passini E, Mincholé A, Coppini R, et al. Mechanisms of pro-arrhythmic abnormalities in ventricular repolarization and anti-arrhythmic therapies in human hypertrophic cardiomyopathy. J Mol Cell Cardiol 2016;96:72–81.

20. Locati E, Schwartz PJ. Prognostic value of QT interval prolongation in post myocardial infarction patients. Eur Heart J 1986;7(Suppl A):393–8.

21. Betensky BP. Dixits: Sudden cardiac death in patients with nonischemic cardiomyopathy. Indian Heart J 2014;66:s35.es45.

22. McNally EM, Mestroni L. Dilated cardiomyopathy: genetic determinants and mechanisms. Circ Res 2017;121:731–48.

23. Johnson JN, Grifoni C, Bos JM, et al. Ackerman MJ Prevalence and clinical correlates of QT prolongation in patients with hypertrophic cardiomyopathy. Eur Heart J 2011;32(9):1114–20.

24. El-Sherif N, Caref EB, Chinushi M, et al. Mechanism of arrhythmogenicity of the short-long cardiac sequence that precedes ventricular tachyarrhythmias in the long QT syndrome. J Am Coll Cardiol 1999;33(5):1415–23.

Arrhythmias in Patients with Implantable Devices

Luigi Sciarra, MD[a],*, Martina Nesti, MD[b], Zefferino Palamà, MD[c], Jacopo Marazzato, MD[d], Giuseppe Bagliani, MD[e,f], Fabio M. Leonelli, MD[g], Roberto De Ponti, MD, FHRS[d]

KEYWORDS

- Cardiac arrhythmias • Pacemaker • Implantable cardioverter-defibrillator
- Implantable loop recorder • Pacemaker-mediated tachycardia

KEY POINTS

- Many patients with implantable devices may experience atrial or ventricular arrhythmias.
- These devices can help clinicians improve diagnosis of cardiac arrhythmias by recording and store electrical signals during arrhythmias, as well as the modalities of their onset and termination.
- Intracardiac electrograms by recording local potentials from different programmable electrodes or far- and near-field signals provide different information helping in the analysis of the ongoing rhythm.
- Surface electrocardiogram (ECG) looks different from an electrogram, but both illustrate cardiac activity in the form of tracings and both can be analyzed to detect and interpret arrhythmias or device malfunctions.
- Correct ECG interpretation may be sometimes prevented by pacing artifacts or paced beats that may mask atrial waves on surface ECG, interfering with discrimination of atrial flutter, tachycardia, or fibrillation.

INTRODUCTION

Many patients with implantable pacemaker or implantable defibrillator (ICD) may experience atrial or ventricular arrhythmias. Thanks to progressively more sophisticated diagnostic capabilities, these devices provide detailed information presented in numeric or graphic format displayed at the touch of a button. Despite the availability of these numerous data, many clinicians use little or none of the information stored in these devices.

Extensive information can be difficult to interpret and sometimes it is hard to decide how to select the useful information from the great deal of presented data.

The Role of Intracardiac Electrogram

The most important tool available in device diagnostics is the intracardiac electrogram, commonly known as EGM. Although the surface ECG records a trace of cardiac rhythm based on electrical

Disclosure Statement: L. Sciarra, M. Nesti, Z. Palamà, J. Marazzato, G. Bagliani, and F. Leonelli have no conflict to disclose. R. De Ponti has received lectures fees from Biosense Webster and Biotronik and his institution has received educational grants from Biosense Webster, Biotronik, Medtronic, Abbott, and Boston Scientific.
[a] Cardiology Unit, Policlinico Casilino, Via Casilina 1049, Rome 00169, Italy; [b] Cardiovascular and Neurological Department, Ospedale San Donato, Via Nenni, 20/22, Arezzo 52100, Italy; [c] Cardiology Unit, Ospedale SS. Annunziata, Via Bruno 1, Taranto 74100, Italy; [d] Department of Heart and Vessels, Ospedale di Circolo and Macchi Foundation, University of Insubria, Viale Borri 57, Varese 21100, Italy; [e] Arrhythmology Unit, Cardiology Department, Foligno General Hospital, Via Massimo Arcamone, Foligno, Perugia 06034, Italy; [f] Cardiovascular Disease Department, University of Perugia, Piazza Menghini 1, Perugia 06129, Italy; [g] Cardiology Department, James A. Haley Veterans' Hospital, University of South Florida, 13000 Bruce B Down Boulevard, Tampa, FL 33612, USA
* Corresponding author.
E-mail address: lui.sciarra@gmail.com

cardiacEP.theclinics.com

signals recorded from body surface, an intracardiac EGM relies on the sensing capabilities of the lead electrodes located in the heart. An EGM is an "inside look" at what is going on in the heart and can be recorded from any programmable electrode (anode and cathode) or using far- or near-field signals, analyzing the heart rhythm from different points of view.[1] The storage of arrhythmic events, with the relative atrial and ventricular EGMs recorded by the device, may consistently help reach a correct diagnosis.[2,3]

Electrocardiogram and Electrogram: Two Sides of the Same Coin

The EGM is definitely different from surface ECG, yet there are many similarities between the two. Like an ECG, the EGM illustrates the cardiac activity in the form of a tracing, which describes electrical variations from baseline. Therefore, moving from EGM to ECG and vice-versa should be easy. The device offers the possibility of a real-time EGM taken at the same time of a surface ECG during follow-up and this also allows discrimination between arrhythmias and device malfunctions. Some ICDs can record a signal between the device and the shocking coils, therefore recording a bipolar far-field EGM resembling a surface ECG able to improve rhythm analysis. In fact, some algorithms are based on these far-field signals to improve discrimination between supraventricular and ventricular arrhythmias.

Electrocardiogram Interpretation in Patients with an Implantable Device

If on one hand implantable devices can help in arrhythmia diagnosis, on the other pacing can interfere with correct ECG interpretation, particularly when pacing artifacts and/or ventricular paced beats are superimposed to atrial waves on surface ECG, making the electrocardiographic diagnosis of atrial arrhythmias difficult. In this situation, by temporarily modifying the device pacing mode, for example, by decreasing the pacing rate, it is possible to unmask atrial activity and reach the correct diagnosis.

From Arrhythmia to Device

As mentioned, EGMs help diagnose the heart rhythm disturbances by providing information that can be integrated with surface ECG.[4] For example, discrimination of supraventricular and ventricular tachycardia become possible thanks to the simultaneous detection of atrial and ventricular activity.[5] These tracings can be analyzed real-time or stored in the device memory.[6,7] The information are more accurate with a dual-chamber

than a single-chamber device,[8] but both provide a wealth of information on the mechanisms of the patients' arrhythmias. It is also possible to detect events that initiate or terminate an arrhythmia, evaluate response to therapy, and assess device function and accuracy of programmed parameters. For correct interpretation, it is necessary to know the device's company-specific capabilities and programming parameters, as well as the different symbols used to mark intracardiac events.

From Device to Arrhythmia

In patients with dual-chamber implantable devices, a pacemaker-mediated tachycardia (PMT) can occur. PMT or endless-loop tachycardia is a reentrant arrhythmia, possible only in patients with preserved ventriculoatrial conduction, initiated by a device-sensed retrograde P wave occurring outside the post-ventriculoatrial refractory period (PVARP). Once a retrograde P wave is sensed, ventricular pacing is delivered (antegrade limb) after the programmed atrioventricular interval, causing in turn a ventriculoatrial conduction (retrograde limb), with a new retrograde P wave perpetuating reentry.[9] Once established, this reentry continues until it is spontaneously interrupted or until the retrograde P wave is blocked. This arrhythmia can be terminated or prevented by reprogramming the device to extend the PVARP or to switch to DDI mode.[10]

Other Implantable Devices

New devices without implantable leads in the heart chambers can detect the heart rhythm using a pure "electrocardiographic" technology. In the past, an entirely subcutaneous ICD (s-ICD) was designed and it has been made available in clinical practice in the recent years.[11,12] The device detects the heart rhythm recording as a far-field signal of cardiac electrical activity using 2 subcutaneous sensing electrodes (in xiphoid and subjugular areas) or either the subcutaneous sensing electrodes and the pulse generator. The device automatically selects an optimal vector to detect heart rhythm and avoids double counting of the QRS complex and T-wave.[13,14] This recording arrangement is different from the one of standard ICDs. In fact, the morphology of the recorded signal is different from standard ICDs using intracardiac leads, but both systems can accurately detect the occurrence of ventricular tachyarrhythmias with a high degree of sensitivity.[15,16]

Long-term ECG recording is made possible also by implantable loop recorders.[17] Unlike pacemakers and ICDs, implantable loop recorders are inserted under the skin without intracardiac leads and the electrical activity of the heart is recorded using subcutaneous electrodes. They are able to record cardiac events with a loop memory, as they continuously analyze the electrical signal and store information pertaining to relevant cardiac arrhythmias, automatically detected according to predefined algorithms. Recording begins before the onset of arrhythmia, because analysis of onset and termination of a rhythm disorder can help clinicians to understand its underlying mechanism.[18] They can be patient-activated during symptoms, so that a cause-effect relationship between heart rhythm disorders and symptoms can be established.[19,20]

Arrhythmia detection by implantable loop recorders can be very useful also to guide patient's management by demonstrating clinical response to antiarrhythmic therapy. Moreover, subclinical atrial fibrillation more frequently occurring in elderly patients can be detected by implantable loop recorders and also by using remote monitoring[21] that allows early diagnosis. As a consequence, an appropriate anticoagulation therapy is timely started and thromboembolic events reduced.[22–24]

Detailed description of the capabilities of implantable loop recorders and their clinical use is given elsewhere in this issue. In the following paragraphs, some paradigmatic cases of arrhythmia occurring in patients with an implantable device are presented and described.

PRESENTATION OF CLINICAL CASES
Case 1: Discrimination Between Ventricular and Supraventricular Tachycardia

A 78-year-old woman with ischemic heart disease and low left ventricular ejection fraction (35%) was referred for episodes of wide QRS complex tachycardia. The patient had been previously implanted with a dual-chamber ICD. The wide QRS complex tachycardia had a right bundle branch block morphology and its origin was unclear (**Fig. 1**). In fact, careful analysis of the surface ECG identifies a notch just after the QRS complex more evident in leads II and V5 that can be interpreted as a retrograde P wave. However, the morphology of the QRS complex is not very typical for aberrancy, and 1:1 ventriculoatrial ratio, if confirmed, does not exclude per se a ventricular tachycardia. Moreover, on the right-hand side of **Fig. 1**, a

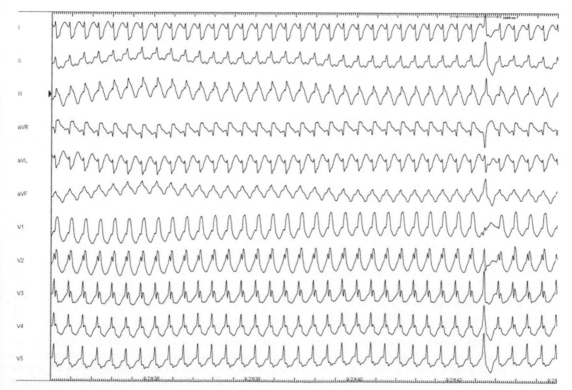

Fig. 1. Case 1. Wide QRS complex tachycardia with right bundle branch block morphology. Based on the final diagnosis of atrioventricular nodal reentry tachycardia, the narrower QRS complex has to be interpreted as a premature ventricular beat, possibly arising from the right ventricle and therefore originating a narrower fusion QRS complex.

beat with a narrower QRS complex and a shorter R-R interval could be a fusion beat, if, opposite to what suggested by leads II and V5, ventriculoatrial dissociation is actually present.

At device interrogation, EGMs showed detection of 2 arrhythmia episodes terminated by antitachycardia pacing. The tachycardia cycle length was 345 ms, the onset and stability criteria were satisfied, and the arrhythmia was treated as a ventricular tachycardia with a single effective burst. However, analysis of the arrhythmia onset showed initiation of the arrhythmia by a premature atrial contraction recorded by the atrial lead and conducted with a longer atrioventricular interval (**Fig. 2**), and therefore, this highly suggests a supraventricular tachycardia, possibly an atrioventricular node reentry tachycardia based on the onset modality. Diagnosis of slow-fast atrioventricular node reentry tachycardia was confirmed at electrophysiologic study and the patient was successfully treated by slow pathway ablation. In this case, the EGM proved to be of key importance for the correct

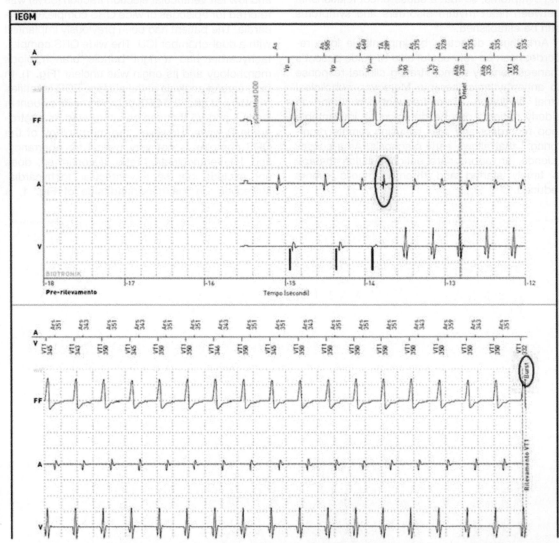

Fig. 2. Case 1. EGM continuously recorded from the atrial and ventricular leads (*second and third line*) together with the far-field recording (*first line*). At tachycardia onset, a premature atrial contraction (*upper red circle*) is conducted to the ventricle with a longer atrioventricular interval and induces a tachycardia with a 1:1 regular ventriculoatrial conduction. The ventriculoatrial interval is not <60 ms, a diagnostic criterion for atrioventricular node reentry tachycardia at electrophysiologic study, but in this case the atrial electrogram is recorded from the right atrial lead located in the right atrial appendage. A jump in atrioventricular conduction at arrhythmia onset highly suggests the presence of a slow pathway favoring the hypothesis of an atrioventricular node reentry tachycardia. The lower red circle indicates the time when antitachycardia pacing starts.

interpretation of the arrhythmia that led to appropriate arrhythmia treatment by catheter ablation.

Case 2: False Arrhythmia Detection due to Double Counting of QRS Complexes and T Waves

The s-ICD adopts a morphology-based detection algorithm to accurately discriminate supraventricular from ventricular arrhythmias on the analysis of cardiac electrical signals recorded subcutaneously and therefore more similar to a surface ECG than to an EGM. For this reason, before implantation, the patient undergoes screening to assess that cardiac electrical signals recorded with this modality allow correct interpretation of cardiac rhythm avoiding under- or oversensing. In fact, it has been reported that the accuracy of the s-ICD in arrhythmia detection is very high.[15,16]

A young competitive cyclist of 26 years of age, affected by arrhythmogenic right ventricular cardiomyopathy, was referred for poorly tolerated episodes of sustained monomorphic ventricular tachycardia. The patient, informed of the advantages and disadvantages of transvenous and subcutaneous ICD, preferred s-ICD implantation. Despite medical prescription, he continued practicing of amateur cycling. Two months later, the patient was referred again for device intervention during cycling with no loss of consciousness.

At device interrogation, tracings of this episode show double counting of the QRS complex and T wave occurring when premature ventricular beats alternate to sinus tachycardia with R waves of decreased amplitude (**Fig. 3**), which triggered inappropriate therapy. Because the clinical event occurred while the patient's torso was forward flexed, a sensing test was performed during mild exercise stress test in supine and sitting-up position. The forward flexion of the torso reproduced the amplitude reduction of the R wave in the alternate and secondary sensing vectors (**Fig. 4**A, B), whereas the R-wave amplitude was preserved in the primary vector (**Fig. 4**C). The device was then programmed with detection in primary vector and the patient had an uneventful follow-up.

Case 3: Discrimination of Atrial Arrhythmia in Case of Ventricular Pacing

Correct ECG interpretation may be sometimes prevented by pacing artifacts or paced beats. Particularly, a continuous sequence of paced ventricular beats can mask waves related to atrial activity on surface ECG. In this context, discrimination of an atrial arrhythmia can be difficult based only on surface ECG. On the other hand, correct diagnosis of typical or atypical atrial flutter, atrial fibrillation, or atrial tachycardia is of key importance in some cases, because therapeutic options and invasive approaches are different.

Fig. 5 shows the ECG of a male patient aged 72 years referred for several episodes of recurrent sustained palpitations. This patient was affected by ischemic dilated cardiomyopathy with severe depression of left ventricular ejection fraction and a dual-chamber ICD was previously implanted. Two years before, the patient also underwent ablation of typical atrial flutter for recurrent episodes of this arrhythmia requiring electrical cardioversion.

In the presenting ECG (see **Fig. 5**), P waves are barely visible and more evident in leads II and V1, with a variable relationship with paced QRS complexes, suggesting atrioventricular dissociation. Moreover, P (or F depending on the atrial rhythm) waves seem mainly positive both in lead II and V1. However, the presence of paced ventricular rhythm prevents a detailed analysis of atrial activity on surface ECG. Therefore, the pacemaker function was temporarily reprogrammed to VVI at a very low rate and a second ECG recorded (**Fig. 6**). After reprogramming spontaneous ventricular complex at a rate of 30 beats per minute with a ventricular escape beat and F waves related to the atrial activity are now more evident. Based on the morphology of the atrial waves (mainly positive in the inferior leads and V1, negative in aVL, and flat in almost all the other leads) atypical left atrial flutter with a cycle length of 340 ms was diagnosed. Electrophysiologic study and mapping confirmed the diagnosis and identified the critical

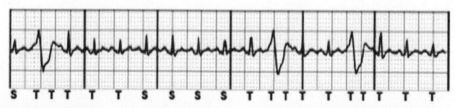

Fig. 3. Case 2. Electrocardiographic recording from an s-ICD. Double counting of the QRS complex and T wave during sinus tachycardia and ventricular premature beats resulting in oversensing (see text for further explanation) is observed. S stands for sinus rhythm detected and T for tachycardia detected.

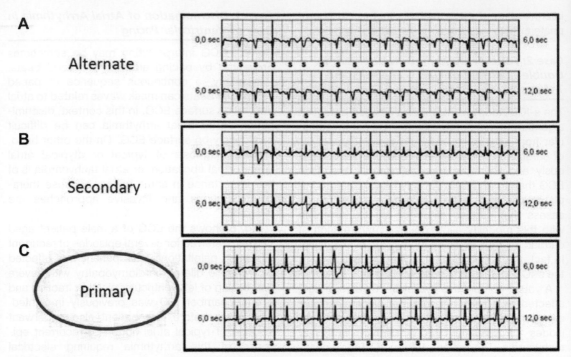

Fig. 4. Case 2. Electrocardiographic recordings from an s-ICD during effort stress test. Reduction in the R-wave amplitude is reproduced in the alternate (between xiphoid and subjugular electrodes) and secondary (between subjugular electrode and can) sensing vectors (A and B, respectively) in the flexed position of the torso, whereas the amplitude of the R-wave is preserved in the primary (between xiphoid electrode and pulse generator) vector (C).

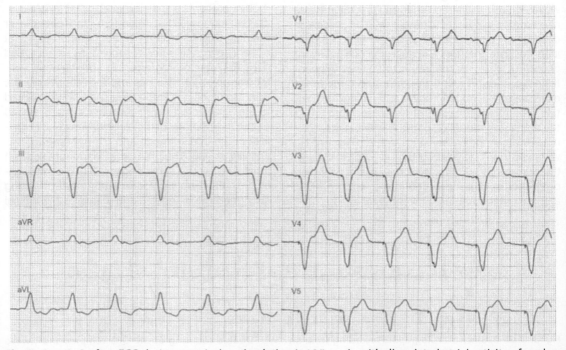

Fig. 5. Case 3. Surface ECG during ventricular stimulation in VVI mode with dissociated atrial activity of unclear origin.

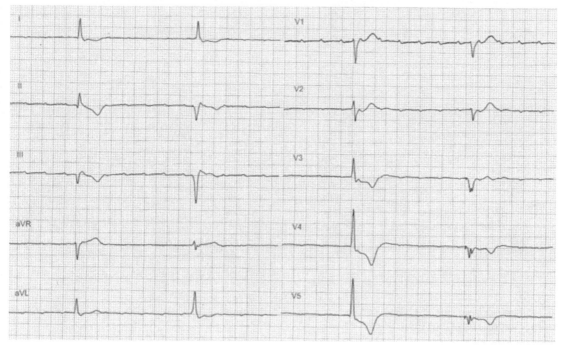

Fig. 6. Case 3. Surface ECG after reprogramming of the pacing modality at a lower rate. Flutter waves consistent with a left atrial flutter are now clearly evident.

isthmus of the reentry circuit in the left atrial roof. Radiofrequency energy ablation in this site suppressed the arrhythmia and sinus rhythm was stably restored.

In this case, transient pacemaker reprogramming favored an accurate interpretation of the surface ECG allowing correct diagnosis of the arrhythmia and appropriate decisions on the best patient management.

Case 4: Irregular Wide QRS Complex Tachycardia: What Is the Diagnosis?

A 70-year-old male patient, who had been previously implanted with a dual-chamber pacemaker for sick sinus syndrome, presented with palpitations and dizziness. The surface ECG showed short and iterative runs of wide QRS complex tachycardia with irregular R-R intervals alternated to sinus rhythm (**Fig. 7**). The genesis of this tachycardia is unclear. During tachycardia, the QRS complex has a limited duration and shows a right bundle branch block morphology. Despite the limited duration of the QRS complex, a monophasic R wave in lead V1 and a superior axis deviation are consistent with a ventricular origin, likely from the posterior left fascicle. The R-R interval during tachycardia varies from 280 to 600 ms with no variation in the QRS complex morphology, which corroborates the hypothesis of a ventricular origin and is against aberrancy. No aberrant conduction is

present in the only sinus beat, but this occurs after a very long pause, longer than any tachycardia cycle recorded in this sequence. However, during QRS complex tachycardia, neither clear atrioventricular dissociation nor retrograde P waves are clearly seen, so that one could suspect that disappearance of P wave is due to occurrence of self-limiting runs of atrial fibrillation. The irregularity of the R-R interval could reinforce this suspect. Moreover, prolonging the observation (**Fig. 8**), a premature P wave with apparently aberrant conduction is noted.

The diagnosis of a ventricular tachycardia with irregular cycle length eventually came from the EGM recordings of the dual-chamber pacemaker (**Fig. 9**). Therefore, therapy with calcium antagonists was started with arrhythmia suppression.

This case further demonstrates that "a look inside the heart" by analyzing the pacemaker EGMs helps the physician in appropriate diagnosis. However, once the final diagnosis was made, the 12-lead ECG also contributed in identifying the origin of the tachycardia from the posterior left fascicle and therefore oriented the pharmacologic treatment.

Case 5: Pacemaker-Mediated Tachycardia

A 50-year-old male patient with nonischemic cardiomyopathy and depressed left ventricular ejection fraction underwent dual-chamber ICD

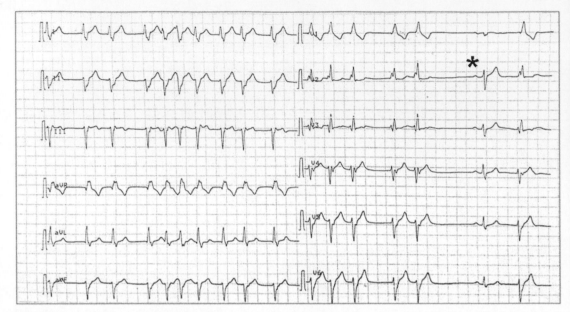

Fig. 7. Case 4. Continuous 12-lead ECG showing wide QRS complex tachycardia with irregular R-R intervals. *Asterisk* indicates the only sinus beat.

implantation. During postimplant monitoring, the electrophysiologist was again asked for intervention because of short but frequent episodes of symptomatic wide QRS complex tachycardia at 100 beats per minute, which turned out to be runs of ventricular pacing occurring after ventricular ectopic beats. All episodes were similar and all elements were in favor of PMT.

The analysis of EGMs stored in the device (**Fig. 10**) confirmed PMT, because retrograde

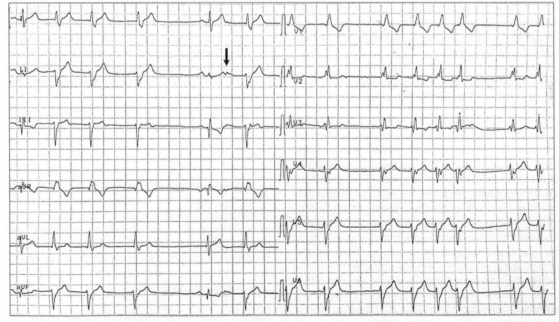

Fig. 8. Case 4. Another 12-lead ECG of the same patient. The *vertical arrow* indicates a premature atrial beat that might have been conducted with aberrancy, supporting the hypothesis of atrial fibrillation with aberrant conduction. After confirmation of the ventricular origin of the tachycardia, this has to be interpreted as a blocked atrial ectopy.

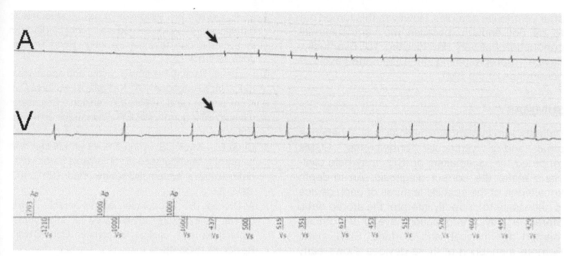

Fig. 9. Case 4. EGM from the atrial (A) and ventricular (V) leads of the dual-chamber pacemaker. After the first 3 atrial paced beats, the tachycardia starts with cycle length ranging from 351 to 617. In the first tachycardia beat, the ventricular electrogram (arrow in the ventricular tracing) precedes the atrial electrogram (arrow in the atrial tracing) and this is diagnostic of a ventricular beat with retrograde conduction to the atrium. In the following beats, the same pattern is invariably observed and this not only confirms the ventricular origin of the tachycardia but also explains why no atrioventricular dissociation is observed.

ventriculoatrial conduction was constantly present after the ventricular ectopies initiating the PMT. The PMT required appropriate intervention to avoid both patient's discomfort and further depression of the left ventricular function related to the right ventricular pacing. Therefore, the first intervention was device reprogramming with extension of the PVARP to avoid atrial sensing

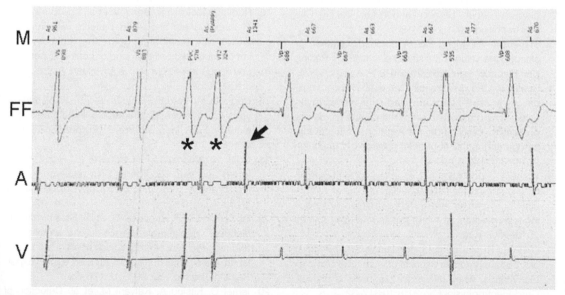

Fig. 10. Case 5. EGM at device interrogation shows from top to bottom: device markers(M), far-field electrogram (FF), atrial (A) and ventricular (V) bipolar electrograms. After 2 sinus beats, a ventricular couplet (asterisks) results in a late retrograde atrial activation (arrow) with a very long ventriculoatrial interval (1341 ms) due to decremental retrograde conduction over the atrioventricular node in this patient. This sensed atrial signal triggers ventricular pacing as shown by the pacing artifacts in the following beats and a pacemaker-mediated tachycardia starts. Ventriculoatrial conduction is maintained also in premature ventricular beat (second last beat), so that the pacemaker-mediated tachycardia goes on. In this patient, prolongation of the post-ventriculoatrial refractory period was not enough to avoid this arrhythmia, because the ventriculoatrial conduction was very slow. Therefore, reprogramming of the device mode was required.

after ventricular ectopies. However, this turned out to be not enough, because the ventriculoatrial conduction was very slow (see **Fig. 10**). Eventually, device reprogramming in DDI-mode avoided occurrence of the PMT.

SUMMARY

Patients with implantable devices may experience atrial and/or ventricular arrhythmias. EGMs recorded by pacemakers or ICDs may help clinicians make the correct diagnosis. An in-depth knowledge of the specific features of each device is necessary to correctly interpret the stored data. Moreover, device information have to be complemented by clinical and surface ECG data. Remote monitoring of these devices allows early arrhythmia detection and favors prompt intervention by the physicians. In some cases, the device itself can be responsible for arrhythmic events, known as PMTs.

REFERENCES

1. Kenny T. SVT discrimination. In: Kenny T, editor. The nuts and bolts of ICD therapy. Maden (MA): Blackwell Futura; 2006. p. 62–9.
2. Pollak WM, Simmons JD, Interian A Jr, et al. Clinical utility of intraatrial pacemaker stored electrograms to diagnose atrial fibrillation and flutter. Pacing Clin Electrophysiol 2001;24:424–9.
3. Stevenson IH, Mond HG. A coroner's request for closure: the value of the stored electrogram. Pacing Clin Electrophysiol 2006;29:670–3.
4. Swiryn S, Orlov MV, Benditt DG, et al. Clinical Implications of brief device-detected atrial tachyarrhythmias in a cardiac rhythm management device population: results from the registry of atrial tachycardia and atrial fibrillation episodes. Circulation 2016;134:1130–40.
5. Yoshida K, Liu TY, Scott C, et al. The value of defibrillator electrograms for recognition of clinical ventricular tachycardias and for pace mapping of post-infarction ventricular tachycardia. J Am Coll Cardiol 2010;56:969–79.
6. De Ponti R, Marazzato J, Bagliani G, et al. Peculiar electrocardiographic aspects of wide QRS complex tachycardia: when differential diagnosis is difficult. Card Electrophysiol Clin 2018;10:317–32.
7. Shandling AH, Castellanet MJ, Messenger JC, et al. Utility of the atrial endocardial electrogram concurrent with dual-chamber pacing in the determination of a pacemaker-mediated arrhythmia. Pacing Clin Electrophysiol 1988;11:1419–25.
8. Zimetbaum P, Goldman A. Ambulatory arrhythmia monitoring: choosing the right device. Circulation 2010;122:1629–36.
9. Ip JE, Lerman BB. Validation of device algorithm to differentiate pacemaker-mediated tachycardia from tachycardia due to atrial tracking. Heart Rhythm 2016;13:1612–7.
10. Huizar JF. Pacemaker timing cycles and special features. In: Ellenbogen KA, Kaszala K, editors. Cardiac pacing and ICDs. 6th edition. Chichester (United Kingdom): WILEY Blackwell; 2014. p. 211–71.
11. Chue CD, Kwok CS, Wong CW, et al. Efficacy and safety of the subcutaneous implantable cardioverter defibrillator: a systematic review. Heart 2017;103:1315–22.
12. Al-Ghamdi B. Subcutaneous implantable cardioverter defibrillators: an overview of implantation techniques and clinical outcomes. Curr Cardiol Rev 2019;15:38–48.
13. Bardy GH, Smith WM, Hood MA, et al. An entirely subcutaneous implantable cardioverter–defibrillator. N Engl J Med 2010;363:36–44.
14. Mesquita J, Cavaco D, Ferreira A, et al. Effectiveness of subcutaneous implantable cardioverter-defibrillators and determinants of inappropriate shock delivery. Int J Cardiol 2017;232:176–80.
15. Gold MR, Theuns DA, Knight BP, et al. Head-to-head comparison of arrhythmia discrimination performance of subcutaneous and transvenous ICD arrhythmia detection algorithms: the START study. J Cardiovasc Electrophysiol 2012;23:359–66.
16. Rudic B, Tülümen E, Berlin V, et al. Low prevalence of inappropriate shocks in patients with inherited arrhythmia syndromes with the subcutaneous implantable defibrillator single center experience and long-term follow-up. J Am Heart Assoc 2017;6:e006265.
17. Brignole M, Vardas P, Hoffmann E, et al. Indications for the use of diagnostic implantable and external ECG loop recorders. Europace 2009;11:671–87.
18. Galli A, Ambrosini F, Lombardi F. Holter monitoring and loop recorders: from research to clinical practice. Arrhythm Electrophysiol Rev 2016;5:136–43.
19. Di Cori A, Lilli A, Zucchelli G, et al. Role of cardiac electronic implantable device in the stratification and management of embolic risk of silent atrial fibrillation: are all atrial fibrillations created equal? Expert Rev Cardiovasc Ther 2018;16:175–81.
20. Israel C, Kitsiou A, Kalyani M, et al. Detection of atrial fibrillation in patients with embolic stroke of undetermined source by prolonged monitoring with implantable loop recorders. Thromb Haemost 2017;117:1962–9.
21. Chen-Scarabelli C, Scarabelli TM, Ellenbogen KA, et al. Device-detected atrial fibrillation: what to do with asymptomatic patients? J Am Coll Cardiol 2015;65:281–94.

22. Israel CW, Grönefeld G, Ehrlich JR, et al. Long-term risk of recurrent atrial fibrillation as documented by an implantable monitoring device: implications for optimal patient care. J Am Coll Cardiol 2004;43: 47–52.

23. Bettin M, Dechering D, Kochhäuser S, et al. Extended ECG monitoring with an implantable loop recorder in patients with cryptogenic stroke: time schedule, reasons for explantation and incidental findings (results from the TRACK-AF trial). Clin Res Cardiol 2019;108:309–14.

24. Simantirakis EN, Papakonstantinou PE, Chlouverakis GI, et al. Asymptomatic versus symptomatic episodes in patients with paroxysmal atrial fibrillation via long-term monitoring with implantable loop recorders. Int J Cardiol 2017;231:125–30.

Complex Arrhythmias Due to Reversible Causes

Andrea Pozzolini, MD[a], Teresa Rio, MD[a], Margherita Padeletti, MD[b], Roberto De Ponti, MD, FHRS[c], Fabio M. Leonelli, MD[d], Giuseppe Bagliani, MD[e,f],*

KEYWORDS

- Complex arrhythmias • Cardiac rhythm • Bradycardia • Tachycardia • Antiarrhythmic drugs
- Electrolytes imbalance

KEY POINTS

- Abnormalities in cardiac rhythm are caused by disorders of impulse generation, conduction, or a combination of the 2, and may be life-threatening because of a reduction in cardiac output or myocardial oxygenation.
- Cardiac arrhythmias are commonly classified as tachycardias (supraventricular or ventricular) or bradycardias.
- Bradycardias are uncommon in the critically ill patient and often are caused by an underlying reversible disorder (eg, hyperkalemia, drug toxicity).
- Supraventricular and ventricular tachycardias are more often encountered in the critically ill patient and often have underlying treatable disorders that precipitate their development (eg, hypokalemia, hypomagnesemia, antiarrhythmic proarrhythmia, myocardial ischemia).
- The initial management of an arrhythmia must focus on correcting precipitating or reversible causative disorders.

TACHYCARDIAS CAUSED BY DRUGS, ELECTROLYTE DISTURBANCES, AND TREATABLE NONCARDIAC CONDITIONS
Supraventricular Arrhythmias Induced by Reversible Causes

Atrial fibrillation

Atrial fibrillation (AF) is an arrhythmic disorder leading to stroke, heart failure, and death. Several cardiac and noncardiac conditions are risk factors of AF, such as, among others, heart failure and hypertension (**Box 1**).

Most common causes are addressed in later discussion.

Thyroid diseases Thyroid hormones directly affect the chronotropism and bathmotropism and the lusitropic effect of the heart and change the preload and afterload conditions. Thyroid hormones have widespread effects on cellular function, including expression of several ion channels and induction of hypertrophy and increased contractility.

Hyperthyroidism Hyperthyroidism is a well-known cause of AF with 16% to 60% prevalence.[1] The risk of AF is increased in clinical and subclinical hyperthyroidism.

Thyrotoxicosis has a deep impact on electrical impulse generation and conduction. Several

---

[a] Department of Cardiology, Azienda Ospedaliera Marche Nord, Piazzale Cinelli, 4, Pesaro 61121, Italy; [b] Cardiology Unit, Mugello Hospital, Viale della Resistenza, 60, 50032 Borgo San Lorenzo, Firenze, Italy; [c] Department of Cardiology, School of Medicine, University of Insubria, Viale Borri, 57, Varese 21100, Italy; [d] Cardiology Department, James A. Haley Veterans' Hospital, University South Florida, Tampa, FL, USA; [e] Arrhythmology Unit, Cardiology Department, Foligno General Hospital, Via Massimo Arcamone, Foligno, Perugia 06034, Italy; [f] Cardiovascular Disease Department, University of Perugia, Piazza Menghini 1, Perugia 06129, Italy

* Corresponding author. Arrhythmology Unit, Cardiology Department, Foligno General Hospital, Via Massimo Arcamone, Foligno, Perugia 06034, Italy.
E-mail address: giuseppe.bagliani@tim.it

Card Electrophysiol Clin 11 (2019) 375–390
https://doi.org/10.1016/j.ccep.2019.03.002
1877-9182/19/© 2019 Elsevier Inc. All rights reserved.

Box 1
Risk factors of atrial fibrillation

- Thyroid diseases
- Alcohol intoxication
- Drugs: amphetamines, caffeine, theophylline
- Pulmonary embolism
- Chronic obstructive pulmonary disease
- Postoperative
- Hypoxia
- Cerebrovascular accident
- Electrolyte abnormalities
- Trauma
- Pneumonia
- Sepsis

cardiac effects of thyroid hormone are possibly related to development of AF, including elevation of left atrial pressure secondary to increased left ventricular mass and impaired ventricular relaxation, ischemia resulting from increased resting heart rate, and increased atrial ectopic activity. Hyperthyroidism is also associated with a shortening of the atrial effective refractory period and action potential duration, which may also contribute to AF (**Figs. 1** and **2**).

Treatment of hyperthyroidism results in conversion to sinus rhythm in up to two-thirds of patients Hypothyroidism is frequently associated with sinus bradycardia and chronotropic

incompetence as a direct result of the absence of the thyroid's hormone-stimulating effect on sinus node (SN) and on body temperature, which, being decreased, favors the sinus bradycardia.

The role of hypothyroidism in atrial arrhythmogenesis, however, is less recognized and is not fully understood. AF patients with hypothyroidism have elevated risk of atrial tachyarrhythmia recurrence after catheter ablation of AF.

Alcohol intoxication Acute and chronic alcohol consumption has been associated with arrhythmias, in particular, AF. *"Holiday heart syndrome,"* considered as greater than 5 drinks consumed in only 1 occasion, is a common emergency department presentation, with AF precipitated by alcohol in 35% to 62% of cases. Cellular effects, such as damage of the gap junction of the intercellular channels, direct injury/inflammation of the myocyte, and acute oxidative stress, along with autonomic effects, such as sympathetic activation, vagal inhibition, and reduced heart variability, result in formation of the electrophysiological milieu for the onset of AF, by shortening atrial and pulmonary vein action potential, shortening the atrial effective refractory period, slowing of intra-atrial and interatrial conduction, and enhancing AV nodal conduction.[2]

Chronic obstructive pulmonary disease and risk of atrial fibrillation Chronic obstructive pulmonary disease (COPD), when stable or during exacerbations and its therapy, is a common risk factor that often triggers AF by altering cardiopulmonary physiology. Smoking, airway inflammation,

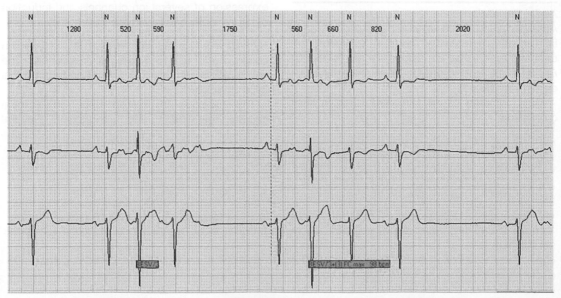

Fig. 1. Recurrent episodes of non-sustained atrial fibrillation and isolated sinus rhythm beats.

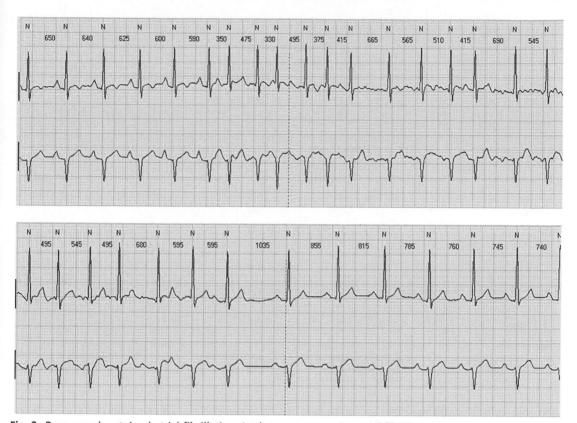

Fig. 2. Paroxysmal sustained atrial fibrillation. In the upper ecg strip: atrial fibrillation induction after five beats of sinus rhythm. In the inferior ecg, recorded after four minutes, sinus rhythm restores.

hypoxia, hypercapnia, pulmonary hypertension, β-adrenergic agonist, and steroids all contribute to ultimately causing or worsening AF.

P pulmonale (P wave ≥0.25 mV in the inferior leads; **Fig. 3**) is common on electrocardiograms (ECGs) of COPD patients. A digital analysis of ECGs in a 25-year period showed that P-wave duration and PQ interval were found significantly longer in the AF group than in the non-AF group. The PQ interval resulted in the strongest risk factor for AF development in patients with P pulmonale. The P-wave dispersion (PwD), which is the difference in the maximum and minimum duration of the P wave, was also found to be an independent risk factor associated with the development of AF, and the PwD was found to be increased more in the acute phase than in the stable phase and is greater in patients with more frequent exacerbations, which may explain the increased incidence of AF in these patients.[3,4]

Postoperative atrial fibrillation and supraventricular arrhythmias Postoperative AF is the most common perioperative cardiac arrhythmia, in both cardiac and noncardiac surgery. AF develops in 3% of unselected adults aged 45 years undergoing

noncardiac surgery, but it is much higher (30%) following thoracic surgery[5,6] and increases to 40% for patients undergoing cardiac surgery.

Following surgery, AF may be triggered by the following multiple mechanisms:

- Activation of the sympathetic system due to stress increases heart rate and catecholamines release.
- Clinical circumstances, such as hypovolemia, intraoperative hypotension, anemia, trauma, and pain, can also affect the sympathetic activity.
- Hypoglycemia or electrolytes disturbances: both can alter the arrhythmic atrial substrate increasing automaticity.
- Hypoxia can result in pulmonary vein vasoconstriction, increasing right ventricular pressure and right atrial stretch and ischemia of the myocardial atrial cells, altering the cardiac conduction system.
- Hypervolemia can increase intravascular volume and stretching of the right atrium.

During anesthesia's induction, secondary to hypotension, autonomic imbalance, or airway manipulation, patients with underlying structural

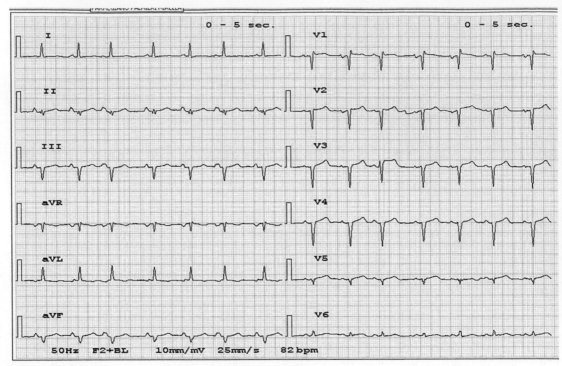

Fig. 3. P pulmonale (P wave ≥0.25 mV in the inferior leads).

heart disease are at greatest risk for developing supraventricular tachycardia (SVT).[7]

In addition, during cardiac or major vascular surgery, patients may experience SVT during dissection of the pericardium, placement of atrial sutures, or insertion of the venous cannulas required for cardiopulmonary bypass.

Risk stratification and reversible causes of ventricular arrhythmias In the assessment of the risk of recurrence, it is very important to identify a transient or correctable cause for the ventricular tachycardia/ventricular fibrillation (VT/VF): when the cause can be eliminated, there is a low risk of recurrence.

Transient triggers (ischemia, heart failure, hypokalemia) may cause ventricular arrhythmias in a substantial proportion of patients. Ventricular premature beats can trigger VT in the setting of structural heart disease.[8]

Psychological stress may also be an important trigger.

Sympathetic activity is important in electrical stability as demonstrated by a decreased baroreflex sensitivity in patients with clinical VT.[9]

Assessment of transient arrhythmia triggers at the time of the arrhythmic event requires a complete clinical and laboratory evaluation, including serum electrolyte assessment, echocardiography, and coronary angiography.

Transient or correctable cause of VT/VF includes the following:

- Acute myocardial ischemic event (including myocardial infarction or unstable angina)
- Proarrhythmic drug reaction
- Worsening of heart failure
- Electrolyte imbalance (hypokalemia or hypomagnesemia).

The concept of risk stratification is very important for patients who have ventricular arrhythmias: patients at high risk for recurrence need to be aggressively treated, and patients at low risk do not need specific treatment.

Ischemia, myocardial infarction, and ventricular tachycardia/ventricular fibrillation reversibility Myocardial ischemia or scarring is the most common setting for life-threatening ventricular arrhythmias.[10] Patients with coronary artery disease without myocardial scarring who have a cardiac arrest at the onset of ischemia are thought to be at low risk for recurrent arrhythmias when the ischemia is successfully treated.[11]

Patients with a myocardial scar from a previous myocardial infarction who have sustained VT might be at higher risk for recurrent arrhythmias because at least a part of the underlying cause (the myocardial scar) cannot be completely eliminated.[12]

Myocardial ischemia was proven to be the trigger for electrical instability (**Fig. 4**), and VF can be its arrhythmic manifestation (**Fig. 5**). VF and myocardial ischemia are inseparable. Transmural heterogeneities in myocardial action potential and ionic currents produce transmural asymmetry in conduction during acute ischemia. Acute ischemia depresses the excitability and velocity of conduction more rapidly in the epicardium than in the endocardium, leading to increased dispersion.

Other triggering factors include the development of electrolyte disturbances, such as hypokalemia.

Electrical instability is enhanced in patients in whom drug therapy for congestive heart failure often acts to further increase electrolyte disturbances.

Antiarrhythmic drugs and ventricular tachycardia/ ventricular fibrillation reversibility Another cause of transient arrhythmic event is the proarrhythmic effects of antiarrhythmic drugs[13]: patients treated for minor arrhythmias can develop life-threatening arrhythmias because of the antiarrhythmic drug itself; these patients might present underlying abnormalities of sodium or potassium channel function, unmasked or exacerbated by the antiarrhythmic drug. In these patients, the simple elimination of the antiarrhythmic drug will remove the propensity to life-threatening ventricular arrhythmias.

Patients with cardiac disease who are treated with diuretics occasionally develop serious electrolyte abnormalities that can precipitate ventricular arrhythmias.[14] It is less well known whether correction of the electrolyte abnormalities sufficiently removes the risk for arrhythmia recurrence.

Hypoglycemia and ventricular arrhythmias Insulin-induced hypoglycemia can causes abnormal QT prolongation and dispersion and can be associated with hypokalemia and sympathoadrenal activation, increasing the potential risk for ventricular arrhythmias, particularly in individuals with preexisting long QTc. The sympathoadrenal discharge induced by hypoglycemia alters cardiac repolarization by both direct and indirect (by reducing extracellular potassium) mechanisms.[15] These abnormalities in cardiac repolarization indicate a risk of VT and sudden death in other conditions, including ischemic heart disease and congenital long QT syndrome.

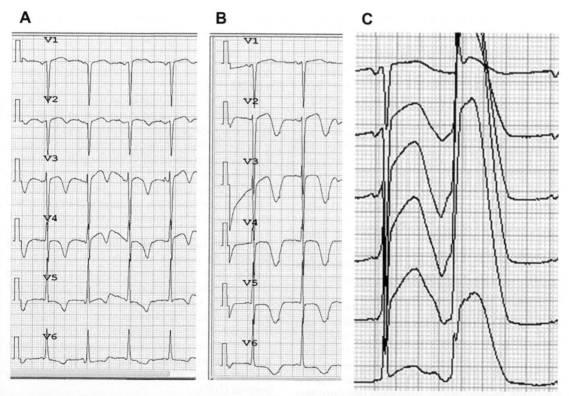

Fig. 4. Myocardial ischemia was proven to be the trigger for electrical instability. Ischemic T wave. Panel A: in V1–V5 diffuse negative T wave. Panel B: more evident negativity of the T wave. Panel C: in the same leads, QT prolongation and the trigger of an ectopic beat. (see the same case in **Fig. 5**).

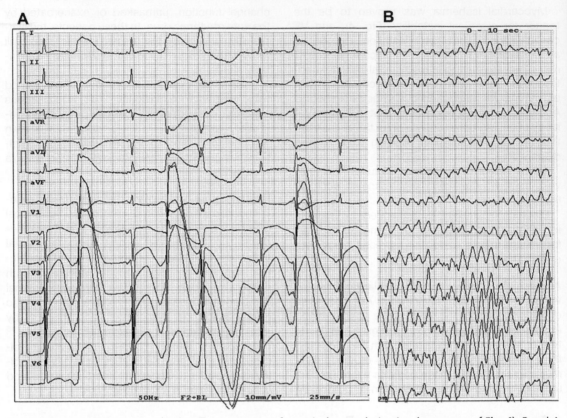

Fig. 5. VF as a manifestation of ischemic impairment of ventricular repolarization (same case of **Fig. 4**). Panel A: bigeminal ventricular ectopic beats, bigeminism and couplets, as expression of a further impairment of repolarization. Panel B: VF development.

Hypothermia Hypothermia is present when the core temperature decreases to less than 35°C from its normal value of 37°C. Hypothermia is considered mild at 32°C to 35°C, moderate at 28°C to 32°C, and severe at less than 28°C.

Several risk factors may favor hypothermia, such as exhaustion, very young age, mental problems, alcohol and drug use, and some health disorders affect the body's ability to regulate body temperature, like hypothyroidism, poor nutrition or anorexia nervosa, diabetes, stroke, severe arthritis, Parkinson disease, trauma, and spinal cord injuries. In addition, some drugs can change the body's ability to regulate its temperature, like antidepressants, antipsychotics, narcotic pain medications, and sedatives.

Hypothermia with a body temperature between 35°C and 33°C reduces the depolarization of cardiac pacemaker cells, resulting in bradycardia. Because this bradycardia is not vagally mediated, it can be refractory to standard therapies, such as atropine. Hypothermia alters several ion channel functions, leading to abnormal early repolarization manifested in the ECG as "Osborne wave." Furthermore, mean arterial pressure and cardiac

output decrease, as a consequence of severe hypothermia.

If the core temperature decreases to 25°C to 28°C, atrial and ventricular arrhythmias may appear and degenerate in asystole and VF.

In the setting of early repolarization pattern, hypothermia leads to VF/VT by exaggerating repolarization abnormalities, leading to the development of phase 2 reentry. Quinidine, cilostazol, and milrinone suppress the hypothermia-induced VT/VF by reversing the repolarization abnormalities.[16]

Association between ventricular arrhythmias and Torsades de pointes and acquired long QT syndrome from stress cardiomyopathy (Takasubo syndrome) Stress cardiomyopathy is a syndrome of transient ventricular dysfunction triggered by severe emotional or physical stress, likely resulting from catecholamine-mediated myocardial toxicity. Repolarization abnormalities associated with other hyperadrenergic states can cause QT prolongation and lethal arrhythmia, including Torsades de pointes (TdP).

Carbon monoxide induces cardiac arrhythmias via induction of the late Na$^+$ current Clinical reports describe life-threatening cardiac arrhythmias after environmental exposure to carbon monoxide (CO) or accidental CO poisoning between mechanism of disruption of repolarization and prolongation of the QT interval.

The proarrhythmic effects of CO arise from activation of nitric oxide (NO) synthase, leading to NO-mediated *nitrosylation* of the Na channels and induction of the late Na current.[17]

BRADYCARDIAS CAUSED BY DRUGS, ELECTROLYTE DISTURBANCES, AND TREATABLE NONCARDIAC CONDITIONS
Drugs

Several cardiac drugs, mainly those used in the treatment of cardiac arrhythmias, and several noncardiac medications, can cause bradyarrhythmias (**Box 2**).

Drugs can depress SN and/or atrioventricular (AV) node (AVN) function either directly or by an effect mediated by the autonomic nervous system. The effect of any given drug on the function of the SN and the AVN is highly variable from subject to subject. Drug-induced bradycardia usually does not appear in patients with normal SN function and normal AV conduction. In the critically ill patient, bradycardias are more rarely encountered than tachycardias, but often are caused by an underlying disorder (eg, hyperkalemia, calcium channel

---

Box 2
Drugs potentially responsible of reversible bradyarrhythmias secondary to sinus node dysfunction and/or atrioventricular block

Cardiac drugs

Digoxin

Ivabradine

Ranolazine

Beta-blockers

Nondihydropyridine calcium channel blockers (verapamil, diltiazem)

Antiarrhythmic drugs

- Amiodarone
- Quinidine
- Flecainide/propafenone

Noncardiac drugs

Lithium

Chloroquine

Carbamazepine

Chemotherapeutic agents

---

blocker toxicity, beta-adrenergic receptor blocker toxicity) that has to be corrected while using catecholamines, atropine, aminophylline, or a temporary pacemaker for initial treatment of complete heart block or asystole.

Cardiac drugs
Digoxin effects Digoxin is one of the oldest drugs for the heart, which is extracted from a plant called *Digitalis purprurea.*

Digoxin inhibits the sodium-potassium ATPase pump, causing intracellular calcium accumulation. The augmented intracellular calcium causes an increase in myocardial contractility but also Ca overload and Ca waves capable of triggering spontaneous depolarizations. With an unclear mechanism resembling vagomimetic and antiadrenergic effects, digitalis causes depression of the SN and AVNs as well as shortening of atrial refractory period and dispersion of atrial depolarization. The use of digitalis generates changes in the ECG at therapeutic doses, with a mild PR increase due to increased vagal tone; the morphology of QRS-T segment is typically described as "sagging" or "scooped." The T wave is biphasic with an initial negative and fast positive wave; U wave may also be present. These particular features are present due to shortening of the atrial and ventricular refractory periods that result in a short QT interval with secondary repolarization abnormalities affecting the ST segments, T waves, and U waves and increased vagal effects at the AVN, which cause a prolonged PR interval to slow the rate during AF (**Fig. 6**). Therapeutic digoxin serum level is 6 to 1.3 to 2.6 ng/mL.

Digoxin toxicity often occurs in particular conditions, and acute toxicity may be accompanied by hyperkalemia, whereas chronic toxicity may be accompanied by hypokalemia and hypomagnesemia.

Digoxin toxicity may cause almost any dysrhythmia, due to increased automaticity and increased AVN concealed conduction.

Sinus bradycardia and AV conduction blocks are the most common ECG changes along with ventricular ectopy. Nonparoxysmal atrial tachycardia with heart block and bidirectional VT is particularly characteristic of severe digitalis toxicity.

Beta-blockers Beta-blockers act as competitive inhibitors of catecholamines, slowing heart rate and AVN conduction. They do not depress conduction at the His-Purkinje level. The occurrence of a bradyarrhythmia following beta-blockers administration is more likely in the case of underlying SN dysfunction or AV conduction disturbances.[18]

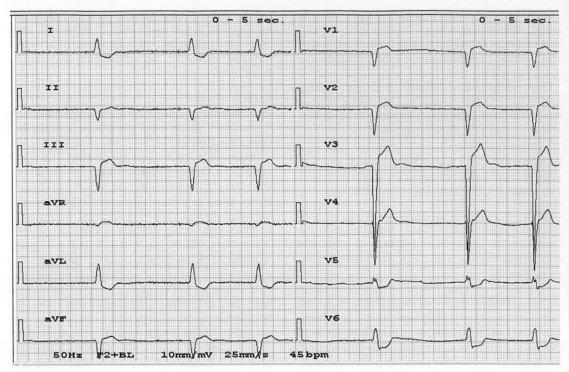

Fig. 6. Typical digitalis changes of ventricular repolarization at therapeutic doses. The morphology of QRS-T segment is typically described as "sagging" or "scooped". These particular features are present due to shortening of ventricular refractory periods that results in a short QT interval with secondary repolarization abnormalities affecting the ST segments, T waves, and U waves.

Calcium channel blockers Nondihydropyridine calcium channel blockers (verapamil, diltiazem) share a direct, not neurally mediated effect on the SN and the AVN, with slowing of heart rate and AVN conduction. At high doses, these drugs can cause marked sinus bradycardia and second- and third-degree AV block.[19]

Amiodarone Amiodarone lengthens the action potential and refractoriness of all cardiac myocytes with a direct, only in a minimal part, neurally mediated effect. At normal therapeutic doses, it slows conduction through the AVN and slows SN rate. In the case of underlying SN dysfunction or AV conduction disturbances, amiodarone can cause second- and third-degree AV block and marked sinus bradyarrhythmias (**Fig. 7**).[20]

Quinidine Quinidine has a direct depressant effect on SN and AVN, normally counterbalanced by a vagolytic action. In rare instances, the drug can cause marked sinus bradycardia.[21]

Flecainide/propafenone Flecainide and propafenone are class 1c antiarrhythmic drugs. Both drugs slow the influx of *sodium* ions into the *cardiac muscle* cells, causing a decrease in excitability of the cells, and have a direct depressant

effect on AV conduction at any level of the myocytes, whereas flecainide has little effect on SN function and prolongs the AVN conduction time and His-Purkinje conduction time.

Propafenone, differently from flecainide, has a beta-adrenergic blockade function, which can cause bradycardia and bronchospasm.

Both drugs have indications for treatment of supraventricular arrhythmias, such as of AF, atrial flutter, and for wolf parkinson white, atrioventricular reentrant tachycardia, and atrioventricular nodal reentrant tachycardia.

Flecainide and propafenone share the same adverse cardiac effects, including moderate negative inotropic action and depression of all major conduction pathways, but in different incidences, due to a narrower therapeutic index of flecainide compared with propafenone. Flecainide and propafenone action on conduction pathways is manifested on ECG as an increased PR interval and QRS duration. Toxicity is suggested when a 50% increase in QRS duration compared with baseline ECG or 30% prolongation in PR interval occurs. The QTc interval can also be prolonged in cases of flecainide/propafenone overdose (**Fig. 8**). When flecainide/propafenone toxicity occurs, proarrhythmic effects can

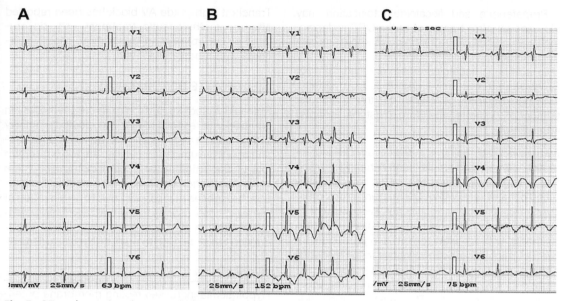

Fig. 7. QT prolongation due to amiodarone therapy.

counteract the antiarrhythmic effects. Symptomatic bradycardia, different degrees of AV block, and VT and TdP due to QT prolongation may occur. Treatment of acute flecainide/propafenone overdose includes administration of activated charcoal, administration of sodium bicarbonate because it reverses the action of sodium channel blockade, pressors as dobutamine if profound hypotension is present, and transthoracic or transvenous pacing.

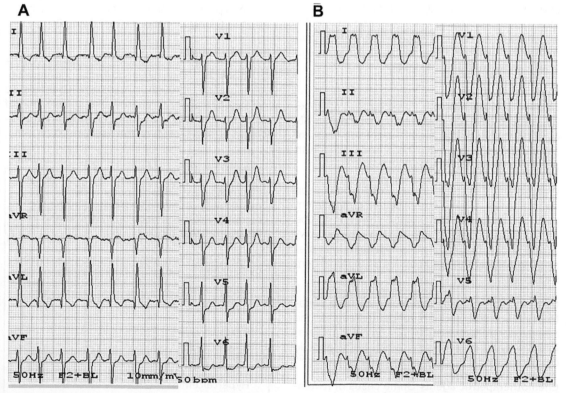

Fig. 8. A case of 1:1 atrial flutter (*A*) and a wide complex tachycardia (*B*) due to left bundle branch block induced by flecainide.

Propafenone and flecainide intoxication may also appear after treatment of the QRS widening, with persistent T-wave inversion as known as cardiac memory.

In addition, flecainide treatment can unmask Brugada pattern I on V1 and V2 lead in patients with susceptible genotype; in this particular setting of patients, the drug must be stopped immediately.

Ivabradine Ivabradine is a selective I_f channel inhibitor, also known as the "funny channel," which has emerged as a novel site for the selective inhibition of heart rate, without decreasing blood pressure, and showed a significant improvement in outcome in patients with heart failure. These I_f channels, with a mixed sodium and potassium inward current, have been identified in the sinoatrial node of the heart, which mediates the slow diastolic depolarization of the pacemaker of the spontaneous rhythmic cells. The most common side effect of ivabradine is symptomatic bradycardia.

Ranolazine Ranolazine is a new, common antianginal drug that may also have potential antiarrhythmic effects. Ranolazine exerts modulatory effects on ion channels that have been similarly observed in amiodarone, such as in reduction of inward current (I) INa^+ and I K^+ slow and rapid and I Ca2. Consequently, ranolazine appears to have beneficial roles in both atrial and ventricular arrhythmias. As for common antiarrhythmic drugs, ranolazine overload may result in symptomatic bradycardia and QT prolongation.

Noncardiac Drugs

Lithium Lithium-induced sodium channel blockade is likely an important mechanism in SN dysfunction. Both therapeutic and toxic levels of serum lithium levels have been associated with SN dysfunction and bradyarrhythmias.[22]

Chloroquine Complete heart block has been described as a rare complication of treatment with chloroquine. This toxicity seems to be restricted to long-term, high-dose treatment; however, it should be kept in mind in patients with pre-existing conduction disturbances during long-term treatment.[23]

Carbamazepine Carbamazepine may have negative chronotropic and dromotropic effects on the cardiac conduction system and can induce reversible SN dysfunction and AV block at therapeutic concentrations, in most cases in elderly women.[24]

Chemotherapeutic agents Some cases of reversible SN dysfunction have been described in patients after chemotherapy for lymphoma. Transient high-grade AV block has been reported after chemotherapeutic treatment with doxorubicin or cyclophosphamide, in most cases in patients with breast carcinoma.

ELECTROLYTE DISTURBANCES

Potassium, sodium, and calcium are the major ion components responsible for the electrical activity of the heart. In circumstances when the concentration of potassium and/or calcium are too high or too low in the extracellular space, disruption of the orderly activation and recovery of electrical excitation through the myocardium due to an alteration of the ionic contributions to the cellular action potential can determine SN dysfunction and/or AV conduction block, leading to bradyarrhythmias (**Box 3**).

Hypokalemia

Hypokalemia increases resting membrane potential and both the duration of the action potential and the duration of the refractory period. It also increases threshold potential as well as automaticity. Slowed conduction is attributed to membrane hyperpolarization and increased excitation threshold. Hypokalemia can rarely promote the appearance of different degrees of AV blocks, usually localized at the His-Purkinje level (**Fig. 9**).[25]

The typical arrhythmia associated with drug-induced QT prolongation is TdP (**Fig. 10**).

Hyperkalemia

In patients with hyperkalemia, potassium conductance through potassium channels is increased, leading to an increase in the slope of phases 2 and 3 of the action potential and therefore to a shortening of the repolarization time.

Box 3
Electrolyte disturbances potentially responsible of reversible bradyarrhythmias secondary to sinus node dysfunction and/or atrioventricular block

Bradyarrhythmias secondary to sinus node dysfunction

    Hyperkalemia

    Hypercalcemia

Bradyarrhythmias secondary to AV block

    Hyperkalemia

    Hypokalemia

    Hypercalcemia

    Hypocalcemia (in newborns)

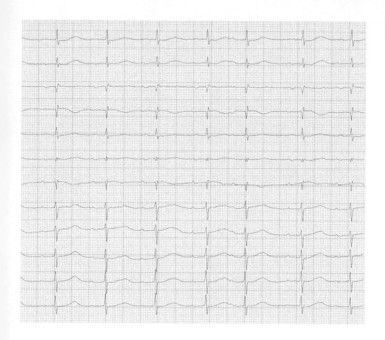

Fig. 9. QT prolongation due to ipokaliemia.

The ECG manifestation of hyperkalemia is characterized by narrow-based peaked T waves, prolongation of the PR interval, widening of the QRS complex, and consequent sine waves. Bradyarrhythmias are usually observed at potassium concentrations ≥ 7 mEq/L. Sinus bradycardia, eventually progressing to sinus arrest, and second and third-degree AV block, usually localized at the His-Purkinje level, have all been described on the presenting ECGs of patients with hyperkalemia (**Fig. 11**). These bradyarrhythmias are more frequent in patients with underlying SN dysfunction and/or AV conduction disturbances, or when there is concomitant acidosis or hypocalcemia.

Hypercalcemia

An increased extracellular concentration of calcium decreases the duration of the action potential by shortening its phase 2. Furthermore, hypercalcemia can slow the impulse conduction, resulting rarely in the appearance of second- and third-degree AV block and of SN dysfunction.[26]

Hypocalcemia

Hypocalcemia increases the duration of the action potential by lengthening its phase 2 and typically prolongs the Q-T interval on the ECG. Hypocalcemia-induced second- and third-degree AV block has been described in the neonatal and pediatric populations.[27]

TREATABLE NONCARDIAC CONDITIONS

Several treatable noncardiac conditions can cause transient bradyarrhythmias, more frequently represented by varying degrees of AV conduction block (**Box 4**) Reversible bradyarrhythmias can be produced with different mechanisms from noncardiac conditions by affecting directly the SN, such as during an infection as in Lyme disease, or by promoting the electrolytes imbalance as in hyperparathyroidism, that increases the extracellular concentration of calcium, or inducing hypothermia, as in hypothyroidism (see earlier in the article), or by increasing the intracranial pressure as, for example, in hemorrhagic stroke or hypertensive hydrocephalus that results in triggering a parasympathetic response via the *vagus nerve* (Cushing reflex).

Pulmonary Embolism

Many ECG abnormalities can be seen during pulmonary embolism (PE) due to acute pulmonary hypertension, hypoxia, and pulmonary vasoconstriction. Right ventricular strain on the ECG has been found to correlate with the degree of pulmonary artery obstruction due to PE, increased pressure, and wall tension on the right heart. The presence of the right ventricular strain pattern on the ECG is associated with an increased risk of all-cause death and clinical deterioration, even with normal systemic blood pressure. In patients with right ventricular dysfunction, T-wave inversions in leads V1–V3 (**Fig. 12**) had greater

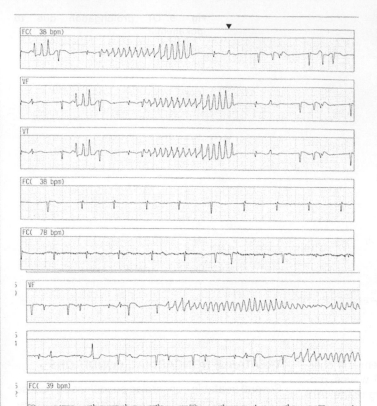

Fig. 10. The typical arrhythmias associated with drug-induced QT prolongation are TdP.

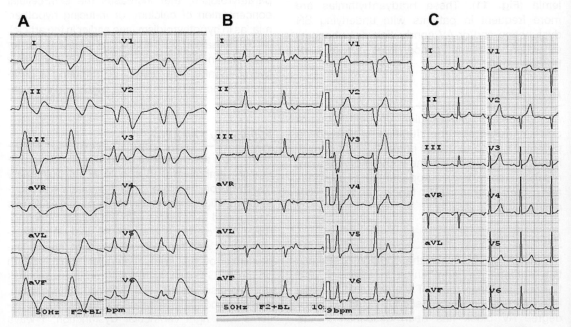

Fig. 11. ECG signs of severe Hyper-kaliemia (*A*) reversed during Hemodialysis (*B–C*). Atrial fibrillation (*B*).

Box 4
Noncardiac conditions potentially responsible of reversible bradyarrhythmias secondary to sinus node dysfunction and/or atrioventricular block

Lyme disease

Lymphoma

Hypothyroidism

Hyperparathyroidism

Intracranial hypertension

Pulmonary embolism

- *Sinus tachycardia* (44% of cases), the most common abnormality
- *Right ventricular strain pattern* (34% of patients), T-wave inversions in the right precordial leads (V1-4) ± the inferior leads (II, III, aVF). This pattern is seen in up to 34% of patients and is associated with high pulmonary artery pressures
- *S_I Q_{III} T_{III} pattern* (20% of patients), deep S wave in lead I, Q wave in III, inverted T wave in III. This "classic" finding is neither sensitive nor specific for PE.
- *Complete or incomplete RBBB* (18% of patients), which is also associated with increased mortality
- *Right axis deviation* (16% of patients), extreme right-axis deviation may occur, with axis between 0° and −90°, giving the appearance of left-axis deviation ("pseudo left axis")
- *Dominant R wave in V1*, a manifestation of acute right ventricular dilatation
- *Right atrial enlargement* (P pulmonale, 9% of patients), peaked P wave in lead II greater than 2.5 mm in height
- *Clockwise rotation*, shift of the R/S transition point toward V6 with a persistent S wave in V6 ("pulmonary disease pattern"), implying rotation of the heart due to right ventricular dilatation
- *Atrial tachyarrhythmias* (8% of patients) AF, flutter, atrial tachycardia

sensitivity and diagnostic accuracy compared with the S1Q3T3 and right bundle branch block (RBBB) features (**Fig. 13**), which had good specificity but only moderate accuracy.

In addition, a novel parameter for diagnosis of PE is the time between the T peak (Tp) and T end (Te) on at least 3 precordial leads. There was a significant increase in Tp-Te results in V1 in PE patients compared with non-PE patients. The Tp-Te interval measured at greater than126 ms is a predictor of mortality and morbidity in PE patients.

- *Nonspecific ST segment and T-wave changes* (50% of patients), including ST elevation and depression

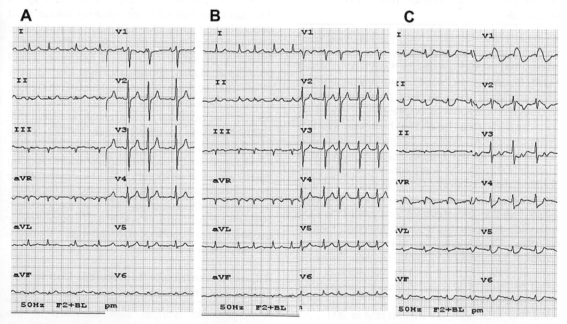

Fig. 12. ECG in pulmonary embolism. (*A*) Right atrial overload and junctional ectopic beats. (*B*) Atrial fibrillation development. (*C*) Right ventricular acute bundle branch block ST elevation and T-wave inversions in leads V1–V3.

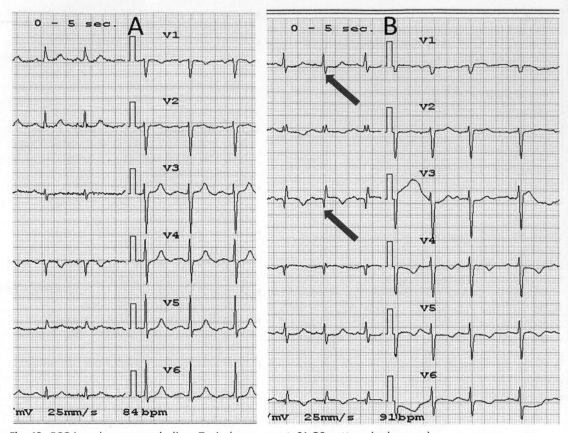

Fig. 13. ECG in pulmonary embolism. Typical, new onset, S1-Q3 pattern (red arrows).

CASE REPORTS
A Case of 1:1 Atrial Flutter Induced by Flecainide

A woman in her 60s with a history of paroxysmal AF and a structurally normal heart was prescribed flecainide 100 mg twice a day for rhythm control (see **Fig. 8**). She presented to the emergency department with complaints of experiencing palpitations for the past several hours. Her blood pressure on presentation was 80/50 mm Hg, and her heart rate was 200 beats per minute (bpm). A 12-lead ECG was performed (see **Fig. 8**B, wide complex tachycardia at a rate of 200 bpm). She was given intravenous bicarbonate, and a second ECG was performed (see **Fig. 8**A, typical atrial flutter at a rate of 200 bpm with 2:1 ventricular response). Analysis of the ECG with wide complex tachycardia: although there is no clear AV dissociation, the presence of an apparent negative concordance in precordial leads, QRS duration longer than 160 milliseconds, and onset to nadir of S wave in lead V1 longer than 100 milliseconds point toward VT. On the other hand, the wide complex rhythm rate is 200 bpm, exactly the same as that of atrial flutter in the second ECG; this raises the possibility of wide complex

rhythm being atrial flutter with 1:1 AV conduction. Flecainide causes rate-dependent slowing of the rapid sodium channel, slowing phase 0 of depolarization, and slows conductance in atrial and ventricular tissues by increasing the effective refractory period. It also has a regulatory effect on atrial fibrillatory activity and may lead to slow atrial flutter, typically at a rate of around 200 bpm, owing to decreased atrial tissue conductance. Flecainide, like quinidine, has a vagolytic action that counterbalances partially the direct effect on the AVN and does not slow AV conduction. As a result, in the absence of a concomitant AV nodal blocking agent, this slow atrial flutter can be conducted to the ventricle in a 1:1 ratio, resulting in extremely rapid ventricular response. This is associated with aberrant conduction and a bizarre QRS morphology caused by rate-dependent exaggerated intraventricular conduction delays.[28]

A Case of Ventricular Tachycardia During Pulmonary Embolism

A 70-year-old woman was admitted to the emergency department for shortness of breath and syncope for the past 2 hours (**Fig. 14**).

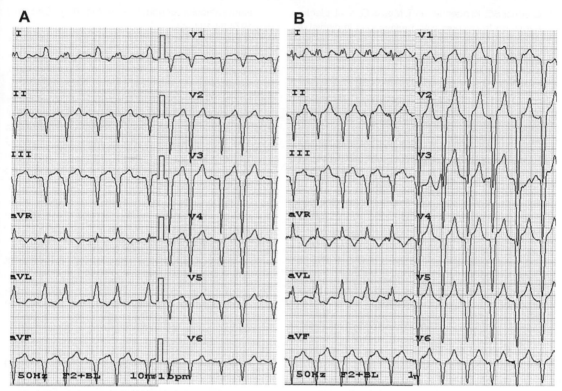

Fig. 14. ECG in pulmonary embolism. A rare case of bigeminal ectopic beats. (*A*) and ventricular tachycardia (*B*) originating from the right ventricle.

Her blood pressure on presentation was 90/60 mm Hg. A 12-lead ECG, echocardiography, and contrast-enhanced computed tomography were performed. Her heart rate was 180 bpm, and the ECG showed wide complex tachycardia at a rate of .... bpm with typical left bundle branch block (LBBB) morphology (see **Fig. 1**). A DC shock restored sinus rhythm. The 12-lead ECG during sinus rhythm was compatible with the diagnosis of PE. Echocardiogram and pulmonary CT scan confirmed the diagnosis of PE.

This case suggests that PE with extremely enlarged right heart should be considered as a cause of VT, syncope, and sudden cardiac death.

A recent case report by Gong and colleagues[29] reported that VT with typical LBBB morphology is not an absolute necessity as a major criterion for the diagnosis of ARVC when the right heart is extremely enlarged.

REFERENCES

1. Reddy V, Taha W, Kundumadan S, et al. Atrial fibrillation and hyperthyroidism: a literature review. Indian Heart J 2017;69:545–50.

2. Voskoboinik A, Prabhu S, Ling LH, et al. Alcohol and atrial fibrillation: a sobering review. J Am Coll Cardiol 2016;68(23):2567–76.

3. Hayashi H, Miyamoto A, Kawaguchi T, et al. P-pulmonale and the development of atrial fibrillation. Circ J 2014;78:329–37.

4. Tukek T, Yildiz P, Akkaya V, et al. Factors associated with the development of atrial fibrillation in COPD patients the role of P-wave dispersion. Ann Noninvasive Electrocardiol 2002;7:222–7.

5. Durheim MT, Holmes DN, Blanco RG, et al. Characteristics and outcomes of adults with chronic obstructive pulmonary disease and atrial fibrillation. Heart 2018. https://doi.org/10.1136/heartjnl-2017-312735.

6. Bhave PD, Goldman LE, Vittinghoff E, et al. Incidence, predictors, and outcomes associated with postoperative atrial fibrillation after major noncardiac surgery. Am Heart J 2012;164:918–24.

7. Thompson A, Balser JR. Perioperative cardiac arrhythmias. Br J Anaesth 2004;93:86–94.

8. Rosman J, Honan S, Shapiro M, et al. Triggers of sustained monomorphic ventricular tachycardia differ among patients with varying etiologies of left ventricular dysfunction. Ann Noninvasive Electrocardiol 2006;11:113–7.

9. Credner SC, Klingenheben T, Mauss O, et al. Electrical storm in patients with transvenous implantable cardioverter-defibrillators: incidence, management and prognostic implications. J Am Coll Cardiol 1998;32:1909–15.

10. Cobb LA, Baum RS, Alvarez H, et al. Resuscitation from out-of-hospital ventricular fibrillation: 4-year follow-up. Circulation 1975;51,52(suppl III):223–8.

11. Morady F, DiCarlo L, Winston S, et al. Clinical features and prognosis of patients with out-of-hospital cardiac arrest and a normal electrophysiologic study. J Am Coll Cardiol 1984;4:39–44.

12. Brugada J, Aguinaga L, Mont L, et al. Coronary artery revascularization in patients with sustained ventricular arrhythmias in the chronic phase of a myocardial infarction: effects on the electrophysiologic substrate and outcome. J Am Coll Cardiol 2001;37:529–33.

13. Roden DM. Mechanisms and management of proarrhythmia. Am J Cardiol 1998;82:49I–57I.

14. Nordrehaug JE. Malignant arrhythmia in relation to serum potassium in acute myocardial infarction. Am J Cardiol 1985;56:20D–3D.

15. Kacheva S, Karges B, Goller K, et al. QT prolongation caused by insulin-induced hypoglycaemia – an interventional study in 119 individuals. Diabetes Res Clin Pract 2017;123:165–72.

16. Gurabi Z, Koncz I, Patocskai B, et al. Cellular mechanism underlying hypothermia-induced ventricular tachycardia/ventricular fibrillation in the setting of early repolarization and the protective effect of quinidine, cilostazol, and milnirone. Circ Arrhythm Electrophysiol 2014;7:134–42.

17. Dallas ML, Yang Z, Boyle JP, et al. Carbon monoxide induces cardiac arrhythmia via induction of the late Na+ current. Am J Respir Crit Care Med 2012; 186:648–56.

18. Bigger JT Jr, Reiffel JA. Sick sinus syndrome. Annu Rev Med 1979;30(1):91–118.

19. Zipes DP, Fischer JC. Effects of agents which inhibit the slow channel on sinus node automaticity and atrioventricular conduction in the dog. Circ Res 1974;34:184–92.

20. Hofmann R, Leisch F. Symptomatic bradycardia with amiodarone in patients with pre-existing conduction disorders. Wien Klin Wochenschr 1995; 107:640–4.

21. Alboni P, Cappato R, Paparella N, et al. Electrophysiological effects and mechanism of action of oral quinidine in patients with sinus bradycardia and first degree A-V nodal block. Eur Heart J 1987;8:1080–9.

22. Oudit GY, Korley V, Backx PH, et al. Lithium-induced sinus node disease at therapeutic concentrations: linking lithium-induced blockade of sodium channels to impaired pacemaker activity. Can J Cardiol 2007;23(3):229–32.

23. Reuss-Borst M, Berner B, Wulf G, et al. Complete heart block as a rare complication of treatment with Chloroquine. J Rheumatol 1999;26:1394–5.

24. Takayanagi K, Hisauchi I, Watanabe J, et al. Carbamazepine-induced sinus node dysfunction and atrio-ventricular block in elderly women. Jpn Heart J 1998;39:469–79.

25. Varess G. Hypokalaemia associated with infra-His Mobitz type second degree A-V block. Chest 1994;105:1616–7.

26. Shah AP, Lopez A, Wachsner RY, et al. Sinus node dysfunction secondary to hyperparathyroidism. J Cardiovasc Pharmacol Ther 2004;9:145–7.

27. Stefanaki E, Koropuli M, Stefanaki S, et al. Atrioventricular block in preterm infants caused by hypocalcemia: a case report and review of the literature. Eur J Obstet Gynecol Reprod Biol 2005;120:115–6.

28. Crijns HJ, Van Gelder IC, Lie KI. Supraventricular tachycardia mimicking ventricular tachycardia during flecainide treatment. Am J Cardiol 1988;62:1303–6.

29. Gong S, Wei X, Liu G, et al. Arrhythmogenic right ventricular cardiomyopathy with multiple thrombi and ventricular tachycardia of atypical left branch bundle block morphology. Int Heart J 2018;59: 652–4.

Hidden Complexity in Routine Adult and Pediatric Arrhythmias Interpretation
The Future of Precision Electrocardiology

Fabio M. Leonelli, MD[a],[*], Roberto De Ponti, MD, FHRS[b],
Fabrizio Drago, MD[c], Anwar Baban, MD, PhD[c],
Daniel Cortez, MD[d], Massimo Griselli, MD[d],
Giuseppe Bagliani, MD[e],[f]

KEYWORDS

- ECG • Precision electro cardiology • Arrhythmias • Genetic testing • Channelopathies

KEY POINTS

- Several pediatric and adult challenging ECGs are presented.
- ECG analysis is able to reach a diagnosis of the arrhythmia mechanism.
- The pathologies inducing the abnormalities triggering an arrhythmia can be suspected only by ECG investigation.
- The article presents several new technological advances, identifying the macroscopic and microscopic abnormalities in each case.
- The current limitations of some of these tools are presented.

INTRODUCTION

The goal of this issue is to illustrate a more comprehensive method of interpreting complex arrhythmias. The Andrea Pozzolini and colleagues' article, "Complex Arrhythmias Due to Reversible Causes," has presented several abnormal ECG tracings, discussed the findings, and deductively explained the abnormalities. Our approach was based on the observation of morphologic variations of the P-QRS complex or on the interpretation of changes in impulse conduction or generation during stable or unstable rhythms. This time-honored method relies on current knowledge of the electrophysiologic properties of normal and abnormal

No relevant conflicts to disclose.
[a] Cardiology Department, James A. Haley Veterans' Hospital, University of South Florida, 13000 Bruce B Down Boulevard, Tampa, FL 33612, USA; [b] Department of Heart and Vessels, Ospedale di Circolo and Macchi Foundation, University of Insubria, Viale Borri, 57, Varese 21100, Italy; [c] Pediatric Cardiology and Cardiac Arrhythmias Complex Unit, Department of Pediatric Cardiology and Cardiac Surgery, Bambino Gesù Children's Hospital and Research Institute, Rome 00165, Italy; [d] Pediatric and Adult Congenital Cardiology, Department of Pediatric Cardiology and Cardiac Surgery, University of Minnesota/Masonic Children's Hospital, Minneapolis, MN, USA; [e] Arrhythmology Unit, Cardiology Department, Foligno General Hospital, Via Massimo Arcamone, Foligno, Perugia 06034, Italy; [f] Cardiovascular Disease Department, University of Perugia, Piazza Menghini 1, Perugia 06129, Italy
* Corresponding author.
E-mail address: Fabio.Leonelli@va.gov

cardiacEP.theclinics.com

myocardial cells and is based on the classic approach of ECG tracing analysis alone. In the past years, several technological advances have greatly expanded knowledge of the electro-physiologic behavior of healthy and diseased cardiac cells. This article presents a snapshot of the new tools available, including cardiac imaging, with detailed analysis of tissue viability, genetic analysis of ion channel function, and implantable device to treat arrhythmias in unusual circumstances. The authors believe integration of these new technologies with ECG analysis will further improve our understanding of arrhythmias and their therapy.

CASE 1: DRUG-RESISTANT VENTRICULAR ARRHYTHMIAS IN A TODDLER

A 27-month-old toddler (weight, 12 kg; height, 88 cm) was referred to the cardiac arrhythmias service of the authors' institution for an alleged drug-resistant paroxysmal supraventricular tachycardia (Fig. 1, leading to multiple admissions and ineffective drug therapy attempts. Investigations performed during this evaluation included cardiac MRI, which showed normal ventricular dimensions (left ventricular end-diastolic volume [LVEDV] index, 59 mL/m²; right ventricular end-diastolic volume [RVEDV] index, 63 mL/m²; RVEDV/LVEDV 1.1) and minimally depressed biventricular function. No evidence of late gadolinium enhancement and/or myocardial edema was observed (Fig. 2).

The patient's conditions gradually deteriorated, due to arrhythmia persistence and secondary heart failure, requiring inotropes and mechanical ventilation, and a combination of antiarrhythmic drugs was attempted without clinical response.

Despite age and weight, an electrophysiologic study with possible radiofrequency ablation (EPS-RFA) of supraventricular arrhythmia was attempted. During the study, the earliest site of local activation was identified in the RV near the bundle of His using a 3-D mapping system.

Restoration of normal sinus rhythm occurred after 13 seconds of radiofrequency (RF) delivery. The day after the procedure, a persistent wider QRS tachycardia reoccurred, leading to rapid hemodynamic deterioration (Fig. 3). A second EPS-RFA was performed, documenting an earliest tachycardia activation site located in the right midseptal area; 9 applications of RF, at 20W of power, at 55°C, delivered at the location, restored sinus rhythm. Two days postprocedure, a new wide complex tachycardia occurred; the ECG consistent with ventricular tachycardia (VT) showed a change in morphology and axis of QRS. Because this arrhythmia was poorly tolerated and the patient's clinical conditions dramatically worsened, the authors decided to attempt a third RF ablation; 3-D mapping of the entire right ventricle (RV) identified a vast low-voltage area sited in the RV free wall, from the posterior infundibular to the inferior part, with evidence of positive pace-mapping. The authors performed scar isolation through a vast lesion, applying 20 W to 25 W, at 48°C to 52°C (Fig. 4).

At 7 months' follow-up, the patient was in good clinical conditions and regular ECG always showed sinus rhythm. Considering the difficulties of patient's clinical presentation and course, a molecular analysis of 150 genes for major cardiomyopathies in a next generation sequences targeted panel. This analysis revealed 2 variants of uncertain significance,

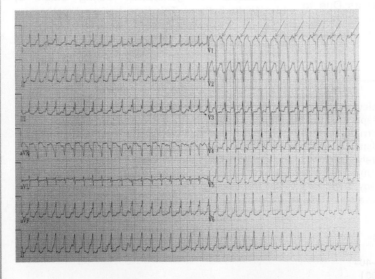

Fig. 1. Narrow QRS tachycardia cycle length, 220 milliseconds, variable QRS duration, prominent intrinsicoid deflection, and 2:1 VA conduction (arrows). VA, ventriculo-atrial.

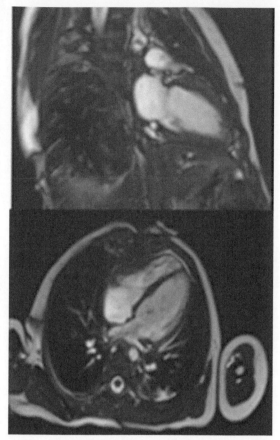

Fig. 2. Sagittal (*upper*) and coronal (*lower*) cardiac MRI view showing no evidence of late gadolinium enhancement and/or myocardial edema.

both heterozygous: c.2054G> C on *XIRP1* (Arg685Pro) and c.2746A > G on *RYR3* (Lys916Glu).

Despite this nondiagnostic result, it is relevant that both XIRP1 and RYR3 are implicated in the genesis of ventricular arrhythmias and sudden cardiac death. In particular, RYR3 encodes proteins for the ryanodine receptor involved in Ca transport within the cell, and mutations in this gene have been associated with catecholaminergic polymorphic VT and arrhythmogenic RV dysplasia.[1] XIRP1 has been linked to Brugada variants and sudden unexplained nocturnal death syndrome.[2,3]

CASE 2: BRADYCARDIA IN A NEONATE WITH SUSPECTED GENETIC SYNDROME

A normal Bangladeshi newborn girl (weight, 2.5 kg; length, 46 cm) with uncomplicated delivery, was referred after an episode of severe bradycardia (heart rate 40–50 beats per minute [bpm]). While monitored, the HR decreased with the development of 2:1 atrioventricular block (AVB) with

persisting long QT and T-wave alternans (**Figs. 5 and 6**). The echocardiogram showed asymmetric septal hypertrophy with RF apical hypertrabeculation, subaortic ventricular septal defect, patent formen ovale, small patent ductus arteriosus, and dysplasia of the pulmonary valve with mild/moderate impairment (**Fig. 7**). Based on the presence of long QT syndrome and multiple cardiac malformations a diagnosis of Timothy syndrome was made. This rare condition was confirmed with demonstration of an heterozygous mutation of CACNA1C NM_000719: c.1216G > A; p.Gly406Arg (rs79891110), de novo. The *CACNA1C* gene encodes for the main cardiac L-type calcium channel, causing a gain of function of the channel. The increased amount of Ca entering the cell causes an extremely prolonged ventricular repolarization and refractory period of the myocytes and the AVN. The ECG faithfully records the consequences of these abnormalities by recording long QT, T-wave alternans, and high-degree AVB.

Patient was treated with β-blockers with improvement of ECG abnormalities (**Fig. 8**). Due to recurrent VT requiring defibrillation and periods of bradycardia, the patient underwent placement of implantable cardioverter defibrillator (ICD) and patent ductus arteriosus ligation (**Fig. 9**). Patient was reevaluated 10 months later having experienced an episode of syncope; ICD interrogation documented 3 ICD shocks for ventricular fibrillation (VF). Antiarrhythmic therapy with mexiletine and propranolol was begun during hospitalization and patient was listed for cardiac transplantation. At follow-up, arrhythmia seemed well controlled with no recurrences of life-threatening VTs.

CASE 3: HIGH-DEGREE ATRIOVENTRICULAR BLOCK AND PRECISION PACING

A 5-year-old patient (female, weight 15.5 kg; height, 103 cm) was admitted to the authors' Pediatric Cardiology and Cardiac Arrhythmias Complex Unit, Bambino Gesù Children's Hospital and Research Institute, Rome, Italy with a diagnosis of third-degree AVB and junctional escape rhythm. The patient experienced only light dizziness without frank syncope. At admission, the patient underwent 24-hour dynamic ECG Holter monitoring, where junctional rhythm was confirmed, with an average HR of 38 bpm (minimum 49 bpm; maximum, 106 bpm); echocardiogram was normal and an exercise test again demonstrated third-degree AVB with bradycardia.

To monitor the HR and eventual life-threatening arrhythmias, an implantable loop recorder (ILR) (Reveal LINQ, Medtronic, Minneapolis, Minnesota)

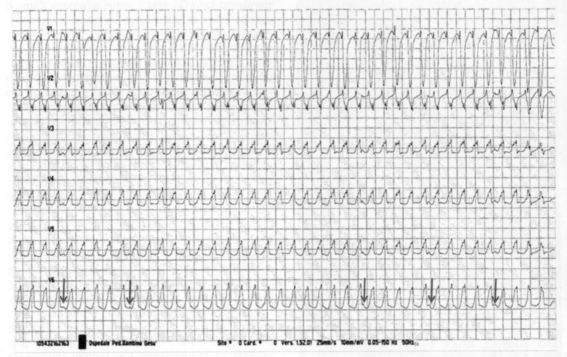

Fig. 3. Precordial leads of a wide QRS tachycardia cycle length, 280 milliseconds, with evidence of VA dissociation (*arrows*). VA, ventriculo-atrial.

was implanted. The child was followed-up with periodic in-hospital evaluations with Holter monitoring, echocardiogram, and exercise testing.

Seven months later, monitoring showed a period of complete AVB with junctional escape (**Fig. 10**), periods of polymorphic ventricular ectopic tachycardia, and prolonged nocturnal pauses.

Consequently, the ILR was explanted and an endocardial single-chamber pacemaker with a

screw in lead in the His position was implanted (Microny II SR + 2525T, Abbot, Lake bluff, Illinois). To guide the placement of the lead, an electroanatomic mapping system (EnSite Precision, Abbott, Lake bluff, Illinois) was used to mark the His potential location and to guide the pacing lead to that site. In detail, a quadripolar deflectable catheter was used to perform a 3-D mapping of the ventricle activation identifying the His potential (**Fig. 11**).

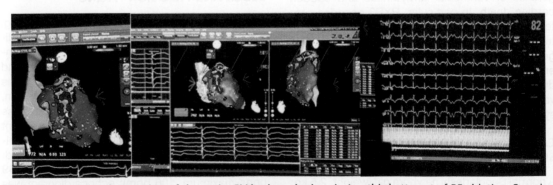

Fig. 4. Electroanatomic mapping of the entire RV in sinus rhythm during third attempt of RF ablation: 3 projections are shown from left to right, respectively: RAO, posterior view, and LAO. Coded voltage mapping is shown with areas in pink showing normal tissue and areas in green areas of low voltage. A vast low-voltage area sited in the RV free wall, from the posterior infundibular to the inferior part, was identified with evidence of positive pace-mapping. Scar isolation through a vast lesion (*red dots*), applying 20 W to 25 W, at 48°C to 52°C *blue arrows* and *red arrows* mark the alternating T wave polarity.

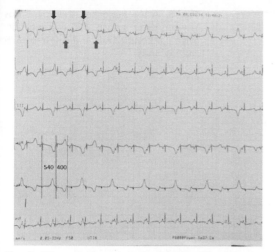

Fig. 5. Sinus rhythm at cycle length 600 with alternating QT duration between 400 milliseconds and 540 milliseconds and T-wave alternans (*arrows*).

Pace-mapping from the same catheter identified an area with the narrowest paced QRS in the parahisian bundle (QRS stimulated 120 ms). Then, a percutaneous puncture of left axillary vein was made and a guide wire placed in the inferior vena cava. A ventricular screw in lead (Solia S53, Biotronik, Berlin, Germany) was visualized using the

same mapping system and, with its guidance, was placed on the septum, on the same site previously identified by pace-mapping. In this location, paced QRS duration was 115 ms (see **Fig. 2**B). Radiological exposure of this procedure was only 2 mGy (49 μGy/m²). No complications occurred and the patient was discharged in good condition. No arrhythmic therapy was administered or prescribed. Currently, the patient is regularly followed-up without symptoms or complications.

Pacing from the His bundle allows the distribution of the artificial electrical impulse to follow the physiologic His Purkinje system, mimicking the normal left ventricular (LV) and RV activation. Localization of optimal pacing site as previously described, allows the identification of the ideal location, with minimal fluoroscopy exposure a relevant consideration when placing a device in small children.

CASE 4: AN ADOLESCENT WITH TWO RARE CARDIAC CONDITIONS

A 16-year-old girl (height, 163 cm; weight, 51 kg) presented to the authors' service with sudden-onset palpitations and wide complex tachycardia (**Fig. 12**), after an 8-year history of similar but less sustained episodes. Prior to transfer to the hospital, she had been treated with flecainide

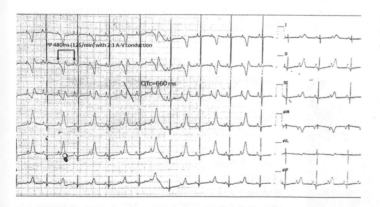

Fig. 6. Sinus rhythm cycle length, 580 milliseconds, with 2:1 AVB and a QTc of 660 milliseconds.

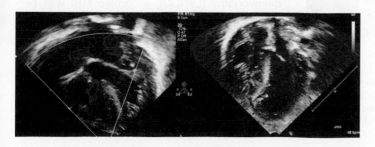

Fig. 7. Five and four echocardiographic view demonstrating asymmetric hypertrophy of IVS with RV apical hypertrabeculation, subaortic ventricular septal defect, patent foramen ovale, small patent ductus arteriosus, and dysplasia of the pulmonary valve with mild/moderate LV impairment. IVS, inter ventricular septum.

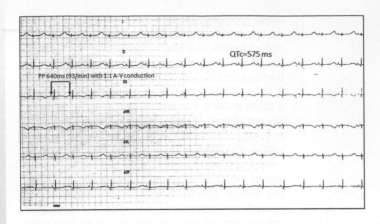

Fig. 8. After β-blocker therapy: sinus rhythm cycle length, 800 milliseconds, with 1:1 conduction and a QTc of 575 milliseconds.

with intermittent conversion of her tachycardia to sinus rhythm. After presentation to the hospital, her tachycardia persisted and was treated with intravenous propranolol with termination of the arrhythmia. Baseline ECG, in sinus rhythm, demonstrated a wide QRS with a morphology similar to the tachycardia QRS (**Fig. 13**).

An echocardiogram was obtained, demonstrating LV hyperlucency, septal thickness of 13 mm (z score 3.3), and posterior wall thickness of 11 mm (z score +2.3), together with apical thickening and low-normal LV function. A cardiac MRI study demonstrated a concentric decreased/nonperfusion subendocardial area in a ringlike distribution demonstrating gadolinium enhancement and hypertrophy of the intraventricular septum and inferior wall, also with LV ejection fraction of 47% (**Fig. 14**). Her myocardial mass at end diastole was 110 g/m^2 (normal range 63–95 g/m^2).

An electrophysiology study was performed with induction of an orthodromic supraventricular tachycardia using a left lateral accessory pathway. Subsequent ablation of the pathway was performed, with no further supraventricular tachycardia induction. Subsequent Holter monitoring demonstrated episodes of nonsustained VT; thus, an internal cardioverter defibrillator for primary prevention was placed. Genetic testing to evaluate her infiltrative cardiomyopathy is pending while she is currently undergoing transplant evaluation.

CASE 5: SIMPLE ARRYTHMIAS IN A RARE CARDIAC DISEASE

A 65-year-old man with previously documented left bundle branch block (LBBB) and ventricular premature contractions (VPCs) (**Fig. 15**) presented with symptoms and signs of congestive heart failure. Previous cardiac echocardiograms were reported as normal. On admission, his ECG showed atrial fibrillation (AF) with rapid ventricular rate and fused VPCs (**Fig. 16**). A new echocardiogram demonstrated a decreased EF and apical dyskinesis. Suspecting an LV noncompaction cardiomyopathy (LVNCC), a cardiac MRI was performed (**Fig. 17**).

The long-standing abnormality in this patient was an abnormal ECG showing an LBBB. This abnormality frequently is accompanied by some abnormality in LV function or structure, but, in this case, repetitive echocardiograms were reported as normal. At follow-up, the patient developed frequent VPCs and later developed AF. All these conditions are common in clinical

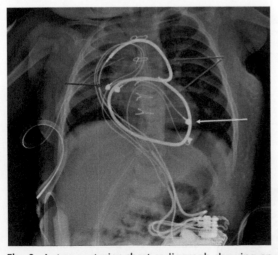

Fig. 9. Anteroposterior chest radiograph showing an abdominally placed ICD generator with a defibrillation coil tracked to the chest and inserted in the pericardial space (*blue arrows*); atrial and ventricular sensing/pacing leads are indicated.

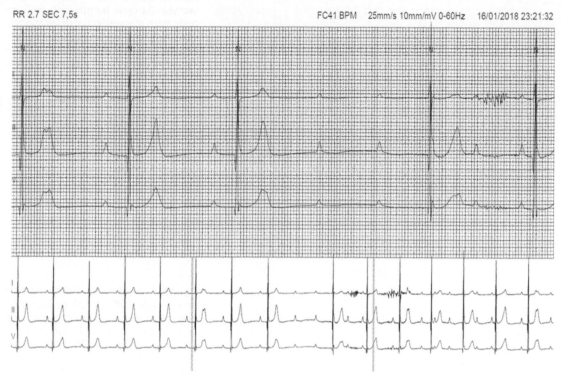

RR 2.7 SEC 7,5s　　　　FC41 BPM　25mm/s 10mm/mV 0-60Hz　16/01/2018 23:21:32

Fig. 10. Holter monitor recording showing Sinus rhythm with periods of high-degree AVB.

practice but the concurrent occurrence in a patient without previously documented cardiac disease should engender the clinical suspicion of an unusual disease. LVNCC is a rare progressive disease due to an arrest of myocardial compaction during embryogenesis, leading to hypertrophic ventricular trabeculations and deep interventricular recesses; abnormal genes encoding for sarcomeric or cytoskeletal proteins are the disease's cause in 50% of cases. This cardiomyopathy initially may be silent or manifest with subtle evidence, such as VPCs, or progress to congestive heart failure, ventricular arrhythmias, or systemic emboli from LV thrombi. When clinically suspected, a cardiac MRI is diagnostic.

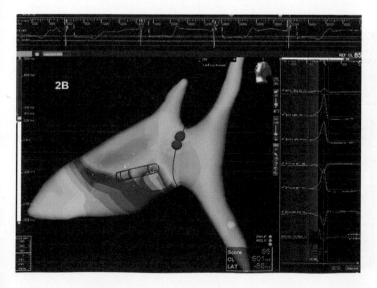

Fig. 11. Electroanatomic reconstruction of the RV interventricular septum shown in left lateral position with recordings of His potential marked by red dots. The stylized catheter represents the pacing lead positioned at the optimal pacing site previously identified (see text).

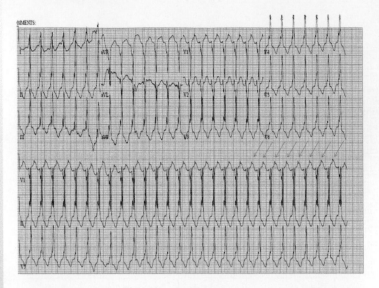

Fig. 12. ECG shows a wide complex tachycardia cycle length, 240 milliseconds, with marked initial delay suggestive of increased intrinsicoid deflection. Retrograde P wave with 1:1 VA relationship is visible in lead V1 (*arrows*). VA, ventriculo-atrial.

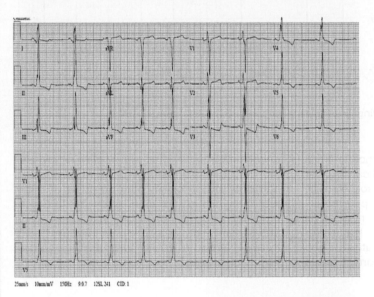

Fig. 13. Sinus rhythm with a short PR and a wide QRS of 120 milliseconds. The initial delay observed during the tachycardia is still present with a similar morphology. The differential diagnosis of this tracing should include Wolff-Parkinson-White syndrome.

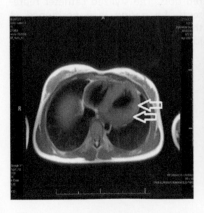
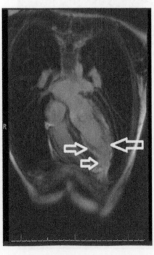

Fig. 14. *Left* sagittal *right* coronal cardiac MRI view demonstrating ringlike area, probably scar/infiltrate (*arrows*) with gadolinium enhancement in the LV.

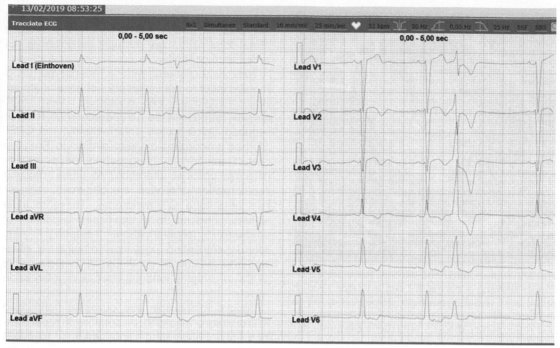

Fig. 15. Normal sinus rhythm with wide QRS and VPCs. The QRS measures 140 milliseconds with evidence of LV conduction delay. The maintained septal vector and a more prominent delay on the descending limb of the R wave in V3-V6 suggest an intramyocardial delay more than proximal LB block/delay. VPCs originate in an infero-lateral LV location. LB, left bundle.

CASE 6: ARRHYTHMIC STORM IN SHORT QT SYNDROME (ECG AS PHENOTYPE OF MULTIPLE LETHAL UNDEFINED CHANNELOPATHIES)

ECG as phenotype of multiple lethal undefined channelopathies.

A 27-year-old man with previous history of syncope, sustained an aborted cardiac arrest during registration of a baseline 12-lead ECG followed by an arrhythmic storm (**Fig. 18**). Previous resting ECGs had demonstrated a short QT (SQT) (**Fig. 19**) and several other QRS-ST

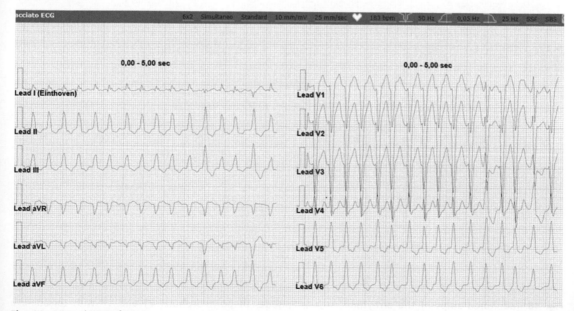

Fig. 16. AF and VPCs fusion.

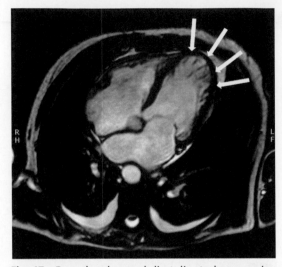

Fig. 17. .Four-chamber end-diastolic study precession frames showing a normal RV and a dilated LV with apical and septal hypokinesis. Hyper-trabeculation (*arrows*) with noncompacted to compacted myocardial ratio greater than 2:1 are criteria diagnostic for LVNCC.

abnormalities (**Figs. 20** and **21**). An ICD was implanted and oral quinidine therapy initiated (**Fig. 22**), with no further recurrences of arrhythmia or VPCs.

This is a patient with a phenotype (ECG manifestations) of multiple channelopathies. Major findings are consistent with SQT known to be related to increased K flow or reduced Ca entrance. Intermittently, the QRS-ST has a morphology very similar to Brugada type 1 abnormality, suggesting the possibility of a Na channel alteration. At times, delayed repolarization potentials are observed, suggestive of a long QT syndrome. These multiple abnormalities led to a significant dispersion of ventricular repolarization, creating early afterdepolarization potentials manifested electrocardiographically as VPCs. VF is induced by VPCs in a highly inhomogeneous repolarization milieu.

Long-term therapy with quinidine normalized QT duration, resolving dispersion of repolarization and preventing spontaneous triggered activity.

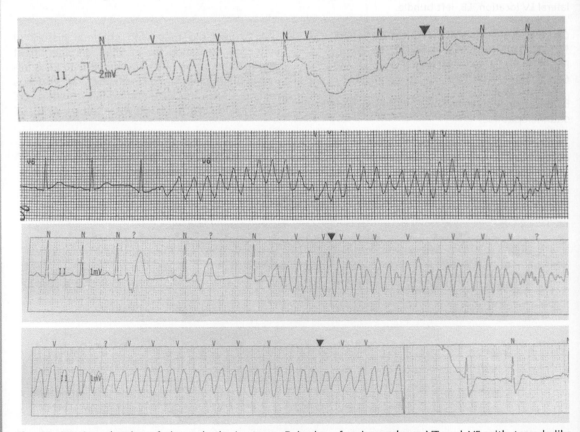

Fig. 18. Monitored strips of the arrhythmic storm. Episodes of polymorphous VT and VF with torsade-like morphology. A DCCV, direct current cardio version terminates sustained episodes.

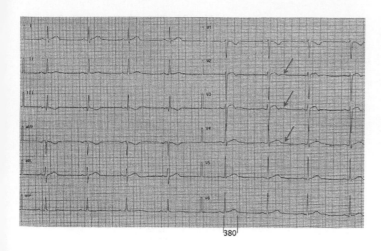

Fig. 19. Sinus rhythm with QT of 380 milliseconds (msec). Predicted QT calculated as follows.[3] QTp (ms) = 65.600/(100 + HR) = 65.600/150 = 437 msec. The minimal QT interval for this HR derived from the gaussian distribution curve of physiologic QT is 385 msec (QTp = 437 msec 88% of QTp = 385 msec). This value defines an SQT for this patient. Despite this SQT, delayed repolarization wave forms are observed in V2-V4 (*arrows*).

Genetic analysis, including high-pressure liquid chromatography and sequencing, failed to identify mutations at the level of the commonest genes (SCN5A, KCNQ1, KCNH2, KCNE1, and KCNE2) causing SQT syndrome. Based on current knowledge, genetic defects can be identified in patients with a suspected channelopathy in approximately 20% of tested

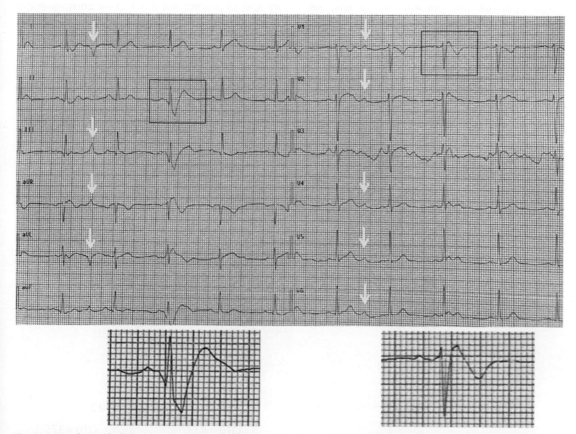

Fig. 20. ECG (recorded during the storm period) showing sinus rhythm with normal conduction and intermittent abnormal QRS-ST (*red squares*). This abnormality in V1 closely resembles a Brugada type 1 with a coved ST elevation, a 2-mm J-point elevation, and a gradually descending ST segment followed by a negative T wave. Two late terminal depolarization waves (*yellow arrows*) are observed as an intermittent long QT.

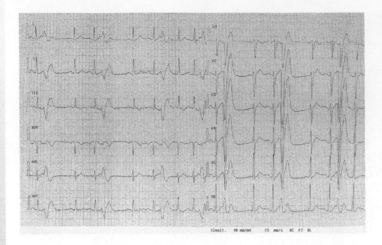

Fig. 21. Sinus rhythm with frequent PVCs; their coupling interval to the previous QRS is fixed at 240 milliseconds, and they appear to originate during the descending T-wave limb.

individuals. A negative test, therefore, does not exclude the presence of a genetic ionic channel dysfunction in patients with clinical manifestations of the disease, especially in cases of patients in whom as-yet unknown channelopathies are present. As genetic sequences become faster, more reliable, and less expensive, several other associations between genetic defects and electrocardiological manifestations will be known. This will allow clinicians to understand the link between an abnormal ECG and the ionic imbalance causing abnormality and to predict the most likely consequences deriving from it.

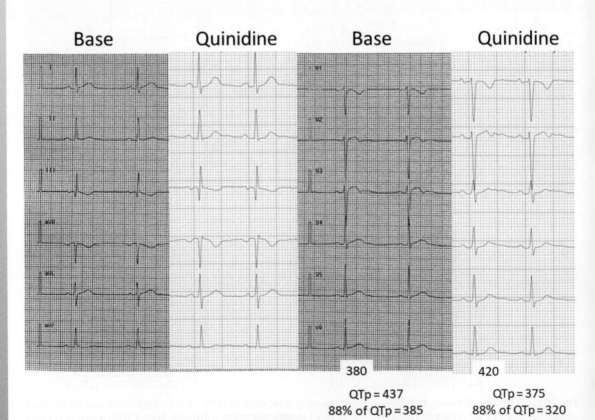

Fig. 22. QT response to chronic therapy with oral quinidine. QT predicted is now normalized at 375 milliseconds, with a minimal value for this rate of 320 milliseconds.

SUMMARY

A 12-lead ECG is one of the oldest clinical test, devised more than a century ago, and has remained in its principles unchanged. At the time the ECG was invented, technology we understand it today, was in its infancy, and clinical observation and deductive reasoning were the primary tools in the armamentarium of the skilled physician. In many ways, 12-lead ECG demonstrated graphically what was suspected from observations of cardiac impulse, venous waves, and cardiac timing. In-depth anatomic observations and animal studies confirmed the electrophysiologic behavior of different cardiac tissues suspected by analyzing the ECG tracings. From these initial observations, the milestones of ECG analysis were built, which withstood the test of time, serving, still today, as the basis of ECG interpretation.

The ECG, therefore, is the graphic representation of multiple electrophysiologic phenomena directly related to basic cardiac cellular properties as they respond to variable stimulations. An ECG tracing cannot be fully understood without knowledge of the interplay of these factors.

Among the most important ECG limitations is the distance between recording electrodes and electrical events, producing a graphic representation of the sum of different depolarization and repolarization cardiac potentials. This distance records only potential of a certain magnitude, and important low voltage events, such as common His depolarization, cannot be registered.

Technological advances over the past 50 years have enabled recording endocavitary electrograms with increasing precision, allowing the mechanisms of the majority of arrhythmias to be understood. Integrating these observations with the ECG has brought a better understanding of the genesis of the waveforms and has helped establish differential criteria for morphologic similar ECGs. Directly studying the myocardial cell action potential was accomplished more than 100 years ago; this research constituted the foundation of understanding of the phenomena of depolarization and repolarization. As technology allowing precise interpretation of ionic channels dynamics became available, understanding of the ionic currents involved in depolarization and repolarization became more precise. Mechanisms behind physiologic impulse generation and conduction, antiarrhythmic drug effect, and channelopathies became clear, greatly advancing diagnostic and therapeutic capabilities.

With new electrical recording techniques, the goal of defining the cellular structures determining the ionic shifts was achieved. ECG patterns suspected of reflecting an abnormality of the AP were clearly explained as a result of malfunctioning ionic channels. When the inherited component of some channelopathies was investigated, with technologies borrowed from genetic analysis, the last link between ECG and genes encoding malfunctioning channel proteins altering the action potential was finally closed.

The ECG records cardiac impulse's genesis and its transmission via specialized tissue to atria and ventricles. This is accomplished by specialized groups of myocardial cells, some of which spontaneously depolarize or conduct impulses at high speed. These properties are determined by variable expression of different ion channels on their membranes. ECG abnormalities depend on destruction of entire cardiac cells or anomalies of the genes encoding the channels' structural proteins. The ECG, therefore, could be considered a phenotype reflecting different degrees of structural abnormalities at the cellular or subcellular level. Evaluation of ECG tracings often allows pinpointing, with a high degree of certainty, the type and level of these variations from the norm. From the morphologic analysis of a resting tracing in normal conditions to the observation of different responses during, for example, increased rate of stimulation or prematurity, deductive analysis of the ECG is always based on a chain of events connected in a logical relationship. The more detailed the knowledge, the more accurate the diagnosis, to the point of reaching a level of precision electrocardiology. The cases presented in this article, together with other sections of this review, demonstrate how it is possible to fully interpret the pathologic behavior of myocardial cells by relating a simple surface tracing to some of the most basic cellular and subcellular cardiac functions. This depth of knowledge will allow correcting abnormalities, using drugs counteracting the dysfunctions; implanting sophisticated devices correcting the physiologic consequences of the pathologies; or, in a not so distant future, directly intervene in genetic mishaps.

ACKNOWLEDGMENTS

The authors would like to thank Dr Maria Mastrantuono and Johny Helou for their help in collecting the ECG shown in cases 3 (MM) and cases 5, and 6 (JH).

REFERENCES

1. Huang L, Kuo-Ho W, Zhang L, et al. Critical roles of X irp proteins in cardiac conduction and their rare variants identified in sudden unexplained nocturnal death syndrome and Brugada syndrome in Chinese han population. J Am Heart Assoc 2018;7:1.

2. Blayney LM, Lai FA. Ryanodine receptor-mediated arrhythmias and sudden cardiac death. Pharmacol Ther 2009;123(2):151.

3. Rautaharju PM, Zhou SH, Wong S, et al. Sex differences in the evolution of electrocardiographic QT interval with age. Can J Cardiol 1992;8:690–5.

Moving?

Make sure your subscription moves with you!

To notify us of your new address, find your **Clinics Account Number** (located on your mailing label above your name), and contact customer service at:

Email: journalscustomerservice-usa@elsevier.com

800-654-2452 (subscribers in the U.S. & Canada)
314-447-8871 (subscribers outside of the U.S. & Canada)

Fax number: 314-447-8029

Elsevier Health Sciences Division
Subscription Customer Service
3251 Riverport Lane
Maryland Heights, MO 63043

*To ensure uninterrupted delivery of your subscription, please notify us at least 4 weeks in advance of move.

Moving?

Make sure your subscription
moves with you!

To notify us of your new address, find your Clinics Account Number (located on your mailing label above your name), and contact customer service at:

Email: journalscustomerservice-usa@elsevier.com

800-654-2452 (subscribers in the U.S. & Canada)
314-447-8871 (subscribers outside of the U.S. & Canada)

Fax number: 314-447-8029

Elsevier Health Sciences Division
Subscription Customer Service
3251 Riverport Lane
Maryland Heights, MO 63043

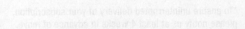

Printed and bound by CPI Group (UK) Ltd, Croydon, CR0 4YY

Printed and bound by CPI Group (UK) Ltd, Croydon, CR0 4YY

03/10/2024

01040308-0004